Sociology of health and health care

Sociology of health and health care

Fourth edition

Edited by

Steve Taylor
BA LL.B MPhil PhD

Senior Lecturer, London School of Economics

David Field
BA MA AM PhD

*Visiting Professor, Department of Health Sciences,
University of Leicester*

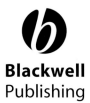

Blackwell
Publishing

Blackwell Publishing editorial offices:
Blackwell Publishing Ltd, 9600 Garsington Road, Oxford OX4 2DQ, UK
  Tel: +44 (0)1865 776868
Blackwell Publishing Inc., 350 Main Street, Malden, MA 02148-5020, USA
  Tel: +1 781 388 8250
Blackwell Publishing Asia Pty Ltd, 550 Swanston Street, Carlton, Victoria 3053, Australia
  Tel: +61 (0)3 8359 1011

First edition published 1993
Second edition published 1997
Third edition published 2003
Fourth edition published 2007

ISBN: 978-14051-5172-6

Library of Congress Cataloging-in-Publication Data
Sociology of health and health care / edited by Steve Taylor, David Field. – 4th ed.
    p. ; cm.
  Includes bibliographical references and index.
  ISBN-13: 978-1-4051-5172-6 (pbk. : alk. paper)
  ISBN-10: 1-4051-5172-2 (pbk. : alk. paper)   1. Social medicine.   2. Social medicine–
Great Britian.   I. Taylor, Steve (Steve D.)   II. Field, David, 1942–
  [DNLM: 1. Great Britain. National Health Service.   2. Delivery of Health Care–
Great Britain.   3. Sociology, Medical–Great Britain.   4. State Medicine–Great Britain.
W 84 FA1 S67 2007]
  RA418.3.G7S636 2007
  306.4′610941–dc22

                                                                    2006030357

A catalogue record for this title is available from the British Library

Set in 10/12pt Sabon
by Graphicraft Limited, Hong Kong
Printed and bound in Singapore
by C.O.S. Printers Pte Ltd

For further information on Blackwell Publishing, visit our website:
www.blackwellnursing.com

Contents

List of contributors

Ellen Annandale BSc, PhD, Senior Lecturer, Department of Sociology, University of Leicester, UK

Daphna Birnbaum-Carmeli BA, MA, PhD, Reader in Medical Sociology, Department of Nursing, University of Haifa, Haifa, Israel

Ken Blakemore BA, MSocSci, PhD, contributed to the 3rd edition, but has now retired from his post of Senior Lecturer, Department of Social Policy, University of Swansea, UK

David Field BA, MA, AM, PhD, Visiting Professor, Department of Health Sciences, University of Leicester, UK

Edwin Griggs BSc, PhD, Senior Lecturer in Social Policy, Open University, UK

Michael P. Kelly BA, MPhil, PhD, Public Health Excellence Director, National Institute for Health and Clinical Excellence and Visiting Professor, London School of Hygiene and Tropical Medicine, University of London, UK

Steve Taylor BA, LL.B, MPhil, PhD, Senior Lecturer in Medical Law and Medical Sociology, Coventry University, UK

Preface

This fourth edition of *Sociology of Health and Health Care*, like its predecessors, aims to provide a clear, easy to understand introduction to the area. As in the previous editions, the book is organised to provide continuity between chapters while also allowing each chapter to be read on its own. Although we have oriented the text and examples towards nursing, the book will also be relevant to students in other health professions.

The book retains the structure of the previous edition, although all chapters have been revised and updated to take account of new research evidence, developments in the sociology of health and illness, and changes in the organisation of health care. The first section introduces sociology and social research and looks at sociological approaches to health and health care. Chapter 1 has been updated to include more material on research designs and methods, reflecting nursing's increasing interest in this area. Chapter 2 examines various approaches to understanding health and illness, including the sick role and identities and illness.

The second section on the social patterning of health and disease uses new information to examine the profound effects upon their health of the social positions of individuals within contemporary British society. Chapter 3 examines the relationship between socio-economic status and the continuing inequalities in health and mortality, discussing the links between the individual lifecourse, socio-economic status and health. It concludes with a consideration of the societal, community and individual level policy strategies to address socio-economic inequalities in health. Chapter 4 examines the complex relationships between ethnicity and health, focusing primarily upon minority ethnic groups. Chapter 5 looks at the narrowing gap between the health and behaviours of males and females in our society and the role of changing gender expectations and definitions. Chapter 6 discusses the relationship between old age and health in contemporary Britain and discusses whether increasing longevity means that older people are in good health for most of their old age or whether their extra years of life mean more years of chronic illness and disability.

Despite the increasing policy emphasis upon health promotion and prevention, the major part of nursing work continues to be the care of people who are sick. Therefore the third section examines patterns and experiences of three important areas of illness. Chapter 7 looks at chronic illness and physical disability and the ways that these are shaped and given meaning in social interaction. Chapter 8 looks at mental disorders, suicide, and contains a new section on eating disorders. It examines changing patterns of hospital and community care and examines ethical issues in the care of mentally disordered people. Chapter 9 considers how and where death and dying are dealt with in contemporary Britain and reviews important new social models of bereavement and issues surrounding euthanasia and end of life care.

The rapid pace of change in the organisation and management of the NHS has had, and will continue to have, profound effects upon those using health services, nurses, health care professionals and others caring for the sick. These are examined in the final section on the social organisation and delivery of health care. Chapter 10, which provides a background for understanding the social context of health and health care in contemporary Britain, has been substantially reorganised and updated. It discusses continuing pressures on the NHS and outlines the main elements of the 'mixed economy' of health care. Chapter 11 has been completely re-written to provide an analysis of the reorganisation of the NHS under New Labour. The final chapter looks at the changing position of nursing in the NHS, paying particular attention to changing work roles and boundaries, and the tensions created by conflicting expectations of nurses and nursing.

Steve Taylor and David Field

Part I

Introduction

Chapter 1

Sociology, social research and health

Introduction

We are living in a world of dramatic and unprecedented social change. New technologies and cultural upheavals are transforming our lives and millions of people in modern societies are confronted by more choices than ever about how they can live their lives. However, greater prosperity and more lifestyle choices come at a price, as rates of crime, mental disorder, drug addiction and self-harm continue to rise.

So how did our world become this way? Why are people's lives today so different from those of their parents and grandparents? What are the possibilities for our lives in the future? These are the questions that sociology asks and attempts to answer. Sociology is about trying to understand the social world, but it is also about trying to understand ourselves, and how we fit into the societies in which we live.

In this chapter we shall introduce you to:

- the meaning of sociology and the idea of sociological problems;
- the aim of sociological research and the main research designs in sociology;
- the major methods of sociological research;
- the role of theory in sociology;
- some applications of sociology to the study of health and health care.

What is sociology?

The study of social relations

There is no clear and simple definition of sociology. The word sociology comes from a combination of the Latin *socius* (meaning companion) and the Greek *logos* (meaning the study of), so the word literally means the study of companionship, or *social relations*. These may be *direct*, face-to-face relationships, such as those we have with people in our family or at our college, or they may be *indirect*, as the actions and decisions of people not known to us personally can have an important influence on our life. For example, decisions of health policy makers can bring about significant changes in nurses' working conditions, their professional practice and the nature of their relationships with patients. The fact that social relationships take many different forms means that the scope of sociology is very wide. For example, the sociology of health and health care can range from things like large-scale social and economic developments that affect the health of millions of people, to the study of organisations like hospitals, right down to nurse–patient conversations on a hospital ward. However, the key idea behind all sociology is that people's lives and behaviour cannot be divorced from the social contexts in which they participate, directly or indirectly.

Social relationships are rarely random. For example, you will know from your own experiences that college life tends to follow certain regular patterns. Sometimes this is the result of the *formal organisation* of the college, such as the demands of the syllabus or the times classes start and end. However, a great deal of social organisation is *informal*. For example, in their free time students tend to socialise with the same people in the same places. Sociologists are interested in describing and comparing different forms of social organisation and exploring how they develop and how they shape individual lives. For example, how do changes in the economy or in cultural values affect things like the organisation and delivery of health care?

Sociological problems

It is often thought that sociology is about studying *social problems*; that is things that people feel are going 'wrong' with society, such as increasing crime, poverty and drug abuse. Sociologists are interested in social problems, but sociology is about much more than this. Sociologists are just as interested in things that are generally seen to be 'good', 'normal' or 'ordinary'. Sociological problems are about how societies, or parts of societies, work in the way they do. *Thinking sociologically* means being curious about the order of everyday social life, how this order changes and its relationship to the behaviour of individuals.

Social order and social change

Next time you find yourself in a place with lots of people, such as a busy street, a shopping mall or crowded hospital waiting area, just take a few minutes to stop and look. Social order is all around you. Cars stopping at a red light, people paying for the goods they take from the shops (most of the time!) and patients waiting for their turn to see the doctor or nurse. Most of us take this order for granted and the only time we notice it is when someone breaks a rule by driving through a red light, taking goods without paying or going straight to the front of a queue. However, for sociologists the regularity of social life is the starting point. Why do most people follow the rules of a society or social group most of the time? Where does this order come from? And are these rules generally agreed, or are some groups imposing their rules on others (Abercrombie 2004, chapter 7)?

Statistical data provide more evidence of the regularities of social life. For example, some societies have consistently better health than others and, even within the same society, there are significant and consistent variations in the health of different social groups. For example, people from poorer socio-economic groups are more likely to have lower expectations of health, have worse health and, on average, die at a younger age.

The social orders studied by sociologists are also constantly changing and sociological research often involves looking back to the past to try to explain these changes. Sociological thinking involves developing ideas that try to describe and explain changing *social processes*. For example, although the terms 'health' and 'illness' seem clear enough, people's views of what constitutes 'health' and 'illness' change over time. Many things that were simply seen as part of everyday life in Britain a century ago, such as pregnancy, long-term unhappiness, disruptive behaviour in school and loss of libido in later life, are now seen as medical conditions requiring treatments. Sociologists use the term *medicalisation* to describe the ways in which the scope of medical diagnoses has expanded to include more and more areas of social life, and they are interested in why this process happens and how it might be affecting our lives.

The individual and society

Common sense thinking holds that societies are all about individuals. Some social scientists and scientists would agree with this, arguing that as societies are clearly created by individuals, it is the study of the individual – through biology, medicine and psychology, for example – that provides the key to understanding human behaviour. In questioning this view sociologists are not, as some claim, rejecting the study of the 'individual' in favour of the 'group'. In fact, sociologists are interested in studying individuals and a great deal of their research involves talking to and observing individuals. However, for sociologists, the relationship between the individual and wider society is a two-way, rather than a one-way, relationship. Individuals obviously create societies but sociologists argue that, in important respects, individuals are also shaped by the societies in which they live.

As societies change, certain ways of behaving become accepted as normal, such as speaking a particular language or people organising themselves into small groups called families. Sociologists use the term *institutionalisation* to describe the processes whereby certain social practices become accepted ways of doing things in a society or social group. These social practices, and the values and beliefs surrounding them, make up the *culture* of a society and these cultural practices and values place expectations on how people should behave. The term *socialisation* describes the various ways people learn about, and generally conform to, these expectations. Socialisation processes begin from the time we are born, but continue in different ways throughout our lives. For example, becoming a student, a nurse or a mother not only involves learning new skills but also behaving in ways that are subject to the social expectations of others.

Sociologists do not, for example, explain the generally negative images of the elderly in modern societies merely in terms of biological decline (see Chapter 6). They also explore social *expectations* surrounding ageing and older people. Most older people are no longer economically productive, and for this reason they are usually seen as less valuable. Their care and welfare is also often seen as a 'social problem' and the media, politicians and policy makers sometimes talk of the 'burden', or 'costs', of providing care for the elderly. Once people become 'old' they are usually expected to dress and behave in ways that are seen as appropriate to their status. For example, older people are not expected to fall in love, kiss passionately in public places, or wear up-to-date designer clothes. Growing old is not, therefore, *just* a product of biology, it is also a product of socialisation. People do not just become old; they also *learn* to be old by adapting their behaviour to the expectations of others. Thus an *individual's* experiences of growing old will inevitably be influenced by the dominant views that a *society* holds about ageing. Similarly, health sociologists have shown that social expectations can play an important part in people's experiences of illness (Chapter 7), mental disorder (Chapter 8) and dying (Chapter 9).

Sociological thinking, then, involves exploring the order and regularity of social life, how this order changes over time and how individual behaviour is shaped by the organisation of wider society. However, sociology has to do more than ask interesting questions, it also has to come up with some answers, and this involves doing research.

Social research

What is research?

Research is simply is a process of gathering information systematically. The aim of sociological research (and indeed all research) is to try to move from a *subjective* and partial understanding of the problem being investigated to a more *objective* and complete understanding of it.

Subjective knowledge refers to individuals' perceptions, including their values, opinions and preferences. There is nothing 'wrong' with subjective knowledge and understanding. Everyone – including the sociologist – draws on their subjective understanding to make sense of the world around them. However, sociologists have to provide knowledge of societies that goes beyond their own opinions and prejudices. This is where objectivity comes in. Objective knowledge is knowledge that it is more than personal perceptions; it is knowledge that is free from bias, opinion and prejudice. This is the goal of all research, although it cannot always be attained in practice.

The scientific laboratory experiment is typically seen as the ideal form of generating objective knowledge. There is little scope for laboratory experiments in sociology and therefore there is debate about whether or not it can provide truly objective knowledge of societies. However, even if sociology cannot be truly objective as most sociologists believe, objectivity remains a *goal* of sociology and there are certain criteria, or benchmarks, against which the objectivity of research can be evaluated. Three of the most important are outlined below.

Key criteria in research

Standardisation

If a group of nurses who work together in the same hospital ward were asked to write an account of a particular working day, their accounts would probably be very different. First, they might write about different things, depending on what they felt was important. Secondly, even when they were writing about the same incident, they would probably interpret it differently. People's accounts of things tend to be different because they are selective reconstructions of some set of real events, and the selection process is shaped by people's *subjective* views of what they consider to be important and interesting. Sociologists also have to *select* evidence, but they try to make this selection process more standardised, systematic and reliable (see below) as their aim is to discover things about the social world rather than simply have their views confirmed. One of the ways they try to achieve more standardised data collection is by using *concepts*.

Concepts are clear definitions, or labels, that sociologists give to aspects of the social world that have common features. For example, one of the ways sociologists study social inequalities is by using the concept of class. Social classes are groups of people who share a similar economic position in a society. Many studies have explored the relationship between social class and health (see Chapter 3). If sociologists want to study this relationship statistically, they have to devise ways of measuring the concepts of class and health in much the same way that the mercury in the thermometer measures the concept of temperature. These measuring devises are called indicators. As occupation is the major source of income for most people, sociologists have used various forms of 'occupational ranking' as indicators of class, while rates of mortality (death) and morbidity (illness) are commonly used as indicators of health. By looking at average death rates and illness rates in each occupational group, sociologists have been able to examine the relationship between 'class' and 'health' in a standardised way that can also be checked and developed by other researchers.

Reliability

Reliability is concerned with the question of whether research is *repeatable*. This is important because people have more confidence in research that can be repeated and the results checked out. A research project is reliable if it can be repeated. Data, or information, *can* be said to be reliable if different researchers using the same research instruments obtain the same results. There are many reasons why one researcher may repeat, or replicate, the research of another. For example, the findings of the original research may be unusual, or the second researcher may want to find out if the same results still apply after a time lag.

Validity

In everyday language something is valid if it is believed to be correct or true. In social research it has a slightly more specific meaning. The issue of validity is concerned with the *correspondence* between a set of data and the conclusions that are drawn from it. In other words, how justified is a researcher in drawing *these* conclusions from *this* data set? Two important types of validity are *construct validity* and *ecological validity*.

Construct validity is concerned with whether data represent what they are supposed to represent. For example, standardised IQ (intelligence quotient) tests are designed to measure people's natural intelligence. Data collected from the administration of these tests may well be reliable but some critics have questioned their validity, arguing that the measurement is flawed as the tests favour middle class children over working class children and abstract thinking as opposed to practical skills.

Ecological validity, or authenticity, is concerned with whether the results of social scientific research actually reflect the reality of people's everyday lives. For example, if people answering interview questions give the answers they think the interviewer wants to hear rather than what they really think, the data will lack ecological validity. In order to fulfil the criterion of ecological validity, researchers may have to get much closer to the subjects of their study and observe them in real life situations over a long period of time.

Doing social research

The process of research usually involves three key stages (Box 1.1) and we shall examine each of them, bringing in the criteria identified above.

Box 1.1 Key stages in the research process

(1) **Research design**: research begins with questions that then need to be translated into a researchable form.
(2) **Data collection**: the research has to be organised and data collected through various research strategies and methods.
(3) **Data interpretation**: the information that is collected has to be presented, analysed and related to the question being investigated.

Research design

What is a research design?

Research always begins with questions. Sociologists ask all sorts of questions about social life, such as *why* social groups within the same society have different life chances, *what* people mean by health and illness or *how* a reform of a health care service has affected the working lives of health care professionals. It is the researcher's questions that give research its sense of purpose and direction.

A *research design* is the process of translating a researcher's original ideas and interests into something that can actually be researched. It involves making a number of strategic decisions about the subject of the research, the questions being addressed and the practicalities of how the data are to be collected given the time and resources available (Bryman 2004). Research designs provide an overall framework for the research, rather like travel itineraries provide frameworks for holidaymakers. There are many different types of research design, but two key distinctions are between quantitative/qualitative and macro/micro designs.

Superficially, the distinction between quantitative and qualitative research designs is that the former involves measurement whereas the latter does not. However, the distinction goes deeper than this and can represent different approaches to a research problem (Table 1.1). Quantitative research designs tend to be closer to the scientific ideal of research. Not only do they produce measurable data, but also as researchers tend to be relatively *detached* from the people they are studying there is less chance of their own personal values and preferences influencing the research process. Quantitative designs also tend to allow more standardised data collection and are more reliable, as they are easier to repeat.

Table 1.1 Quantitative and qualitative research.

Focus	Quantitative research	Qualitative research
Key criteria	Objectivity, measurement, reliability	Construct validity and ecological validity
Role of researcher	Detached observer, minimising subjectivity	Using own subjectivity to understand experiences of subjects
Favoured research designs	Surveys, experiments	Ethnographic case studies
Favoured research methods	Structured interviews and observation, analysis of official statistics	In-depth unstructured interviews, participant observation, analysis of documents
Data analysis	Establishing correlations testing theories through statistical procedures of pre-determined concepts	Developing concepts and theories from narrative reconstruction of data

Quantification is the hallmark of science and there are some social sciences – economics and psychology, for example – that are almost entirely quantitative. However, in sociology there are many questions that simply cannot be answered by quantitative methods alone (Silverman 2004). For example, how have cultural values changed over time? What is it like to live with a long-term illness, such as multiple sclerosis? How do nurses and patients interact with each other, or how do nurses break bad news to patients in hospital wards? These kinds of questions can usually be addressed better by observing people in their natural settings, examining documents or by in-depth interviews that allow respondents to talk at length about their experiences. The data produced by qualitative research are normally more ecologically valid but are not usually measurable.

The macro/micro distinction concerns the scope of the research and is best understood as a continuum. At one end macro, or large-scale, designs focus on large institutions or whole societies, while at the other end micro, or small-scale, designs analyse a particular group or even a few individuals in great depth. Between the extremes there are many middle-range, or meso, research projects that focus, for example, on a particular organisation or social group.

A researcher's choice of designs is usually shaped by the nature of the problem being researched. For example, studying the relationship between poverty and health in a whole society will almost certainly require a quantitative macro research design, whereas an in-depth exploration of people's experiences of a particular illness will almost certainly involve a qualitative micro design. The quantitative/qualitative and macro/micro distinction can be used to identify four of the major research designs used in sociology (Figure 1.1). We shall look at each of them separately below, but it is important to recognise that in practice many sociological research projects involve more than one research design.

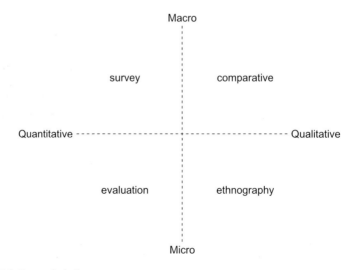

Figure 1.1 Research designs.

Surveys

In everyday language, to survey something is to take a general view. In geography, for example, surveys map out a landscape or a region. Similarly, in social sciences, surveys try to map out aspects of the social world (Williams 2003, chapter 5). Cross-sectional surveys involve the collection of data from more than one group at a specific point in time, while longitudinal surveys follow the same population, or populations, over time. Survey designs are widely used in health research for collecting information about health behaviour, patterns of illness and mortality, testing peoples' opinions or attitudes and mapping out relationships between health and various social factors in a quantifiable form.

Survey data are most commonly collected by asking people questions in postal or internet questionnaires, or in face-to-face interviews using closed questions that require simple yes/no or 'tick the box' responses. However, survey data can be collected through other methods, such as using documents or making observations using pre-determined structured categories.

Sampling

Survey research usually involves studying large populations where data cannot be collected from everyone, so researchers use a sample, or segment, of the population. In quantitative research, it is important that the sample reflects the population being studied as accurately as possible. This is done by *random sampling* where everyone in the population has an equal chance of being selected. *Stratified random sampling* means that every member of a population has an equal chance of being selected in relation to their representation within that population. For example, if women outnumber men by 4 to 1 in a population of nurses, then stratified random sampling will ensure that 80% of those sampled are women. The more the sample surveyed represents the population being studied, especially in terms of key variables such as age, class, ethnicity, gender and occupational status, the more confident the researcher will feel in generalising from the results.

For example, a sociologist interested in exploring relationships between social class and health behaviour could design a survey that takes representative samples from each social class and asks respondents about their health behaviour in terms of a number of indicators, such as smoking, diet, exercise or alcohol consumption. The research should establish whether or not there is a relationship, or correlation, between social class and health behaviour, and the results might then be used to inform health promotion strategies.

Evaluation research

The laboratory experiment is the key design in the natural sciences. In the experiment a possible causal influence, called an *independent variable*, is manipulated under controlled conditions to see if it produces a change in another factor called a *dependent variable*. While laboratory experiments are rare in sociology, 'quasi-experimental' research designs are commonly used in *evaluation research* (Pawson and Tilley 2003). Like the experiment, evaluation designs explore the effect of one variable on another, but they do so in natural, or field, settings. Evaluative research designs are usually policy orientated and one of their aims is to examine social programmes to see if they 'work'.

Control groups

The most common type of evaluative research design uses a *control group*. For example, suppose health policy makers want to know if providing additional information to patients about the nature of their treatment influences patient recovery. Researchers could 'test' this by taking a sample of patients awaiting surgery for a particular condition and randomly allocating them to an 'experimental' or a 'control' group. Patients in the experimental group would be given much fuller information, whereas those in the control group would be given basic information about the procedure. Researchers would then monitor the patients' progress after the operation. If they found significantly 'improved' recovery rates amongst those in the experimental group compared to the control group, it would suggest that the additional information was beneficial.

Comparative research

A major limitation of experimental or evaluative research designs is that they focus on a relatively small number of people in specific settings. This means that larger scale, or macro, questions that interest many sociologists – such as why societies change, why societies are different from each other or why rates of health and illness vary between societies – cannot be studied by evaluative designs. To examine these larger cultural and historical questions, researchers are more likely to use a comparative, or cross-cultural, research design.

Comparative research is much wider in scope than other research designs, for the units of analysis are often large institutions, whole societies or even groups of societies. Comparative research does not *just* mean comparing different societies or the same society over time. It involves using quantitative and qualitative data to search systematically for *similarities* and *differences* between the cases under consideration.

For example, there are many similarities between the health care systems of Britain and The Netherlands. They are both largely state funded, have tiers of primary and secondary care and are organised predominantly around a bio-medical approach (see Chapter 2) to health. However, there are also significant differences. In Britain health care is free to all at point of access but the availability of many treatments is at the discretion of local health authorities or individual doctors. In The Netherlands, in contrast, there is a system of compulsory health insurance that entitles people to a specific package of health care determined by centrally agreed criteria. A comparative research study could look at outcomes of each health care system in terms of specific criteria such as cost per patient, treatment outcomes and patient satisfaction. If one system appeared significantly 'better', the research could be used to advocate reforms of the other.

Ethnographic case studies

Ethnographic research designs involve detailed case studies of particular groups, organisations or individuals, and usually involve researchers being in close contact with the everyday lives of those they are studying (Brewer 2000). The key idea behind ethnographic case studies is to explore the reasoning behind people's actions. This is sometimes referred to as *verstehen*, a German word meaning empathetic understanding, that can perhaps be more easily understood by the phrase 'putting yourself in the shoes' of those you are studying. They are micro in scope, invariably involve a long period of time and the emphasis is on depth rather than breadth. Research reports are in the form of a narrative, with key pieces of evidence, such as detailed descriptions of particular episodes, being reproduced to illustrate the point the researcher is making.

For example, a study examining the educational experiences of student nurses would almost certainly involve an ethnographic research design. It would focus on a relatively small group of nurses and the researcher would spend a lot of time with the subjects, talking to them, sitting in their classes and going with them on placements.

There are two important conclusions to be drawn from this brief review of research designs. First, it has shown that there is not a single sociological approach to research. Rather, the planning and organising of a research project involves making a number of strategic decisions before the research begins. Secondly, it is important to understand that researchers are doing more than *just* giving us information about the social world. They are also shaping and organising it for us. The data generated from a research project are products of the *relationship* between the researcher's design and the intrinsic nature of what is being researched.

Research methods

What are research methods?

Research methods are the techniques used for *collecting* data. It is important that sociologists do not just present their findings but also explain how they were collected, in order to give others the opportunity to make more informed judgements of their value. All aspects of social life are of potential interest to sociologists, and data are gathered from a wide range of sources.

Sociologists may collect their own *primary* data or they may use *secondary* sources; that is, data already in existence.

Two main primary methods of sociological research are talking to people and watching them, while two of the most important secondary methods are the analysis of official statistics and documents. We shall look at each of these in turn and then outline the links between research methods and research designs.

Interview methods

There are many different types of interview methods in sociology (Gillham 2005), but the most important distinction is that between *structured* and *unstructured* interviews.

Structured interviews

In the structured interview respondents are asked a set of identical questions in exactly the same way and are usually asked to select their answers from a limited range of options. Structured interviews have a number of advantages for the researcher. Information from a large number of people can be obtained relatively quickly and cheaply, the data collection is standardised, reliable and can be easily quantified.

However, in spite of their benefits, structured interviews have limitations. They lack flexibility and depth, the questions and range of permitted answers may not reflect the respondents' experiences. In structured interviews it is also difficult to take into account the range of meanings that can be attributed to a word or phrase. To write interview questions and answers the researcher has to use words and the same word can *mean* different things to different respondents. Therefore, if in a survey of patients' views of their health care, respondents interpret the word 'satisfied' in different ways the data will lack construct validity. Sometimes, researchers try to account for this problem of meaning by leaving space or time for respondents to elaborate their answers. However, because the researchers are relatively detached from the subjects in structured interviews it is difficult for them to appreciate how their subjects *really* feel and impossible for them to know how they actually *behave* in real situations. Thus the data may lack ecological validity. The limitations of structured interviews mean that some research questions have to be examined by unstructured interviews.

Unstructured interviews

Unstructured interviews appear to be more like ordinary conversations; there is no set interview structure and interviewees answer in their own words. However, the researcher has an agenda that has to be addressed by the skilful use of conversation. The effectiveness of unstructured interviews often depends on the rapport and trust that is built up between researcher and respondent. The aim of such interviews is to allow respondents to reconstruct their experiences in as much detail as possible, giving the researcher, and ultimately the reader, an insight into how *they* experienced particular events. This is illustrated by the following extract from Field (2001: 344–5) on nursing the dying:

> *I remember very clearly a patient on geriatrics. I had nursed him on nights and I went back on days – he was double sided CVA. He was very incoherent . . . So I just sat with him and held his hand. And I remember the staff nurse coming in asking me if I had nothing better to do. So I said 'No. Not at this moment, no.' So she said 'Would you mind finding something to do?' I really hated her because this man was dying. I'd been with him all this time and why should he die alone?'*

While providing much more depth and validity than structured interviews, unstructured interviews also have important limitations. Data collection is usually not standardised, the method is not reliable as each interview is different and, as there is far too much data to present in full, readers are dependent on the *researcher's* selection of data.

Observational methods

Watching people is another key method sociologists use to find out about social life. Researchers using observational methods do not have to rely on what people *say* they do. They can see for themselves.

Like interviews, observation can be *structured or unstructured*. For example, in structured observation a researcher may use a predetermined list of categories to record the number of times a nurse interacts with a patient. However, the vast majority of observational research studies in sociology are unstructured, and most of them use a method called *participant observation*, where the researcher participates directly in the life of the people being studied. This technique was first used by Western anthropologists who joined tribal societies in order to document ways of life that were disappearing with the relentless advance of industrialisation. Similarly, in the study of contemporary societies, sociologists have to gain access to the groups or organisations they wish to study and, like anthropologists, they have to learn the 'local customs' and make detailed records of the 'ways of life' of those they are studying.

Although observational studies aim to describe things as they 'really are', there is the problem that those being observed may change their behaviour because they are being studied. Sometimes researchers try to get round this 'observer effect' by concealing their true identity from the group being studied. For example, in his classic study of a state mental hospital in the United States, Goffman (1991) worked as a games teacher in the institution. However, such 'undercover' research raises ethical issues, as those being studied have not given their consent to the research. In such cases, researchers have to ask themselves if the potential value of the research findings justifies the deception (Denscombe 2002, chapter 9).

There is a richness of detail in observational research that tends to be lacking in other methods. It is ecologically valid as sociologists are able to see how people behave for themselves, rather than relying on official statistics or what they are told in interviews. However, like all methods, observational research has its limitations. Not only is it time-consuming, but also the data collection is not standardised and the research is hard to replicate. Furthermore, there are many areas of social life – domestic violence, sexuality, suicide and childhood experiences, for example – that cannot usually be studied in this way.

Official statistics

The term 'official statistics' refers to the mass of data collected by the state and other related agencies. For example, a national census is held in Britain every 10 years. This provides information about the composition of the population in terms of factors such as births, marriages, divorces, ethnicity and the structure of families. State sources also regularly produce economic statistics on patterns of employment, unemployment, income and expenditure, as well as rates of crime, illness, suicides and the like. In addition to state generated data, other organisations such as hospitals, economic organisations and child protection agencies can be important sources of statistical information for researchers.

Official statistics are widely used by sociologists. They are readily available, comprehensive and allow for trends to be monitored over time. A great deal of the information used by many of the studies discussed in this book comes from various forms of official statistics, particularly statistics on patterns of health and illness and their relationship to social factors. However, it is important to remember that just because something is 'official' and expressed in statistical form it is not necessarily valid and reliable. Statistics are not self-evident 'facts', they are products of the conceptual categories used by the officials who collect them. For example, we may read that working class people are, on average, twice as likely to die before retirement age than middle class people. However, before we can attach any value to the statistics, we need to know things like what concept of 'class' was being used and what proportions of the population are in those classes.

There may also be problems in the collection of some sets of statistics that make their value for research questionable. A major problem may be under-reporting. For example, it is generally acknowledged that official statistics underestimate the actual levels of income, crime and illness in a society. Therefore, using official statistics in social research not only requires interpreting statistical trends, it also involves understanding *how* the data are produced and evaluating their use for research purposes.

Documents

A document, in its widest sense, simply means anything that contains a text (Prior 2003). Official reports, records from schools, hospitals, law courts, films, photographs, magazines, newspapers, letters, diaries, emails and even graffiti scrawled on a wall are examples of documents.

The analysis of documents is usually the major method for comparative and historical research designs, but documents are also widely used in ethnographic research. For example, the autobiographical accounts of adults who have tried to harm themselves, been anorexic or been abused in their childhood provide an invaluable source of information for sociologists researching these areas. Similarly, those researching patient care (and health care professionals themselves) can learn a great deal about the experience of being a patient from autobiographical and semi-autobiographical works such as Ken Kesey's *One Flew Over the Cuckoo's Nest* or Ruth Picardie's *Before I Say Goodbye*.

Selection of research methods

A researcher's choice of research methods is influenced primarily by the aims of the research design, and there are usually clear relationships between particular research designs and research methods (Table 1.2). Selection of research designs and methods is also influenced by external factors, such as whether or not researchers can get direct access to those they want to study, the time and money available, the nature of the audience they are writing for and the requirements of those funding the research.

While some sociologists have a clear preference for particular methods, most sociologists today favour methodological pluralism; that is using a combination of methods in their research. Evidence gained from several different methods usually gives a much fuller and clearer understanding of a subject. The findings from one method can sometimes also be checked with data from another method. For example, researchers could use structured interviews to elicit the views of a large number of nurses about their working conditions and then carry out observational case studies of some of the same nurses at work. This will give them a much fuller perspective on the research questions. Furthermore, if the things nurses were saying about their work in the survey tended to be confirmed by observing nursing practice, then the

Table 1.2 Research designs and research methods.

Research design	Focus of research	Typical methods
Survey	Samples of large populations	Structured interview, questionnaire
Evaluative	Small groups of subjects	Structured observation
Comparative/cross-cultural	Institutions, societies, groups of societies	Documents, official statistics
Ethnographic	Case studies	Participant observation, personal documents, unstructured interview

researchers would be much more confident about the validity and reliability of their findings.

Data collection is not the end of the research process. From the mass of data they have collected researchers have to select what they think is important, and the remaining data have to be organised and interpreted. This is where theoretical ideas come in, and this is what we shall be looking at in the next section.

Data interpretation: the role of theory

Doing sociological research is not just about gathering data through various research designs and methods, it is also about developing *theoretical* ideas that describe and explain different aspects of social life. The common sense view is that there is a clear separation between theory and research: theories are ideas that are then either 'proved' or 'disproved' by the 'facts'. The problem with this view is that theories and facts cannot be separated that easily (Marsh 2002). First, there are no such things as 'theory-free facts' and, secondly, data never speak for themselves.

Theory-dependent data

Although research seems a purely practical activity, theoretical ideas are still needed to *describe* the aspects of society the sociologist is studying. Suppose sociologists are exploring the relationship between illness and relative poverty. Before any data can be collected researchers have to use a concept, such as 'social class' or 'social deprivation', to describe inequality and these concepts are *theoretical* definitions that are constructed by researchers. In quantitative designs, researchers then have to identify the indicators they are using to measure the concept. They also have to define what they mean by 'illness' and how it is to be measured. For example, is the researcher to include all illnesses – in which case things like having a bout of flu and experiencing heart disease would count in the same figure – or just concentrate on 'serious' illnesses? If it is the latter, what is to be counted as 'serious' illness? Once illness has been defined, how is it to be measured? Researchers could use a subjective definition and ask people if they have experienced illness, or they could use more objective measures, such as medical records or periods in hospital (Bowling 2004). The permutations are endless, but the point is that doing the research involves using *theoretical* notions of 'social class' or 'social deprivation' and 'illness'.

The really important point to take from this is that data are not self-evident 'facts' simply waiting to be collected like apples off a tree. They are *constructed* through researchers' theoretical ideas and research strategies. Different theoretical ideas may well produce different 'facts'. This is not to suggest that there is not *really* a relationship between relative poverty and illness, but rather it can *only* be examined systematically through theoretical ideas. All data are therefore theory dependent.

Data do not speak for themselves

Another mistaken common sense assumption is that truths, or explanations, come from 'facts'. This view is expressed in everyday phrases such as, don't take my word for it, look at the evidence, or the facts speak for themselves. Evidence is clearly an essential component of explanation, but theories are necessary to *explain* why things are the way they are. This can be illustrated by continuing with our example of researching health inequalities.

Suppose the researchers have found reliable and systematic evidence of a relationship between low social class and high levels of illness. This is not an explanation, as 'the facts never speak for themselves'. The reason for this is that the evidence still has to be interpreted, and the same piece of evidence can be interpreted in different ways. For example, health inequalities may be caused by poor living conditions and inadequate health care, or they may be the result of less healthy behaviour amongst the poor, such as higher rates of smoking, or they may be due to genetic influences, with families prone to illness drifting down to lower socio-economic positions (Chapter 3).

This is not to suggest that one explanation is as good as any other. In the example given above, the researchers would try to 'adjudicate' between competing explanations by generating further data to show the extent to which different theories fit the available evidence. However, it is important to recognise the limits of sociological explanation as well as its potential. While sociology offers much more than opinion and common sense, it can never achieve the precision and prediction found in the natural sciences, such as physics or biology, where theories can be evaluated under controlled experimental conditions. As such, sociology offers plausible interpretations of the social world rather than demonstrable and universal truths. As Pawson (1999: 49) observes:

> *Sociological research will always be partial and provisional and never uniform and universal. I figure that certainty requires humility and that sociological research can only help us in choosing between theories rather than proving one. I rest content that good quality research comes with qualifications – our hypothesis will work only for certain people in certain circumstances at certain times.*

Theoretical divisions in sociology

So far we have been looking at things that are common to sociology. However, as with all academic subjects, there are different schools of thought within sociology. Two of the most significant debates in sociology concern *what* societies are (known as an ontological problem) and *how* knowledge of them is generated (known as an epistemological problem).

Social structure and social action

In relation to the question of what societies are, a broad distinction can be made between sociological theories that define societies as social structures and those that define them as the products of the actions of individuals (Parker 2003).

Societies as social structures

Some sociological approaches argue that human societies are best understood as social structures; that is as networks of social institutions and patterns of social relationships that are comparatively long lasting. Sociologists adopting this approach attempt to show the ways that various social structures shape the behaviour of the individuals living within them.

Many of those who founded sociology in nineteenth-century Europe viewed societies as social structures. For example, Durkheim (1858–1917) saw the morals and values of a society, transmitted from one generation to the next, as external forces that constrain individuals by regulating their behaviour and by binding them to each other through shared membership of institutions like families and religion (Lemert 2006). Sociological approaches that see values and beliefs as the 'core' element of societies are called *idealist* theories. Durkheim's sociology was an attempt to demonstrate that different institutional structures produce differences in individual behaviour, and his famous study of suicide attempted to demonstrate that social groups with more integrating social structures have lower suicide rates (Durkheim 1952).

Marx (1818–93), another founder of sociology, viewed social structures in a rather different way. For him, the key to understanding societies lay in their economic structures rather than their values and beliefs. This is known as a *materialist* approach. Marx claimed that social change was caused by changes in the underlying economic structure of societies rather than by cultural values or the decisions of powerful people. He argued that the change from agricultural to industrial production brought about a new type of industrial–capitalist society based on the free exchange of goods and services. Despite the differences between Durkheim's idealist theory, focused on cultural values and beliefs, and Marx's materialist theory, based on economic production, both viewed individual behaviour as the product of the structural organisation of societies.

There are links between a theoretical focus on social structures and the research designs and methods discussed in the previous section. For example, sociologists studying health and illness from a structural perspective would be more likely to use surveys or comparative research designs to examine how things like the culture, class structure or education system of societies influence people's health behaviour, their vulnerability to disease and the organisation of health care.

Societies as products of social action

Social action theory refers to theoretical approaches that focus primarily on the meanings and motives behind the actions of individuals. Action theorists argue that as human societies are produced by the behaviour of people, sociologists should begin by studying individual social action and the meanings behind these actions. Action theorists sometimes accuse structural theorists of reducing people to mere puppets of society. For example, Weber (1864–1920) disagreed with Marx that the rise of industrial–capitalist society in western Europe could be explained merely by changes in the economic structure (Poggi 2006). He argued that this approach did not explain the *motivation* of so many of the early industrial capitalists to work long hours and re-invest, rather than spend, their profits. Weber used statistical and documentary sources to suggest that an important motivating factor in the success of many of the early industrial capitalists was a staunch belief in the Protestant doctrine of predestination, where economic (or worldly) success came to be interpreted as a sign of God's favour. By focusing more on the actions of individuals and the meanings they gave to those actions Weber was able to highlight something that had been absent in Marxism and economic theory, the relationship between religion and the rise of modern capitalism.

Sociologists studying health and illness from a social action perspective would be more likely to use an ethnographic approach to explore things like how people come to define themselves as healthy or sick, individual experiences of health and illness, or day to day interactions between health professionals. This kind of research may reveal certain patterns or regularities that might *then* be linked to structural factors, such as family type or social background. Thus it is not that action theorists ignore structure, or structural theorists ignore action, rather it is that they approach the problem of the relationship between the individual and society in different ways.

Science and sociology

A second key debate in sociology concerns the best way of generating sociological knowledge. Many of the earliest sociologists believed that by diligently applying principles that had been so successful in the natural sciences, sociology would be able to discover 'laws' of social order and social change that could then be used to improve societies. Most contemporary sociologists are neither so ambitious nor so optimistic. However, many believe that it is still possible to study social life in a relatively objective and scientific way. This involves sociologists maintaining a scientific detachment and describing and explaining regularities of social life in terms that can be measured and tested out by other researchers. Sociologists adopting this view are guided primarily by the criteria of objectivity, standardisation and reliability, and usually have a strong preference for quantitative methods. From this point of view, rates of health and disease, for example, are seen as objective realities, the statistical distribution of which can be correlated with other factors, such as social background, housing or type of employment.

Other sociologists are more sceptical about the application of scientific methods to the study of societies. This approach is sometimes called interpretivist, or subjectivist. Interpretivists emphasise the differences between the study of the natural and social worlds. Unlike the atoms studied by physicists, for example, people engage in conscious intentional activity and, through language, attach meanings to their actions (Parker 2003, chapter 7). Thus, as we observed earlier, the meanings of the terms 'health' and 'illness', are products of social definition; that is, their meaning is given by social values and these values vary between different social groups and change over time. Interpretivist sociologists argue that the essentially subjective nature of social life effectively precludes the possibility of a science of society. Sociology is, therefore, about interpreting the different ways that people experience the situations in which they find themselves.

Sociologists studying health and illness from this point of view would be more interested in exploring how certain states of being come to be defined as healthy or unhealthy, and how these social definitions have influenced people's experiences of particular conditions. Interpretivist sociologists try to transcend their subjectivity by understanding the experiences of the subjects of their research. Their key criterion is ecological validity and therefore they have a strong preference for qualitative research methods that bring them into closer contact with those they study.

Some sociologists have rather entrenched views about the relative merits of structural and action theories and scientific or interpretative approaches. However, for most sociologists, and for those such as health professionals looking to apply sociological ideas to practice, it is more useful to view them as complementary, each with their own insights and limitations. In practice most researchers will use a combination of theories and methods, depending on the topics they are researching. For example, a structural approach may have to be employed in exploring something like variations in health care provision, while a social action approach may be helpful in making sense of something like nurse–client interactions. Similarly, studying the social factors that appear to make disease and premature death more or less likely lends itself to something closer to a natural science approach, while patients' experiences of illness and disability may be usefully understood by an interpretive approach.

Sociology applied to health and health care

The working lives of most health care professionals consist of a series of cases presenting a succession of specific problems. Patients, or clients, present with specific symptoms and health professionals give advice and usually offer some form of personalised treatment based on their specialist understanding of the human body. Success is usually judged in terms of improvements in the patient's health or, where cure is not possible, in their comfort. Sociology provides a different way of looking at health and illness. Instead of focusing on factors within the human body, sociology explores the social contexts in which people live and their relationship to health issues. Chapter 2 identifies some key approaches to health, and the other sections of the book illustrate the *application* of sociological approaches to three main areas:

- the distribution of health and illness in societies;
- illness and disabling conditions;
- the organisation and delivery of health care.

Part II focuses on research showing the extent to which people's health is influenced by social and cultural factors. Using research based mainly on structural theories and quantitative methodologies, it examines the relationship between health and the 'core' social variables of socio-economic background (Chapter 3), ethnicity (Chapter 4), gender (Chapter 5) and age (Chapter 6). One of the important implications of this work for health professionals is that improving the health of populations involves looking beyond individual cases and personalised health care to the social contexts that may be producing better health for some and worse health for others.

Part III looks at sociological analyses of illness and death. For sociologists, becoming sick is more than a series of biological changes. It also involves a set of social and psychological changes that are shaped by social organisations and social relations. In this context, sociologists have examined the cultural meanings of illness, the settings of care and the various ways that people's experiences of illness are linked to social interaction. We examine chronic illness (Chapter 7), mental disorders (Chapter 8) and death and dying (Chapter 9). The implication of this work for health care professionals is that the care of the sick is about more than management of symptoms. It also involves taking account of the social and psychological aspects of sickness.

Part IV examines the organisation and delivery of health care. Professional – patient/client interactions take place in various organisational settings that are influenced directly by government health policy decisions and indirectly by social and organisational change in wider society. This section begins by looking at changes in contemporary British society that have brought about changes in the organisation and culture of health care (Chapter 10). It then documents changes in government health policies and their effects on the delivery of care (Chapter 11). Finally, it examines the position and practice of nursing in contemporary UK health care (Chapter 12).

Summary

Sociology is the study of social relationships. It begins by asking fundamental questions about the nature of social order, social change and the relationship between individuals and societies. Sociological research involves planning, data collection and data interpretation. It uses a variety of research designs and methods that have advantages and limitations, and research often involves using a combination of approaches. There is no such thing as theory-free data as social research is collected and interpreted in terms of theoretical ideas. Sociologists have different ideas about how societies are best conceived and the extent to which the principles of scientific research are applicable to sociology. However, all sociological research explores the relationship between individuals and societies and strives to transcend subjective or common sense understanding of societies. Sociological ideas have been widely applied to the distribution of health and disease, experiences of illness and the organisation of health care.

References

Abercrombie, N. (2004) *Sociology*. Polity Press, Cambridge.

Bowling, A. (2004) *Measuring Disease*, 3rd edition. Open University Press, Buckingham.

Brewer, J. (2000) *Ethnography*. Open University Press, Buckingham.

Bryman, A. (2004) *Social Research Methods*, 2nd edition. Oxford University Press, Oxford.

Denscombe, M. (2002) *The Good Research Guide*, 2nd edition. Open University Press, Buckingham.

Durkheim, E. (1952) *Suicide: A Study in Sociology*. Routledge, London.

Field, D. (2001) 'We didn't want him to die on his own' – nurses' accounts of nursing dying patients, in B. Davey, A. Gray and C. Seale (eds) *Health and Disease: A Reader*, 3rd edition. Open University Press, Buckingham.

Gillham, W. (2005) *Research Interviewing*. Open University Press, Buckingham.

Goffman, E. (1991) *Asylums, Essays on the Social Situation of Mental Patients and Other Inmates*. Penguin, London.

Lemert, C. (2006) *Durkheim's Ghosts*. Cambridge University Press, Cambridge.

Marsh, I. ed. (2002) *Theory and Practice in Sociology*. Prentice Hall, Harlow.

Parker, J. (2003) *Social Theory: A Basic Toolkit*. Palgrave, Basingstoke.

Pawson, R. (1999) Methodology, in S. Taylor (ed.) *Sociology: Issues and Debates*. Palgrave, Basingstoke, 19–49.

Pawson, R. and Tilley, N. (2003) Go forth and experiment, in C. Searle (ed.) *Social Research Methods: A Reader*. Routledge, London.

Poggi, G. (2006) *Weber: A Short Introduction*. Polity Press, Cambridge.

Prior, L. (2003) *Using Documents in Social Research*. Sage, London.

Silverman, D. (2004) *Doing Qualitative Research: A Practical Handbook*, 2nd edition. Sage, London.

Williams, M. (2003) *Making Sense of Social Research*. Sage, London.

Further reading

Abercrombie, N. (2004) *Sociology*. Polity Press, Cambridge.
An excellent introduction to the subject, linking key sociological ideas to everyday life experiences in a lively and informative way.

Denscombe, M. (2002) *The Good Research Guide*, 2nd edition. Open University Press, Buckingham.
A very readable and clear account of the major research strategies and methods.

Video/DVD

Introducing Sociology (Halovine 2004: www.halovine.com)

Websites

www.sociolo.com
www.sociology.org.uk
www.socresearchonline.org.uk
www.statistics.gov.uk

Chapter 2

Approaches to health and illness

For many people the idea of health care still conjures up images of doctors and nurses working in surgeries and hospitals, with increasingly complex technology. This is hardly surprising, as the major focus of health care systems in modern societies has been to try to restore people to health through treatments of one sort or another. However, the activities of health care professionals now go well beyond treating the sick. An increasing number of doctors and nurses are focusing on the 'well' rather than the 'sick'. Screening programmes set out to discover signs of disease before they are presented in the surgery, and people are bombarded with information about what they could, and should, be doing to lead healthier lives. To many observers, this represents a fundamental shift in the ways that contemporary societies approach health and illness.

This chapter will:

- explain what is meant by a bio-medical model of health;
- discuss socio-medical models of health and their implications;
- introduce the idea that illness is a distinct social role;
- introduce the key concepts of sickness, identity, stigma and socialisation.

The bio-medical model of health

The development of medicine is usually described in terms of series of spectacular breakthroughs, such as Pasteur's development of vaccinations, Fleming's discovery of penicillin or the first heart transplant by Christian Barnard. In this 'heroic' view of medicine, the struggle for better health is seen as a 'war' waged by doctors and medical scientists against an impersonal enemy called disease on the 'battleground' of the human body. The idea that people's health, at least in a relatively affluent society like Britain, is predominantly a reflection of science's understanding of the body, the disease process and the development and availability of effective treatments reflects *a bio-medical model* of health. In this model:

- health is the absence of biological abnormality;
- diseases have specific causes;
- the human body is likened to a machine to be restored to health through personalised treatments that arrest, or reverse, the disease process;
- the health of a society is seen as largely dependent on the state of medical knowledge and the availability of medical resources.

Although under increasing challenge in recent years (see Chapter 10), the bio-medical model of health still underpins the organisation and delivery of health care in contemporary societies. Medical research is focused primarily on biochemical or genetic processes underlying disease. Most medical work involves diagnosing and treating abnormalities within the body, and the education and training of most health professionals, particularly doctors, revolves around understanding the human body and intervening in the disease process.

Bio-medical dominance over health and healing was consolidated in the nineteenth and early twentieth centuries, with the movement of medicine from the bedside to the hospital and the laboratory. During this period there were great advances in medical science, such as the discovery and treatment of bacterial infections, new and safer surgical techniques and developments in pharmacology. It was generally assumed that these advances in clinical medicine played a significant part in the great improvement in health standards that occurred around the same time. This led to the expectation that it was only a matter of time before scientific medicine overcame the diseases of modern society, such as cancer, heart disease, arthritis and mental illness. It was widely anticipated in industrial societies around the middle of the twentieth century that much greater investment in medical research and health care would produce further dramatic improvements in levels of health. In advanced industrial societies, such as Britain, life expectancy has increased dramatically, but how much of this was due to clinical intervention and treatment? This question is considered in the following section.

Infectious diseases: the role of medicine

Britain, like the rest of the Western world, has become much 'healthier' over the past 150 years. In 1851 the annual death rate was 22.7 per 1000 and average life expectancy at birth was around 40 years. By 1950 average life expectancy had increased to over 60 and in the early twenty-first century it is around 80 years (Figure 2.1) (see also Chapter 6).

The dramatic decline in the death rate from the middle of the nineteenth century to the middle of the twentieth century was due mainly to the decline in deaths from infectious diseases (Table 2.1). It was widely believed that clinical measures, in the form of therapy and later immunisation, played a major part in this decline. However, this view was challenged by McKeown (1979). By tracing the history of specific infectious diseases, he was able to show that most of them were declining well *before* effective medical treatment was

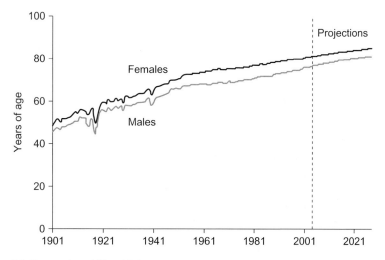

Figure 2.1 Expectation of life at birth.
Source: Social Trends 2006, Figure 7.1. National Statistics website: www.statistics.gov.uk. Crown copyright material is reproduced with the permission of the Controller of HMSO.

available (Figure 2.2). The only exceptions to this general pattern were small-pox, diphtheria and polio, where immunisation was an important factor. Programmes of immunisation against infection are obviously an important safeguard against the spread of infections, but the fact that clinical intervention seemed to play only a relatively small part in the decline of most infectious diseases suggested that there must be other explanations.

Important public health reforms implemented in the nineteenth century, particularly those leading to cleaner water supplies, were the main reason in reducing exposure to water- and food-borne infections such as cholera and typhoid. However, these reforms do not explain the decline in deaths from air-borne infections, such as tuberculosis (TB), that accounted for 40% of the total decline (Table 2.1).

Table 2.1 Reduction of mortality 1848–54 to 1971: England and Wales.

	Percentage of reduction
Conditions attributable to micro-organisms	
(1) Airborne diseases	40
(2) Water- and food-borne diseases	21
(3) Other conditions	13
Total	74
Conditions not attributable to micro-organisms	26
All diseases	100

Source: McKeown T. (1979) *The Role of Medicine*. Blackwell Publishers, Oxford. (Reproduced by permission of Blackwell Publishers and the University Press of Princeton.)

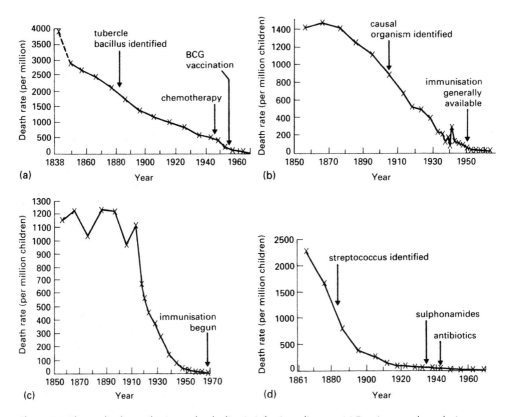

Figure 2.2 The medical contribution to the decline in infectious diseases. (a) Respiratory tuberculosis: death rates, England and Wales. (b) Whooping cough: death rates of children under 15, England and Wales. (c) Measles: death rates of children under 15, England and Wales. (d) Scarlet fever: death rates of children under 15, England and Wales.
Source: McKeown, T. (1976) *The Modern Rise of Population*. Arnold, London. © Thomas McKeown (reproduced by permission of Hodder Arnold).

According to McKeown, the major reason for the declining death rate was that people became stronger, and thus more resistant to infectious disease, due to better nutrition, improvements in public health and changes in their behaviour, especially greater use of contraception and improved personal hygiene. McKeown used his research to criticise the organisation of health care in modern societies. He suggested that modern medicine's preoccupation with the treatment of established diseases was a misuse of health care resources and that the best prospects for improving health in modern societies lay with trying to prevent, or reduce, environmental causes of disease.

McKeown's analysis has been criticised. Szreter (1988) argues that McKeown underestimated the role of medicine in bringing about the public health reforms that, amongst other things, improved the standard of nutrition that helped make people more resistant to disease. It has also been observed that McKeown ignored the fact that thousands of TB patients were incarcerated in institutions, thus limiting the spread of the infection and contributing to the declining death rate (Le Fanu 1999). Critics have also argued that by basing his analysis on *life expectancy* and focusing only on mortality rates, McKeown failed to take into account the contribution of clinical medicine to improving *health expectancy*, that is the *quality* of people's health while they are alive by, for example, controlling pain, improving eyesight and restoring mobility. Bunker (2001) suggests that many new developments in clinical medicine since McKeown's research have made a significant contribution to longevity as well as to quality of life. He cites evidence suggesting that almost 20% of the increase in longevity in the United States and Britain in the twentieth century can be attributable directly to clinical measures. However, despite these reservations, McKeown's research did demonstrate beyond reasonable doubt that health in the past was influenced more by environmental changes than by developments in clinical treatment.

Medicalisation and iatrogenesis

While McKeown was suggesting that clinical medicine has an important, but limited, part to play in improving health, other critics went much further, arguing that modern medicine's preoccupation with technology and drug therapy has led to an 'epidemic' of *iatrogenic* (i.e. medically caused) disease. Medical accidents, infections acquired in hospital, adverse reactions to drugs and complications following surgery are all examples of iatrogenic disease. For example, in Britain, it has been estimated that 10% of hospital admissions suffered some form of iatrogenic complication, equating to more than 850,000 events annually (Stryer and Clancy 2005).

In a radical critique of modern medicine, Illich (1990) extended the concept of iatrogenesis by arguing that the detrimental effects of medicine go beyond *direct* clinical harm. He accused the 'medical establishment' – by which he meant health care professionals, health administrators, pharmaceutical companies and the suppliers of medical equipment – of creating *social iatrogenesis*; that is, sponsoring sickness by creating unrealistic health demands that can then only be met by more health care and greater consumption of medical products. The process of medicalisation means that not only are more and more treatments being found for long established diseases, but more and more aspects of life are also becoming subject to the scrutiny and control of health professionals. Experiences once seen as a normal part of the human condition, such as pregnancy and childbirth, long-standing unhappiness, loss of sexual function in later life, ageing and dying have now been brought under medical jurisdiction.

Illich claimed that these processes of medicalisation produced *cultural iatrogenesis* where people 'unlearn the acceptance of suffering' and 'learn to interpret every ache as an indicator of their need for padding and pampering'. He argued that people should fight back against medical dominance over their lives. Medicine's monopolistic control over health and healing should be abolished, leaving people freer to take more responsibility for their health and health care and, ultimately, for their own lives.

Illich's critique was directed primarily against *bio-medicalisation*; that is the increasing influence of *clinical* treatments, such as surgery and pharmacological products, over people's lives. However, some of his criticisms can also be applied to what may be called *psycho-medicalisation*, a process where increasing numbers of people are now encouraged to see life problems, such as relationship difficulties, antisocial behaviour, inability to cope at work, dietary problems or bereavements, as if they were 'diseases' that can only be 'managed' with the help of expert therapists or counsellors.

It is important to put the critique of the growth of medical influence into context. First, not only have rates of medical cure increased spectacularly in some areas, such as heart disease, skin cancer and leukaemia, but, as we have already observed, many medical treatments contribute a great deal to improving the quality of people's lives. Secondly, Illich's view of the public as the 'passive consumers' of medicines and treatments has been questioned. Developments such as widening educational opportunities, increasing health related media output and the internet have resulted in a process of 'lay skilling', where more people are better informed about health issues and feel more able to question doctors and other experts about their diagnoses and treatment programmes. Thirdly, even if the medicalisation thesis is accepted – as it is by most sociologists – the increasing consumption of medicines and treatments cannot simply be explained in terms of the 'imperialism' of the 'medical establishment' or counselling. It does not explain why so many people in contemporary societies *actively* seek out and even demand bio-medical or psycho-therapeutic solutions to the management of their daily lives.

Some insight into this question may be gained from developing the ideas of Emile Durkheim (Chapter 1). He argued that the process of industrialisation tends to be accompanied by a decline in the influence of social institutions, such as the family, community and organised religion, that had the effect of 'binding' people to each other and giving them a sense of common identity and purpose. While this has resulted in giving people more choice and freedom, in times of personal difficulty and crisis increasing numbers of people have fewer sources of help and social support within their immediate environment. From this perspective, the tendency of more people to seek professional help and medication in coping with their lives is not a *consequence* of medicalisation, as Illich argued, but rather a *cause* of medicalisation that has its origins in the changing fabric of modern societies.

Socio-medical models of health

Bio-medicine and the health care practices arising from it occupy a paradoxical position in contemporary societies. On the one hand, there is continued enthusiasm for new medical breakthroughs as people seek treatment for a broader range of conditions. On the other hand, there is also some disillusionment with clinical medicine and growing distrust of doctors and nurses (Chapter 10). Despite massively increased investments in medical research and health care, most of the diseases of modern society remain stubbornly resistant to effective treatment, let alone cure. As the resources for research-ing and treating disease have become squeezed, the attention of governments and a growing number of health professionals has turned to the social and environmental influences on health, thus giving rise to an alternative socio-medical approach to health based on disease prevention and health promo-tion. In the socio-medical model:

- health is more than the absence of disease, it is a resource for everyday living;
- diseases are caused by a combination of factors, many of them environmental;
- the focus of inquiry is on the *relationship* between the body and its environment;
- significant improvements in health are most likely to come from changes in people's behaviour and in the conditions under which they live.

Three inter-related approaches can be distinguished in the socio-environmental model. The first focuses on individual behaviour and lifestyle choices. The second explores people's immediate social environment, particularly their relationships with others. The third is more concerned with general socio-economic and environmental influences.

Behavioural approaches

An argument that has become increasingly influential in recent years is that health depends less on what doctors and nurses do for patients and more on what people do for themselves. There is now a mass of evidence linking many of the diseases of modern society to 'behavioural factors', such as sedentary lifestyles, poor diet and widespread use of drugs such as alcohol and tobacco. Smoking, for example, is estimated to contribute to 111,000 deaths a year, while alcohol abuse accounts for a further 10,000. Nurses have been at the forefront of campaigns to educate people about the risks of 'unhealthy' behaviour.

In this context it has been argued that health professionals are taking over some of the social control functions previously associated with organised reli-gion, and this helps to explain the strong moral component in much health education. Whereas religious institutions once warned of the punishments waiting in the afterlife for sinful behaviour, health professionals now warn people of the dangers waiting in this life for unhealthy behaviour. Sociological research has suggested that while health care professionals today are more likely to emphasise (positive) 'risk reduction' as opposed to (negative) blame, a lot of health education is still underpinned by a moralistic message linking disease to unhealthy lifestyles (Wheatley 2005). .

The 'health targets' set by government's *The Health of the Nation* (Secretary of State for Health and Social Services 1992) also followed an essentially beha-vioural approach. While stating in principle that better health requires a com-bination of governmental and individual responsibility, in practice the report placed most emphasis on lifestyle factors. For example, the main 'strategies' for combating heart disease and stroke, which together accounted for 38% of deaths in England, were 'to encourage people to stop smoking, increase physical activity and reduce consumption of saturated fatty acids, sodium and alcohol' (Secretary of State for Health and Social Services 1992: 47).

The Health of the Nation also recognised a special role for nurses in health education and health promotion, and recent reforms in nurse education and practice have put more emphasis on health education. *Primary* health education is concerned with encouraging people to behave in ways that will help them avoid disease or injury. This involves nurses helping to educate individual patients and, working in schools, colleges and other community institutions, developing programmes of education about things such as diet and misuse of drugs. *Secondary* health education aims to halt or reverse the development of a disease or a condition. This may include the nurse encouraging high-risk groups to make use of screening services, or spotting signs of disability or developmental delay in children. *Tertiary* health education involves nurses trying to prevent further complications where disease already exists, such as giving guidance about diet to diabetics or helping people adjust to irreversible disability.

While not disputing the influence of behavioural factors on health, sociologists have questioned the value of many health education programmes. From a sociological point of view all human behaviour, including health related behaviour, has to be understood in terms of the social contexts within which it takes place. When studied from the point of view of the people concerned, behaviour that may appear to be 'irrational' from a distance may have a rationality of its own when studied more closely. Smoking behaviour amongst working class women provides a good example of this.

For many years smoking has been identified as the major preventable cause of death in the developed world, resulting in the death of one in four smokers. In general, people from the working classes have been less responsive to antismoking campaigns than people from the middle and upper classes. Working class women with children have become a priority for health educationalists not only for the harm they may be doing to their own health but also because their children are affected directly by passive smoking and indirectly by socialisation into smoking. Research into women in low income families with pre-school children shows that smoking has to be set in the context of both poverty and motherhood, with smoking as part of the 'strategy' for coping with stress and helping to maintain their caring role when their calm breaks down. In a study of over 8000 young women, Graham *et al.* (2006) found that domestic circumstances more commonly associated with low socio-economic position, such as early motherhood, non-cohabitation and lone motherhood, all increased the odds of smoking.

This type of research suggests that behavioural factors cannot easily be separated from the material and domestic circumstances of people's everyday existence. Without such understanding it is all too easy to blame people for unhealthy behaviour that may have deeper roots than individual fecklessness or ignorance. Health education is clearly very important as the information and guidance it provides can give people more autonomy to make informed decisions about their health. However, a sociological perspective suggests that health education programmes, or the efforts of individual primary health care workers, such as community nurses, are more likely to be effective if they place people's behaviour into a social context and take into account the *meaning* that it has for the individuals concerned.

Social relationships and social support

Stress has been described as the epidemic of modern societies. Since the 1960s a number of studies have shown that exposure to stressful life events, such as bereavement, divorce, unemployment or occupational change, financial problems or migration, can make people more vulnerable to disease and even premature death. There is now increasing evidence from the biological sciences suggesting that prolonged exposure to stressful life events produces biochemical changes in the body that weaken its immune system and leave the individual more vulnerable to disease. However, while stressful life events are associated with a higher *risk* of disease, they do not *necessarily* cause it, and there has been a great deal of research, particularly in biology and psychology, into factors that influence people's ability to adapt to stress. In this context sociologists have explored the ways in which people's social relationships might mediate between exposure to stressful life events and health.

More than a century ago, Durkheim (1858–1917) showed that even such an apparently 'individual' act as suicide could be explained sociologically (Durkheim 1952). His research showed that the more people are integrated into the social groups around them, by the way that their lives are woven into those of others through kinship and shared membership of organisations, the less vulnerable they are to suicide. In a pioneering longitudinal study in the United States of America, Berkman and Syme (1979) followed a group of 5000 adults over 9 years. They operationalised the concept of integration by using four indicators (see Chapter 1): marriage, regular contact with friends and relatives, church membership and membership of voluntary organisations. After controlling for health status and health behaviour, such as smoking, they found that morbidity and mortality rates for poorly integrated adults were between two and three times higher than for those who had high levels of integration. In the past two decades a growing body of sociological and social psychological literature has reinforced this finding, showing that people with strong and supportive family and friendship networks tend to remain in good health longer and make better recoveries from illness than those with weaker support networks (Camic and Knight 2004).

Social support operates at different levels. *Emotional support* can reassure individuals that they are still cared for and give them the opportunity to vent worries and negative feelings. *Instrumental support*, such as physical care, financial assistance or help with responsibilities like child care or shopping, is often essential in helping people get through day to day living after a stressful experience. Emotional and, to a lesser extent, instrumental support also have the effect of showing people that they are still valued and worthy of the concern of others, and thus help maintain, or re-establish, their sense of self-esteem. Finally, as stressful life events often place people in situations that are unfamiliar to them, *informational support* can be crucial. For example, if a person has become ill, information about diet and medication is often vital to successful adaptation, coping and recovery. However, it is very important that nurses do not overload patients with too much information, or information that they cannot understand, as this can increase feelings of helplessness and dependency.

It is perhaps ironic that so many people in contemporary societies seem to be turning their backs on traditional sources of social support when sociologists have discovered how important they are for health. Nurses and other health workers cannot change societies, but they have to try to mitigate some of the adverse consequences as best they can. One way of doing this is to develop health promotion initiatives that improve social support networks, especially for clients or patients from vulnerable and marginalised social groups, such as the elderly, certain ethnic minorities, lone mothers and groups with particular social and psychological problems. Within this perspective, the emotional, instrumental and informational support traditionally given to patients by nurses in hospital is not simply to 'service' biomedical treatment, but is itself a crucial part of the healing process and should be valued as such. In the community care of people with long-term illnesses and disabilities, attention is increasingly turning to the social support networks surrounding the patient, following findings that level of social support was a significant predictor of mortality (Temkin-Greener *et al.* 2004).

Most support for people with chronic illnesses or disabilities is provided by families (Chapter 10) and this can be a potential source of stress for those providing it. In addition to the burden of caring, family members may also be confronted by financial strain, reduced opportunities for recreation and increased isolation. The main caregivers in particular, may experience depression, a lack of opportunity to express their distress, inadequate support from other family members and a lack of information from other health professionals, all of which have been found to undermine their health and continued ability to provide effective support for the patient (Hirst 2005).

In the management of long-term illness and disability, support from health professionals for carers can be as important as support for the patient. A number of studies have shown that social support for carers can mitigate some of the stresses of caring. Nurses, in particular, are well placed to provide emotional support by encouraging carers, listening to their problems and allowing them to express their feelings about the patient's condition. This may also result in more open communication between caregivers and patients. Informational support may focus on discussing the nature of the illness with family members and helping to plan strategies for some of the problems most likely to be encountered. By identifying the specific help that can most effectively be provided and the progress that can be realistically expected, nurses may help carers avoid feeling overwhelmed by the extent of their responsibilities and demoralised by the patient's lack of progress. Instrumental support for the family may involve, for example, helping to obtain financial or domestic support, arranging respite care or helping to make contacts with support groups.

Socio-environmental approaches

Socio-environmental approaches to health are aimed at creating social and environmental conditions that are more conducive to health, and are the social responsibilities of governments and other organisations rather than just individual citizens. This involves joint action from communities, government, voluntary agencies and the health service to create 'healthy alliances'. Socio-environmental health initiatives operate at many different levels. For example, there is now a mass of evidence linking health status to socio-economic position (Chapter 3). People living in the poorer sections of society are more at risk of illness and tend to die younger. In this context, health promotion work involves identifying the causes of these health inequalities, developing policies and strategies to try to reduce them and incorporating them into the education and practice of health professionals (Fairnington 2004). Another set of strategies involves encouraging government policy and legislation to confront a corporate 'disease promoting' industry that uses seductive images to persuade people, particularly young people, of the pleasures of things like smoking, fast food, alcohol and fast cars. Recent examples of this approach in Britain include legislation banning smoking from many public areas; measures to reduce traffic speed, especially in built-up areas; and plans to reduce the sale of 'junk food' in schools (Chapter 3).

As well as developing national strategies, many health promotion campaigns are targeted at specific social groups or communities, such as a workforce, a minority group or people living in a particular area. The aim is to help a community, or social group, increase its control over environmental conditions that may be affecting their health. For example, the health education provided by nurses can go beyond informing people of the implications of their own behaviour and include information about the social or organisational factors that may be undermining their health. It could also involve targeting people who have the power to bring about change in an area, such as employers, local government representatives or people in the media. In this respect health workers are encouraged to use a wider definition of health care that incorporates social and political influences on health. This might involve protest action, setting up self-help groups or arranging meetings with the representatives of the council or health services.

There is clearly great scope for improving health by reforming social and environmental conditions, but these approaches are also open to criticism. First, there is rather more rhetoric than reality, with grandiose ideals of social change, empowerment and partnerships not matched with/by concrete and testable strategies for health professionals to follow in their day to day work. Secondly, in their desire to distinguish themselves from individualistic behavioural approaches, socio-environmental writers appear to see solutions to health problems solely in terms of political and environmental factors, and tend to depict people as rather passive victims of 'unhealthy' social arrangements. Sociological analysis suggests that approaches that neglect the complexity of the relationship between the individual and society, and depict people as the helpless victims of social arrangements, are less likely to be successful (Chapter 1).

While behaviourist approaches are based on the idea of individual choice and responsibility, socio-environmental health promotion advocates are more likely to view the state as responsible for the nation's health. Their aim, to convince governments that more unhealthy activities should either be banned or put out of people's reach by price increases, can raise ethical issues. For example, while high taxation on tobacco can be justified on public health grounds, it can create injustice for those who continue smoke, particularly those living in the poorer sections of society.

Surveillance and social control

The growth of preventative and promotional health care has resulted in increasing numbers of health professionals monitoring apparently healthy people for evidence of risk factors in their bodies, their behaviour or in their social environments. This has been described as *surveillance medicine* (Armstrong 1995). The shift in focus from 'sickness' to 'health' has some important implications for health professionals, and for nurses in particular.

First, surveillance health care can give rise to ethical problems, as nurses become more involved in managing people's lives rather than just their illnesses. For example, many community nurses advise and support families, especially where there are young children. The relationship is based on trust and consent. However, community nurses are also expected to engage in surveillance of families, not only for clear-cut evidence of harm to a child but also for any signs of risk that *may* compromise a child's future safety and welfare. They are then expected to pass on their concerns to multi-disciplinary teams that may include representatives of social services, NSPCC and the police. This potential violation of families' rights – for example, the consent they give is not an informed consent – is legitimised by the fact that child care has become medicalised and certain forms of parenting are seen as early symptoms of disease. The surveillance of families without their knowledge or consent not only raises important ethical issues for community nurses, but also threatens the basis of trust on which much of their general work rests (Cowley *et al.* 2004).

Secondly, some criticise what they see as a tyranny of health promotion where, often on the flimsiest evidence, more and more health hazards are being identified in everyday life. They argue that health promotion activists create 'health panics' that cause unnecessary worry and make people scared of daily life. This institutionalised paranoia is captured by Reinharz:

> *I would like to get through a day without being assaulted by warnings. I find this barrage of dire information intrusive, pervasive and depressing . . . the signs, newspaper articles, radio reports and labels tell me to watch*

out. They let me know that life is dangerous. It's almost foolhardy to be in the sun, to be in a car, or to take food (poison?) from a supermarket shelf (Reinharz 2001: 438–41).

It would be ironic if health promotion professionals, in their reaction against the biomedical model and its limitations, succeed in transforming life itself into a disease.

Thirdly, the key idea behind surveillance medicine is that prevention is better than cure. This is a sensible attitude, but it can also be misleading. While some diseases are clearly preventable, disease and disability, like death, can never be prevented, only postponed. Everyone who lives long enough is going to become ill at some time and the majority of health professionals, including the majority of nurses, are going to be involved in one way or another in the treatment and care of the sick. It is thus very important that in its enthusiasm for focusing upon 'health nursing' rather than 'nursing the sick', nurse education does not follow the biomedical model in overlooking its crucial role in the care of long-term sick and disabled people.

Social aspects of sickness

As societies modernise, the burden of disease shifts from acute to chronic (long-term) illness and disability (Chapter 7). Non-communicable chronic diseases are now the major causes of death and disability worldwide and account for nearly 60% of deaths. While clinical medicine can treat many of these conditions, it cannot usually cure them, and this has led to what Frank (1995) has called the 'remission society' where increasing numbers of people are spending a greater proportion of their lives either living with long-term illness or coping with its consequences. Sociologists have explored the social contexts that contribute to shaping people's experiences of illness and demonstrated that the transition from health to illness involves not only biological change, but also significant changes in social status and identity.

The sick role

Parsons (1951) was one of the first sociologists to conceptualise sickness as a social state. He saw sickness as a potential threat to social order, as people were not complying with the work-centred norms of modern societies. Allocating people to a distinct sick-role helped manage this challenge to social and moral order. In Parsons' model the sick role consists of privileges and obligations. Sick people are:

- exempted from their everyday responsibilities;
- not held responsible for their sickness;
- expected to define sickness as undesirable and be motivated to get better;
- expected to seek professional help and comply with medical advice.

Failure to comply with the obligations may result in a loss of the privileges. Parsons also identified a corresponding medical role of privileges and obligations. Doctors and nurses have intimate access to patients, who therefore have to be protected by professionals':

- formal education and training;
- objectivity and detachment;
- professional standards and collegiate control;
- ethical obligations to act in the patients' best interests.

Although Parsons developed his analysis in terms of doctor–patient relations, it can also be used to help make sense of nurse–patient relations. Nurses have less power than doctors but most of them also work with people who have entered the sick role and, like doctors, they have privileged, and often intimate, access to patients. Nurse training, the definition of their work as 'patient centred' and their rules of professional conduct also function to regulate professional relations and protect patients from exploitation.

The concept of the sick role has been subjected to a number of criticisms. First, it has been argued that Parsons' model cannot be applied to many chronic illnesses from which patients cannot recover. However, as Parsons observed in a later re-evaluation of the sick role, many people with chronic illnesses are still expected to follow medical advice to control symptoms in a way that mirrors recovery from acute illness.

Secondly, and more significantly, it has been shown that access to the sick role is rather more problematic than Parsons' model assumes. Studies of *illness behaviour* – that is, the processes by which people come to define themselves as ill – have shown that only a minority of symptoms, including some quite serious ones, are brought to medical attention (Young 2005). Therefore, it has been suggested that what Parsons is really talking about is *a patient role* rather than a sick role.

Thirdly, Parsons' conceptualisation has been criticised for being one dimensional. For example, it is purely Western in orientation and fails to look at alternative forms of healing, it does not recognise a range of possible doctor–patient relationships, and it assumes an unduly consensual model of the doctor–patient relationship. In fact there are differences between the knowledge, interests and expectations of doctors and their patients that may lead to tension and conflict. This is equally true for nurse–patient/client relationships, with the additional complication that these are also influenced by relationships between nurses and doctors, which have their own tensions and conflicts (Chapter 12).

Despite these valid criticisms of Parsons' formulation of the sick role, it is still seen as a major contribution to the sociology of health and illness. The bio-medical model focuses on management of the sick person, and their body in particular, and Parsons' recognition of sickness as a social state with distinct cultural expectations draws attention to the important *role of others* in the processes of becoming and being ill. It also helps to explain differential access to health care and also how certain categories of patients are treated differently by health care staff. For example, in a study of a casualty department, Jeffery (2001) found staff referring to some patients, such as those who had been hurt while drunk, drug takers and the repeated overdosers, as the 'rubbish'. What characterised the 'rubbish' was that, like the heavy and unrepentant smokers who are pushed to the back of waiting lists for cardiac surgery, they were seen to have been largely responsible for their own condition and therefore not legitimately sick.

Experiences of sickness and disability

A large number of sociological studies, using largely ethnographic research designs and qualitative methods (Chapter 1), have pursued the original insights provided by the sick role to document the social expectations surrounding illness and disability and to explore their consequences for individuals.

Sickness and identity

One of the major consequences of having a long-term illness or disability is that it can change a sufferer's sense of identity; that is, their image of who they are and how they are seen. As we saw in Chapter 1, it is through social interaction that people develop a sense of identity. Sociologists exploring these processes sometimes distinguish between social and personal identity, reflecting the idea that people are both members of social groupings and also unique individuals.

Social identities describe characteristics that are ascribed to individuals by others and define them as members of a particular category, such as their age, appearance, ethnicity, gender or occupational role. Self-concepts or *personal identities* refer to those qualities that mark a person out as a distinct individual and set them apart from others. For example, while the label 'nurse' maybe part of someone's social identity, the fact that different nurses may see themselves as a '*successful* nurse', a '*fulfilled* nurse' or a '*disillusioned* nurse' reflects a more personal identity.

Personal identities arise from processes of self-development where an individual builds up a sense of themselves and their relationship to other people and to the world. It develops from people's ability to reflect on and evaluate their actions and to construct biographies of how they came to be the person they are. Whereas social identities describe relatively enduring features of a person's life, personal identities are much more fluid and precarious and have to be negotiated and renegotiated in everyday life. For example, a change in staff or policy at a hospital could result in a 'fulfilled nurse' becoming a 'disillusioned nurse'.

The concept of identity is important in helping to understand people's experiences of sickness, because illness and disability are not only assaults on the integrity of the body, they also assault people's social and personal identity. The sick person's place in the world and sense of who they are can become compromised or even lost.

Because illness and disability labels (particularly if the condition is severe and visible) are usually seen as a dominant source of a patient's social identity, there is a tendency for people, including nurses, to view their behaviour in terms of their condition. For example, an outburst of anger by a person with severe physical disabilities may be rationalised by staff as an understandable consequence of the frustration of being disabled, even though the anger may be caused by something else. It is therefore important for nurses to try to distinguish between the *person* and the *condition* rather than assuming that one is simply a consequence of the other.

Long-term illness can compromise or even destroy a person's social and personal identity by affecting their sense of autonomy and control over their lives. Health care professionals may unintentionally undermine a patient's sense of autonomy and reinforce the break with their former selves by withholding information from them. They may also stereotype them, for example, talking to older patients as if they were children. The playwright Alan Bennett (2005) described visiting his elderly mother in hospital and finding the nurses were calling her Lily. Bennett explained to them that this might be adding to his mother's confusion because she had always been called either Lillian or Mrs Bennett, but never Lily. Nonetheless, the nurses persisted in calling her Lily, thus taking from her one of the last vestiges of her personal identity, her name.

Stigma

Sickness and disabling conditions are often *stigmatising*. People are socially stigmatised when they are seen by others to be in some way unacceptable or inferior, and are thus denied full social acceptance (Goffman 1968). In stigma there is a discrepancy between what Goffman calls people's 'virtual social identity' (they way they should be if they were normal) and their 'actual social identity' (the way they are). Those who are stigmatised are confronted with a series of decisions about their 'spoiled identity', both in terms of their interactions with others and their own self-concept. People are more likely to experience stigmatised reactions from others when their impairment is visible. In Goffman's terms, they are 'discredited' and this may lead to withdrawal from social participation, especially in public areas. When the condition is not visible, as in epilepsy or HIV, for example, and people are potentially 'discreditable', they have to decide whether to be open about their condition or try to 'pass' as 'normal'.

The implications of stigma thus go well beyond public reaction. For example, Scambler and Hopkins (1986) found that very few of the epileptics they interviewed had actually experienced any stigmatising reactions from others (enacted stigma). However, the shame of being epileptic (felt stigma) led most of them to conceal their condition, even from those close to them. For example, two-thirds of those experiencing epilepsy at the time of their marriage concealed it from their partners, while three-quarters had not disclosed their condition to their employers. The authors found that, paradoxically, this felt stigma was more disruptive to their lives than enacted stigma.

In some conditions, such as Parkinson's disease or multiple sclerosis, there may be a long time between initial experiences of symptoms and medical diagnosis. In such circumstances diagnosis can be a relief as it both legitimises the patients' complaints and confirms the reality of their symptoms, while failure to obtain a diagnostic label can be stigmatising. In her study of ence-phalomyelitis (ME) Cooper (1997) found a great deal of conflict between patients, who felt ill, and their doctors, who could find no evidence of disease. Consequently, many were not allowed access to the sick role and, as a result, 'their social position was to some extent eroded, their social identity devalued and stigmatised, and they found it difficult to obtain absence from work or disability benefit' (Cooper 1997: 203).

Socialisation

In Chapter 1 we described socialisation as a process where people learn about the behaviour that is expected in given social situations. Becoming sick or disabled also involves processes of socialisation. Most of the earliest soci-ological studies of socialisation into illness or disability focused on the 'crisis' brought about by a person's comparatively sudden transition from 'health' to 'sickness'. Some of this work suggested that others' reactions to illness or disabling conditions, particularly the reactions of health care professionals, created a self-fulfilling prophecy where the sufferer's personal identity comes to correspond to the social identity given by the expert.

Scott's (1969) classic study of the newly blind provides a good example of this approach. Scott argues that there is nothing inherent in the condition of blindness itself to produce the stereotyped view of the 'blind personality' as passive, docile and compliant. From his observations of interactions between experts and their blind clients, Scott argued that the 'blind personality' is a product of socialisation where experts emphasise to clients the importance of coming to terms with lost sight and accepting themselves as blind. This 'putative social identity' is gradually internalised by clients as a basis for their own personal identity. Thus, according to Scott, blindness is a 'learned social role' because experts create for blind people the experience of being blind. Similarly, sociological studies have suggested that mental hospitals socialise patients into seeing themselves as mentally ill and playing a 'mentally ill role' (see Chapter 8).

More recent sociological studies have tended to look at the transition to sickness as a series of gradual transformations of social and personal iden-tity and experience. This change of focus arose partly from the realisation that specific conditions do not create a unified experience for sufferers, and partly as a result of sociologists' increasing interest in chronic illnesses, such as arthritis, that develop slowly and inconsistently (Chapter 7). Bury (1997) has argued that chronic illnesses involve a series of *adaptations* to illness rather than the single *adoption* of a new illness identity. New ways of living and changes in self-concept have to be negotiated and renegotiated as the disease progresses, and sufferers have to readjust their patterns of work, leisure and personal relationships.

Adaptation to long-term illness requires managing both its physical and psy-chological aspects. The management of the physical aspects involves the develop-ment of new skills, such as operating machinery, administering medication and learning new daily routines. For example, sufferers from debilitating conditions, such as respiratory disorders, have to learn very quickly what they can do before chronic fatigue sets in, and plan their day accordingly. The management of the physical aspects of illness is well described by Parsons' notion of the sick role, where people can be seen to be conforming (or not conforming) to the 'obligations' involved in being ill.

A feature of chronic illnesses and disabilities is that they create a 'biographical disruption' bringing a fundamental break between past and present selves. Frank (1991), a sociologist who suffered both heart disease and cancer relatively early in life, describes the break he felt with his past pre-illness identity by likening it to leaving a place where he had once lived and been happy. Part of the process of adapting to illness involves sufferers trying in various ways to 'repair' the biographical disruption to their lives by developing 'explanations' for the illness. For example, Williams *et al.* (1996) showed how people with rheumatoid arthritis engage in a 'narrative reconstruction' in which their biography is reorganised in order to 'make sense' of the onset of illness. Narratives may also be used to explain sudden fluctuations in symptoms; for example, an increase in symptoms may be 'explained' by having had a stressful experience or 'overdoing things' the day before. While these 'lay theories' and 'narrative reconstructions' may have little or no clinical validity, they are often crucial in helping people restore a sense of order and meaning to their lives.

Sociological work on sickness suggests, amongst other things, that patient care could be improved by nurses and other health professionals recognising the importance of trying to maintain aspects of patients' social and personal identities, trying to adopt practices that help to de-stigmatise a patient or a condition, and understanding the social as well as physical adaptations involved in coping with long-term illness. In recent years, nursing and medicine have moved towards a more patient-centred approach to health care, partly in response to criticisms of the dominance of the bio-medical approach that effectively saw patients as machines to be repaired by technical experts. A patient-centred approach means giving more weight to patients' viewpoints and experiences and changing the balance of power away from professionals towards patients.

Summary

The bio-medical model of health focuses on how the human body works and how disease can be prevented, arrested or cured through treatment. Bio-medicine continues to dominate the organisation of health care in contemporary societies, but the capacity of a medically based health care system to influence overall patterns of health significantly is being increasingly questioned as many of the major determinants of health are environmental. This perspective has given rise to an alternative socio-medical approach to health, and a greater number of health professionals are now engaging in surveillance medicine, monitoring general populations with the idea of preventing disease and promoting better health. In the management of ill-health sociological research has shown that becoming ill and being ill involve social and psychological as well as biological change, and that effective nursing of the sick involves understanding these social processes. In recent years, health care has been moving towards a more patient-centred approach and health care professionals have been encouraged to take greater account of social and psychological aspects of sickness.

References

Armstrong, D. (1995) The rise of surveillance medicine. *Sociology of Health and Illness*, 17, 393–404.

Bennett, A. (2005) *Untold Stories*. Faber & Faber, London.

Berkman, L. and Syme, S. (1979) Social networks and host resistance and mortality: a nine year follow-up study of Almeda County residents. *American Journal of Epidemiology*, 109, 186–204.

Bunker, J. (2001) Medicine matters after all, in B. Davey, A. Gray and C. Seale (eds) *Health and Disease: A Reader*. Open University, Buckingham.

Bury, M. (1997) *Health and Illness in a Changing Society*. Routledge, London.

Camic, P. and Knight, S. eds (2004) *Clinical Handbook of Health Psychology*. Hogrefe & Huber, Ohio.

Cooper, L. (1997) Myalgic encephalomyelitis and the medical encounter. *Sociology of Health and Illness*, 19, 186–207.

Cowley, S., Mitcheson, J. and Houston (2004) Structuring health needs assessments: the medicalisation of health visiting. *Sociology of Health and Illness*, 26(5), 503–26.

Durkheim, E. (1952) *Suicide: A Study in Sociology*. Routledge, London.

Fairnington, A. (2004) Communities that care. *Critical Public Health*, 14(1), 27–36.

Frank, A. (1991) *At the Will of the Body: Reflections on Illness*. Houghton Mifflin, New York.

Frank, A. (1995) *The Wounded Storyteller: Body, Illness and Ethics*. Chicago, University of Chicago Press.

Goffman, E. (1968) *Stigma: Notes on the Management of Spoiled Identity*. Penguin, London.

Graham, H., Francis, B., Inskip, H. and Harman, J. (2006) Socioeconomic lifecourse influences on women's smoking status in early adulthood. *Journal of Epidemiological Community Health*, 60, 228–33.

Hirst, M. (2005) Carer distress: a prospective, population-based study. *Social Science and Medicine*, 61(3), 697–708.

Illich, I. (1990) *Limits to Medicine: Medical Nemesis: The Expropriation of Health*. Penguin, London.

Jeffery, R. (2001) Normal rubbish: deviant patients in casualty departments, in B. Davey, A. Gray and C. Seale (eds) *Health and Disease: A Reader*. Open University, Buckingham.

Le Fanu, J. (1999) *The Rise and Fall of Modern Medicine*. Little, Brown & Co., London.

McKeown, T. (1979) *The Role of Medicine*. Blackwell, Oxford.

Parsons, T. (1951) *The Social System*. Free Press, New York.

Reinharz, S. (2001) Enough already! The pervasiveness of warnings in everyday life, in B. Davey, A. Gray and C. Seale (eds) *Health and Disease: A Reader*. Open University, Buckingham.

Scambler, G. and Hopkins, A. (1986) Being epileptic: coming to terms with illness. *Sociology of Health and Illness*, 8, 26–43.

Scott, R. (1969) *The Making of Blind Men*. Russell Sage, Hartford.

Secretary of State for Health and Social Services (1992) *The Health of the Nation*. HMSO, London.

Stryer, D. and Clancy, C. (2005) Editorial: Patients' safety. *British Medical Journal*, 330, 553–4.

Szreter, S. (1988) The importance of social intervention in Britain's mortality decline. *Social History of Medicine*, 1, 1–38.

Temkin-Greener, H., Bajorska, A., Peterson, D., Kunitz, S., Gross, D., Williams, T. and Mukamel, D. (2004) Social support and risk-adjusted mortality in a frail older population. *Medical Care*, 42(8), 779–88.

Wheatley, E.E. (2005) Disciplining bodies at risk: cardiac rehabilitation and the medicalisation of fitness. *Journal of Sport and Social Issues*, 29(5), 198–221.

Williams, G., Fitzpatrick, R., MacGregor, A. and Rigby, A. (1996) Rheumatoid arthritis, in B. Davey and C. Seale (eds) *Experiencing and Explaining Disease*. Open University, Buckingham.

Young, J. (2005) Illness behaviour: a selective review and synthesis. *Sociology of Health and Illness*, 26(1), 1–3.

Further reading

Bury, M. (2005) *Health and Illness*. Polity Press, Cambridge.
Provides a clear account of the distribution of health and illness, the developing field of the sociology of the body and explores the changing context of health care.

Davey, B., Gray, A. and Seale, C. eds (2002) *Health and Disease: A Reader*, 3rd edition. Open University Press, Buckingham.
A useful collection of articles and extracts from major studies on health, sickness and health care.

Part II

Social patterns in health and disease

Chapter 3

Socio-economic inequalities in health

Introduction

Inequalities in health between social groups are a resilient feature of British society and continue to be part of the social and political landscape of the twenty-first century. This chapter will provide an overview of the evidence about socio-economic inequalities in health and the explanations of these. It will:

- place (locate) socio-economic health inequalities in an historical background;
- discuss the measurement of socio-economic status and health;
- discuss the widening gap in socio-economic health inequalities;
- examine explanations of socio-economic health inequalities;
- consider policies addressing socio-economic health inequalities.

Historical background

Despite significant improvements in the overall health of the UK population, there has been little reduction of the 'health gap' between rich and poor since the 1800s. Current explanations and arguments about these inequalities also echo more than century-old debates. For example, the recent emphasis on individual responsibility for ill health parallels debate in the 1800s about whether poverty and related ill health arose from 'the failings of individuals or from the failings of society' (Davey Smith *et al.* 2001: xxxv). Questions of whether poverty causes ill health or ill health causes poverty also stem back to this time. We can also see continuity between the eugenics movement of the early twentieth century, which stressed that heredity had a greater influence upon health than social environment, and present day socio-biological and genetic accounts for differences in health (Davey Smith *et al.* 2001).

Research from the middle of the twentieth century showed that, although British society as a whole was getting both richer and healthier, health inequalities between people in different social strata were increasing. In 1980 a government commissioned review, the Black Report (Townsend *et al.* 1988), concluded that the main explanation for inequalities in health was material deprivation. However, this conclusion did not match up with the views of the incoming Conservative government, which placed less emphasis on societal factors and more on personal responsibility for health, wealth and opportunity, and so was disregarded in government policy.

A new inquiry into health inequality commissioned by the incoming New Labour government in 1997, the Acheson Report (1998), endorsed the Black Report's conclusion that the origins of health inequalities lay in the social environment. It concluded that, although the previous 20 years had brought a marked increase in prosperity to the country as a whole, the gap between the top and bottom social strata had widened at all stages of the life course, reflected in growing inequalities in health. The most recently commissioned government review of the research evidence (Wanless 2003) suggested a 'layers of influence' model for understanding the causes and patterning of health, combining individual (lifestyle and behaviours) and environmental explanations. This has now been adopted to guide UK health policy (Bajekal *et al.* 2006), and will be discussed later.

Measuring inequality and health

Before we look at research evidence we will consider briefly how researchers have conceptualised and measured socio-economic status and health.

Socio-economic status

Socio-economic status is a widely used concept that derives from the sociological conceptualisation of social class, first proposed by Marx. The two main aspects of social class are the 'material differences' between different occupational groupings (e.g. in income, housing) and the social relationships that people form in earning their living (e.g. the relationships nurses have with doctors, managers, other nurses and patients) (Miers 2003). Social class is most frequently measured by the indicator of occupational ranking (Chapter 1) while socio-economic status is a wider concept than social class, combining occupational status with an array of other factors such as income, education, housing and social status to produce a composite measure (Bartley 2004).

Occupation is the foundation of the widely used British Registrar General's measure of social class, which has been in use since 1921, based on five groups defined by occupational skill (depicted in Tables 3.1 and 3.2). Changes in the labour market and the nature of work, such as increases in information technology, service sector work, home working and call centre work, led to a new measure, which came into use with the 2001 census. This is called the National Statistics Socio-economic Classification (or NS-SEC). The seven main classes are based on job responsibilities, including degree of control over the content and pace of work, and supervisory duties. An eighth class includes the long-term unemployed and those who have never worked (Miers 2003).

Some researchers have questioned the use of occupation as the main measure of socio-economic status. One important weakness is that many people are excluded because they do not have jobs. Also, as we now live in a society defined as much by *consumption* and status as by work and production, measures such as home ownership, car ownership, education, income and deprivation are sometimes more useful. Importantly, these measures also allow us to examine differences *within* occupationally defined groups, and provide a more detailed analysis of health and mortality. People's lives are significantly shaped by where they live. Indeed, as we will see later in this chapter, the characteristics of their *area of residence* may have a greater effect on their health than personal characteristics such as occupation. For this reason *deprivation indices*, based on small area statistics from the census have been used for many years. Much recent research on inequality in health has been geographically based using such measures.

Health

Although it may seem rather strange to use death as a measure of health, mortality statistics are the most reliable way of measuring health inequalities (Chapter 1). Most importantly, since they have been available for many years, we can track changes in life expectancy over time. However, age at death and the causes of death tell us little about the experience of health and illness during life.

Researchers use a large number of different indicators to try to measure morbidity (illness) and consistent socio-economic differences in health have been found using most of these measures. Researchers have found that the simple overall self-assessment of health as 'good' or 'poor' is usually the single best predictor of health status. At the present time, the most frequently used measures in official surveys such as the decennial census and the annual General Household Survey (GHS) are self-reported prevalence of long-standing illness and global self-assessments of overall health. However, it must be remembered that the way that people define their health can itself be influenced by their socio-economic status.

When a large amount of survey data are analysed it is often possible to adjust for the effects of such factors as age and gender by a technique called standardisation. For example, people in higher socio-economic occupational groups are likely to live longer than those in lower socio-economic occupational groups. 'Age standardisation' adjusts for the effects of any such differences between the groups, thus allowing a more precise analysis of mortality and morbidity data.

The widening gap in socio-economic health inequalities

The authors of the Black Report were forced to rely on mortality figures because of the lack of available population-level data that tracked patterns of health – as opposed to death – over time. In the intervening period there has been a massive expansion of research on ill health and inequality, but, since most data on health status cannot be reliably collected retrospectively, data looking at changes in health over long periods of time are still rather limited. Nevertheless, research subsequent to the publication of the Black Report confirms a consistent relationship between social inequalities and ill health: 'Wherever we are in the hierarchy, our health is likely to be better than those below us and worse than those above us' (Marmot 2004: 4).

Mortality

Over time there has been a widening gap in mortality between people at the 'top' and the 'bottom' of the social hierarchy in Britain because, even though mortality rates are improving for all socio-economic groups, improvement has been faster among those at the 'top' than among those at the 'bottom'. Tables 3.1 and 3.2 highlight this change. Table 3.1 shows that while life expectancy has improved for both men and women in all occupational groups between 1972–1976 and 1997–2001, the gap between those in 'professional/managerial' and those in 'partly skilled and unskilled' occupations has grown. Those at the top of the occupational scale live longer than those at the bottom, at both time periods. However, for men only, there is an increasing gap between 1972–1976 and 1997–2001. It is also evident that men have gained more years than women (see Chapter 5).

Table 3.2 also shows that mortality rates have declined (i.e. improved) for men and women in all social class groups over the period, with greater improvement for men than for women. We can also see that for men the mortality gap between classes IV + V and I + II widened over the period, from a ratio of 1.69 to 1.75. By contrast, for women there was a narrowing of the gap from 1.54 to 1.41.

Table 3.1 Life expectancy at birth by social class, England and Wales.

Occupational social class		1972–1976		1997–2001		Differences between 1972–1976 and 1997–2001 at birth	
		Men	Women	Men	Women	Men	Women
I	Professional	71.9	79.1	79.4	82.2	7.5	3.1
II	Managerial and technical/intermediate	71.7	76.9	77.8	81.7	6.1	4.8
IIINM	Skilled non-manual	69.4	78.0	74.6	81.3	7.4	3.3
IIIM	Skilled manual	69.3	75.1	73.3	79.3	5.0	4.2
IV	Partly skilled	68.3	75.0	73.3	78.6	5.0	3.6
V	Unskilled	66.4	73.8	71.0	77.6	4.6	3.8

Source: derived from ONS Longitudinal Study (tables 1–4), available at website www.statistics.gov.uk

Table 3.2 Trends in all-cause mortality by social class 1986–1999, men and women aged 35–64 (directly age-standardised rates per 100,000 person years).*

Social class	1986–1992		1993–1996		1997–1999	
	Men	Women	Men	Women	Men	Women
I and II	460	274	376	262	347	237
IIINM	480	310	437	262	417	253
IIIM	617	350	538	324	512	327
IV and V	776	422	648	378	606	335
Ratio	1.69	1.54	1.71	1.44	1.75	1.41
IV + V : I + II						

*Age standardisation adjusts for the effects of any differences in age distributions of different occupational groups.
Source: derived from White, C., van Galen, F. and Chow, Y.H. (2003) Trends in social class differences in mortality by cause, 1986 to 2000. *Health Statistics Quarterly*, 20, 25–37 (tables 1 and 2).

Geographical location is another important source of health inequality. Shaw *et al.* (2005) examined the relationship between poverty and life expectancy by comparing affluent and poor areas of Britain over the 10-year period 1992–2003. They concluded that at the start of the twenty-first century health inequality is increasing, with life expectancy continuing to rise faster in the most advantaged areas of the UK. They sorted local authority districts into 'poverty groups' by using a version of the 'Breadline Britain' index of poverty (Box 3.1). Over these 10 years, life expectancy rose for all 'poverty groups', but the absolute difference in life expectancy between the top and bottom groups also increased to more than 4 years. The difference between the district with the lowest life expectancy (Glasgow city) and the highest life expectancy (east Dorset) was 11 years for men and 8.4 years for women.

Box 3.1 The Breadline Britain index of poverty

- Lack of basic amenities
- Access to a car
- Unskilled and semiskilled manual occupations
- Unemployment
- Non owner-occupied households
- Lone parent households

Source: derived from Shaw *et al.* (2005) Health inequalities and New Labour: how the promises compare with real progress. *British Medical Journal*, 330, 1016–21.

Morbidity

Figure 3.1 depicts significant differences in *self-assessed general health* by occupational groups as reported in the 2001 national census. The gradients are remarkably clear: as we go down the occupational hierarchy self-assessments of health consistently worsen. While over 80% of the top group see themselves in good health, this reduces to just over 60% among those in routine occupations. About half of those who never worked or were unemployed for a long time reported they were in good health. This group includes people who are classified as permanently disabled or sick; unsurprisingly these reported the lowest rate of good health (11%) and the highest rate of 'not good' health (63%).

Among those who were 'economically active', those working full-time and those who were self-employed were more likely to report themselves as in good health than those working part-time. Overall, economically active men reported higher rates of good health than economically active women (77 : 74%). For those who were economically inactive, women reported higher rates of good health than men (54 : 43%). Within each socio-economic group men consistently reported higher age-standardised rates of good health than women, but there was little difference between them for those reporting their health was not good (Bajekal *et al.* 2006: 12).

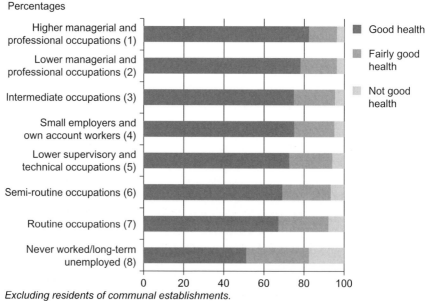

Excluding residents of communal establishments.
For persons aged 16–64.

Figure 3.1 Age-standardised self-assessed general health.
Source: Bajekal *et al.* (2006) *Focus on Health*, Figure 2.3. National Statistics website: www.statistics.gov.uk.
Crown copyright material is reproduced with the permission of the Controller of HMSO.

There is also a marked *regional health divide* in Britain. Drawing on self-rated health from the 2001 census, Doran *et al.* (2004) found self-rates of 'poor health' for men ranging from less than 49/100 in the South-East of England to more than 80/100 in Wales and the North-East. For women the range was from less than 52/100 in the South-East to more than 81/100 in Wales. Using the NS-SEC occupational classification, Doran *et al.* also found that the health of people in each class varied considerably depending on where they lived. For example, women in class 1 in Wales fared worse than women in class 4 in the South-East and men in class 4 in the North-West fared worse than men in class 7 in the South-East. This suggests that the areas in which people live can have an effect on their health over and above their individual circumstances (here occupational class), an issue we take up in the next section.

Given their impact upon health, it is important to consider how '*health behaviours*' such as diet, exercise and cigarette smoking within the population are related to socio-economic status. Since it is seen as the greatest single cause of preventable disease in the UK (Wanless 2003), and because there are reliable data available over time, cigarette smoking can be used as an example. Although overall smoking rates for those over age 16 have declined over time, the differential between the highest and lowest occupational groups in Britain widened between 1974 and 1994. In 1974, men from manual backgrounds were 24% more likely to smoke than men from non-manual backgrounds; by 2000 this had risen to 52%. The equivalent figures for women were 18% and 36% (Babb *et al.* 2004). A further example of current interest is obesity. The prevalence of obesity has increased over time in all social classes, but this has been more pronounced amongst manual social classes (Babb *et al.* 2004).

Explanations for socio-economic health inequalities

A number of explanations for socio-economic health inequalities have been advanced. We review the most influential of these here.

Access to health care

One long-standing explanation of socio-economic inequalities in health is that these reflect access to health care. Indeed, one of the assumptions underpinning the introduction of the NHS in 1948 was that removing financial barriers to access to health services would promote more equitable care and thus improve the health of the worse off in society.

Access to general practice is important because it is typically the 'gatekeeper' to a wider range of services (e.g. hospital care, preventative and screening services, maternity care). Data show that people in lower socio-economic groups are more likely to have consulted a GP in the 14 days before the interview. However, for the large majority of age groups the difference between socio-economic groups is not statistically significant. It is important to bear in mind that even if use *were* equal, this would not necessarily mean that health care needs were being equally met. People in poorer socio-economic circumstances tend to have worse health, thus their *need* is typically greater, and research often points to a reservoir of *unmet need*. In discussions of health service use this is often called the *demand side*. Demand does not simply depend upon clinical need but also involves knowledge about what is available and the economic and social resources available to individuals and families to access care.

Supply side and *demand side* factors often interact to exacerbate disadvantage. Tudor Hart's influential 'inverse care law' describes the situation in which people in deprived areas tend to have greater health care needs, but that services are much less likely to be available to them (and may be of a poorer quality) (Miers 2003). This situation persists in twenty-first century Britain. Poor people experience worse health at younger ages, but the communities in which they live still have fewer GPs. Higher levels of deprivation, lower community incomes per head, high levels of illness and premature death, and higher workload levels in primary care are all associated with lower average consultation times. For example, Bajekal *et al.* (2006) report that for many deprived communities, heart surgery, hip replacements and other services such as screening are less likely to be available than in affluent communities. The prevalence of treated coronary heart disease was about 40% higher in deprived areas than in affluent areas, but it was 25% less likely to be treated with a statin in these areas.

Overall, research suggests that there are socio-economic inequalities in access to health care in the UK on both the demand and supply sides. However, it is important to remember that increases in life expectancy between the mid-eighteenth and mid-twentieth centuries were more to do with improvements in social and economic environment than with developments in medicine, suggesting that health care has a limited role in explaining the health of the population in general (Chapter 2). For these reasons, while unequal access to health care may play a role, it is unlikely to be the major explanation for inequalities in health.

Explanations in the Black Report

The authors of the Black Report (Townsend *et al.* 1988) reviewed the three main explanations of socio-economic inequalities in health that were current at the time (Miers 2003). The first explanation, which they favoured, was that differences in health are socially caused by differences in *material circumstances* such as income, housing and working environment; those in worse material conditions have worse health as a result. It also found some limited support for the '*social selection*' explanation. Here the direction of causation is reversed: it is not material circumstances that influence levels of health and illness, but, rather, levels of health and illness that influence material circumstances. People are *selected* into social positions on the basis of their health; for example, those in poor health are unlikely to hold on to well-paid jobs and are liable to move down the occupational ladder, while those with good health are more likely to be upwardly mobile. Higher social classes tend to recruit the healthiest individuals, while the least healthy 'fall' into the lower classes.

The third explanation focused on differences in *cultures and behaviours* between social classes. People in the lower social classes are more likely to define health as the absence of symptoms and to have low expectations of health, seeing illness as a matter of luck or fate. People from professional and managerial backgrounds have higher expectations about health, believing that their own behaviour can improve it, share medical definitions of health and illness, and are more likely to seek expert help at an early stage in their illness. These different health beliefs are related to differences in health behaviour – such as smoking, exercise, diet – between higher (better informed, with healthier behaviour) and lower (ill-informed, with unhealthy behaviour) social classes.

Layers of influence

Following the Black Report, explanations of health inequality in the 1980s tended to pit structural factors that affect health which are largely outside the individual's control (e.g. pollution, levels of unemployment, access to health care) against factors over which individuals have somewhat more control (e.g. diet, exercise). Government health policy of the time emphasised that 'unhealthy behaviours' which contribute to ill health, such as smoking and eating fatty foods, predominated in working class households and health improvement policies predominantly focused on changing individual behaviour, rather than the wider social environment. However, current research and policy stress the interaction between structural factors and individual behaviours.

Social structural and material factors, individual behaviours and biology interact to produce inequalities in health. Individual lifestyles are likely to be rooted in, and grow out, of particular social contexts. For example, living in an area of high unemployment and being unable to find work causes stress, which in turn provokes unhealthy behaviours like cigarette smoking. In turn, an individual's biological constitution may both influence and be influenced by their lifestyle and social context (see below). Thus, a sociological understanding of health inequalities involves exploring how the socio-economic structure of society influences individuals and how individuals influence the socio-economic structure.

Figure 3.2 is based upon the widely accepted World Health Organisation model of 'layers of influence' that has influenced both the Acheson Report (1998) and current health policy. At the centre of the model are individuals who 'are endowed with age, sex, and constitutional factors . . . which influence their health potential, but which are fixed' (Bajekal *et al.* 2006: 2). Surrounding this are layers of influence, ranging from the macro (societal)-level social, economic and environmental factors to the micro level of individual lifestyles and behaviours.

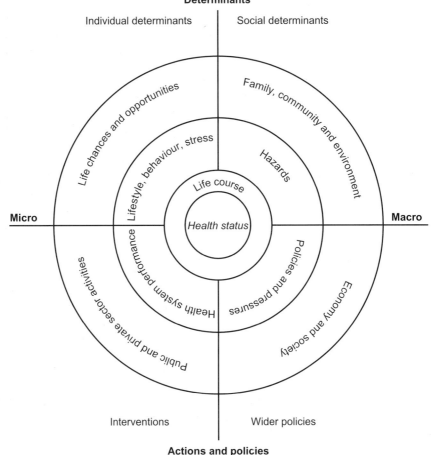

Figure 3.2 Layers of influence on health.
Source: Bajekal *et al.* (2006) *Focus on Health*, Figure 1.1. National Statistics website: www.statistics.gov.uk.
Crown copyright material is reproduced with the permission of the Controller of HMSO.

General socio-economic factors

Large-scale quantitative research has been most successful in tracing the
paths that run from social structure to the individual. In particular, it has
demonstrated the strong association between changes in health and the dyn-
amics of macro-level socio-economic circumstances over time. It is therefore
important to review the kinds of changes that have been occurring.

Income is very important because of its association with access to goods
and services, which in turn is associated with well-being. It is probably the
most obvious and easily understood socio-economic influence upon health.
However, other socio-economic variables can also have an independent effect.
Occupation can have both a direct effect on health (e.g. through industrial
accidents and health hazards at work) and affect it indirectly (e.g. by workers
bringing hazardous substance home on their clothing which affects their

families' health). Another significant influence is *education*. People with higher education qualifications are likely to have better health than those with lower levels of qualifications. This seems to work primarily through increased knowledge and understanding of health and disease and how and when to access appropriate services. *Residence*, both in terms of general area and type of accommodation, is another socio-economic variable that affects health. However, although socio-economic variables may have independent effects upon health, they tend to cluster together and reinforce each other. It is this broad patterning of socio-economic inequalities that is most significant for producing inequalities in health.

During the 1980s and 1990s, and continuing into the early years of the twenty-first century, greater prosperity for the majority of the UK population was accompanied with an increasing gap between the richest and poorest (Shaw *et al.* 2005). Figure 3.3 shows changes in household incomes in the UK since the early 1970s. During the 1970s, income distribution was broadly stable. Inequalities began gradually to decrease in 1973 and 1979, but this was reversed in the early 1980s and the extent of inequality continued to grow throughout the 1990s. Between 1981 and 1989, the average (median) income rose by 27%. However, while income for the top 10% of the population rose by 38%, for the bottom 10% it rose by only 7%. The proportion of the population living in low-income households rose from 12% in 1979 to a peak of 21% in 1991/92, after which it has fallen to reach 17% for 2000/01–2002/03 (Babb *et al.* 2004).

Many researchers have pointed out that these inequalities are driven by significant changes in patterns of employment in contemporary Britain, with more part-time, temporary and flexible work, more self-employment and more long-term chronic unemployment. People living in workless households are

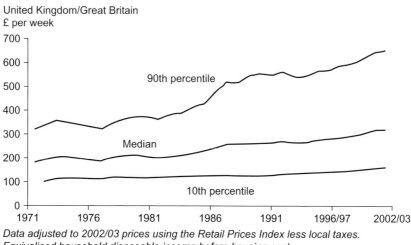

Data adjusted to 2002/03 prices using the Retail Prices Index less local taxes.
Equivalised household disposable income before housing costs.

Figure 3.3 Distribution of real disposable household income.
Source: Babb, P., Martin, J. and Haezewindt, P. eds (2004) *Focus on Social Inequalities*, Figure 4.3. Stationery Office, London. Crown copyright material is reproduced with the permission of the Controller of HMSO.

far more likely to be living below the poverty line (defined as an income below 60% of the population mid point). At the start of the 1980s less than 15% of the population were below the poverty line, increasing to, and remaining at, about 24% of the population in the 1990s.

Although this section has focused upon health inequalities between the top and bottom of the social strata, it is important to recognise that there is a gradient in health. As Bartley (2004: 97) puts it there are 'differences in health and life expectancy between the most advantaged groups and those just beneath them as well as between those who are poor and those who are just "getting by"'. One of the clearest illustrations of this comes from studies of civil servants by Marmot and colleagues (the 'Whitehall Studies'). All of the civil servants were in non-industrial, office-based jobs; that is, none were at the bottom of the class hierarchy. Yet men at the lowest levels of the civil service had, at ages 40–64, four times the risk of death of the administrators at the top. Moreover, the group second from top had higher mortality than those above them, and so on down the hierarchy (Marmot 2004, chapter 1). This suggests that although socio-economic factors exert a powerful influence, they are not the complete explanation for health inequalities.

Social and community networks

Social and community networks are the meeting point between the socio-economic determinants of health (such as income, prosperity and levels of deprivation described above) and individual behaviours or 'lifestyle factors' that influence health.

Although there is substantial evidence that people's health and health behaviour are linked with their socio-economic position, it is important to understand how these are linked. While the way that people view their health, the decisions that they make about their health (such as whether or not to consult a doctor), and the health promoting or health damaging behaviours that they engage in are strongly associated with their socio-economic position, the fit is far from complete. After all, not all middle class people are healthy and not all working class people are unhealthy. Moreover, even if we find a strong *statistical association* between, say, being middle class and good health, this tells us nothing about the complex social mechanisms – such as how people interpret and act on their circumstances – which actually link the two. Thus, social scientists now suggest that we should ground our analysis of health inequalities much more firmly in the social and community networks within which people live out their lives.

This raises important new questions for research and health professionals; such as, what are the health consequences of being an individual living in poor socio-economic circumstances in a relatively prosperous place? How do individuals who live in the most materially disadvantaged areas make sense of and act upon their environments, and with what consequences for health? It is still early days in terms of turning these theoretical questions into empirical research that explores exactly how people and place interact (e.g. Curtis 2004).

Attention has been given to the relative importance for health of inter-personal relationships in an area, and the term *social capital* is increasingly being used to refer to less tangible aspects of community life such as trust, cooperation, a sense of belonging, social support and participation. This concept has similarities to Durkheim's ideas about the positive affects of social cohesion and the integration of individuals into social groups (Chapter 1; Blaxter 2004: 117–21). The social capital that people can 'draw on' is directly related to the types of groups and communities they belong to, and there is considerable interest in the relationship between social cohesion and social networks in government health policy (Miers 2003). While there has so far been little UK research on the relationship between social capital and health (Mohan *et al.* 2004) this is likely to become more important in the future.

Individual lifestyle and the life course

The relationship between individual behaviour and social environments in determining health status is another key area of research. Health status is a product of cumulative experiences built up over a lifetime. However, personal experiences are not static – although it may seem this way when they are conceptualised only in terms of broad socio-economic categories. For example, changing a job (even within the same social class category), or moving to a new home (although in the same census area), may have significant impacts on health, as has been shown in research on the relationship between 'life events' and health (Chapter 2).

Individual biographies

One way that researchers are exploring the link between health-related behaviours and social structures is through biographical research on the life course. That is, to examine how the changing experiences of individuals over time affect their 'lived experience' of health (Williams 2003). The changes in individual lives over time can tell us a lot about how life experience impacts on health.

Blaxter (2000) suggests that it is useful to consider three ways that time is experienced over a lifetime. *Individual biographies* – i.e. the changes in individual lives over time – can tell us a lot about how life experience impacts on health. As their lives unfold, people develop certain understandings and expectations about their lives that are often linked to their socio-economic circumstances, which relate to their health. For example, different socio-economic groups may have different expectations of what counts as health and a healthy life (Blaxter 2004). These expectations may also affect how they interpret symptoms of disease and whether they seek help. *Calendar time* is also important because there are shared expectations about how individual lives should proceed through their life course. These vary by generation; for example, the current generation of new parents in Britain do not expect their children to die in infancy or childhood, and those who do are thought to have died 'before their time'.

Personal biographies are embedded within what Blaxter calls *socio-historical time*. This refers to the experiences of people born into particular generations (age cohorts), each with their own unique social history. Different age cohorts experience quite particular socio-economic vulnerabilities, such as those associated with employment conditions (e.g. the use of asbestos, leading to asbestosis, which peaked in the 1970s) or medical knowledge (e.g. cigarette smoking was not widely known to be dangerous to health until the 1960s). Not only do different generations have different experiences and vulnerabilities, they also have different expectations about their health and differing attitudes towards dealing with illness. For example, older people in the UK appear to be more 'accepting' about illness and to have lower expectations of health care services than those born in the 1960s (Chapter 6). The latter seem to have much higher expectations about their health status, and to be more demanding of health services about the treatment of their illnesses.

Biographical research into the relationships between socio-economic status, individual life courses and health is a relatively new but increasingly important area of activity. It helps us to understand how individual biographies are played out within their wider social context and the implications of this for health. It also has the potential to provide insight into how the health of one generation builds on the health of the generation before it.

The influence of biology

From a life course perspective, a person's biological status is a marker of their past social position, recording a lifetime of accumulated advantage and disadvantage. Age-cohort studies – such as the 1958 British birth cohort study – highlight that longer term health is influenced by factors such as parental disadvantage, low birth weight, financial hardship, poor nutrition, crowded residential accommodation, and delayed growth during childhood (Kuh *et al.* 2002). As Wadsworth (1999) aptly puts it, 'childhood has a long reach'.

Figure 3.4 summarises two main explanations of this socio-biological link between early life and adult disease. The first explanation gives primacy to

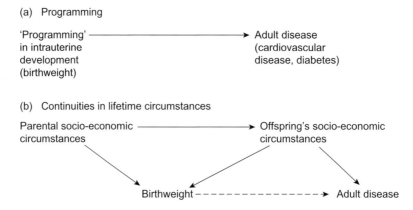

(a) Programming

'Programming' ─────────────────────────▶ Adult disease
in intrauterine   (cardiovascular
development   disease, diabetes)
(birthweight)

(b) Continuities in lifetime circumstances

Parental socio-economic ─────────────────▶ Offspring's socio-economic
circumstances   circumstances

Birthweight - - - - - - - - - - - - - - -▶ Adult disease

Figure 3.4 Pathways linking early life with adult disease.
Source: Power, C., Bartley, M., Davey Smith, G. and Blane, D. (1996) Transmission of social and biological risk across the lifecourse, in D. Blane, R. Brunner and R. Wilkinson (eds) *Health and Social Organisation.* Routledge, London.

events *in utero* or in infancy that 'programme' the individual's ability to respond to risks to health that are encountered later in life. For some infections and negative environmental exposures, it appears that there is a *critical period* during which adverse impacts on health will have a lifelong adverse consequence. Although later life influences play a role, these only operate within the constraints imposed by earlier developmental experiences. One illustration is the groundbreaking research by Barker and his colleagues (Barker 1998) highlighting the impact of a range of pre-natal factors upon fetal growth and subsequent coronary heart disease (CHD) in adults. Direct associations have been made between low birth weight and increased rates of CHD. For example, it seems that if the fetus experiences under-nutrition in late gestation, oxygenated blood is diverted from the trunk to sustain the brain. This affects the growth of the liver, in the process disturbing its regulation of cholesterol and blood clotting, both risk factors for CHD.

The second explanation suggests that there is an *additive or accumulative* general effect upon health over the life course: adverse health events and exposures early in life have an additive effect with adverse influences in later life. For example, there is a relationship between earlier and later negative socio-economic and behavioural factors (excess drinking, smoking) and increased levels of mortality from cardiovascular disease. This explanation highlights continuities in lifetime circumstances and 'biological' factors such as birth weight or height that are influenced by prior social factors and parental circumstances. Thus, for example, low birth weight becomes an indicator for later social disadvantage (such as poor educational attainment) and, consequently, poor health. Petrou *et al.* (2006) followed the mortality and morbidity experience of a large cohort born between 1979 and 1988. The researchers found a 40% increased chance of mortality during the first 10 years of life for children born into social class 5 households as compared to social class 1 households. For each drop in social class the mean number of hospital admissions increased by 5%.

This second explanation suggests that it is not simply a matter of our future health being 'programmed' from birth, but rather of our biology continually interacting with the social environment in which we live. As Wadsworth (1999: 47) puts it, 'biological programming processes require a later-life additional risk to push individuals beyond their biologically programmed safe working envelope'. These additional risks – such as cigarette smoking and obesity – are themselves socially determined.

In summary, this type of research has shown that socio-economic factors may contribute negatively to health by increasing the risk of lifelong adverse health through exposure to negative infectious and environmental hazards at particular points in time, especially in pregnancy and childhood. They may also affect health status cumulatively over the course of a lifetime.

Relative deprivation and psycho-social stress

In the previous section we explored the main determinants of health inequalities in terms of interacting layers of influence. It has been stressed that structural or material factors, individual behaviours and biology interact to produce inequalities in health. One of the most influential and much debated explanations about how these inter-relationships work to produce health inequalities is Wilkinson's (1996, 2005) thesis that there are 'psychosocial pathways' between socio-economic status and health. A similar analysis has also been presented by Marmot (2004).

Wilkinson argues that in contemporary societies such as Britain the psychosocial effects of living in conditions of *relative deprivation* are a more important influence upon people's health than *absolute material deprivation*. Those who are in positions of relative deprivation have less autonomy and control over their lives, have weak social affiliations and experience more stress in their early life.

There are three key stages to this process. First, Wilkinson shows that for wealthy developed countries there is a threshold beyond which the absolute standard of living of the population is no longer associated with improvements in health, measured by life expectancy. He argues that once a country has passed through the epidemiological transition (i.e. the shift away from infectious to degenerative diseases as the major cause of death) 'its whole population can be more than twice as rich as any other country without being any healthier' (Wilkinson 1996: 3). This suggests that there are clear limits on the health returns of a country getting more and more wealthy. Secondly, he argues that although the absolute standard of living is not important for wealthy societies like Britain, differences within society, such as differences in income, are crucial to health inequalities. That is, it is where individuals stand in relation to others (i.e. relative deprivation) that matters most. Thirdly, he argues that the key mechanism linking relative deprivation to health is psychosocial. Simply put, as income differences widened in Britain during the 1980s (as described earlier in this chapter), psycho-social stress increased and we saw a slow down in the improvement in overall mortality rates. Wilkinson argues that many of the biological processes that lead to ill health are triggered by what we think and feel about our material and social circumstances. Therefore it is our subjective experience of life that is important. Those with more power and status, more control over their life circumstances and greater social support fare better in terms of their health. Feelings of hopelessness, anxiety, insecurity and anger amongst those living in relative deprivation leave their mark upon health, directly through biological stress pathways related to weakened immunity and indirectly through negative health behaviours such as smoking, excess consumption of alcohol and eating unhealthy 'comfort foods'. Marmot (2004) argues that striving for status generates hierarchies that, in turn, generate gradients in health. Social hierarchies affect social relations and get under one's skin; that is, they affect the biological body (Wilkinson 2005).

Wilkinson and Marmot support their thesis in two ways. One kind of evidence comes from research into the physiological effects of social status among animals. In studies of macaque monkeys, it is possible to hold factors such as diet and environment (e.g. access to water, food and space) constant while manipulating social status. The research showed that animals in low status groups developed very significant risks to health such as increased atherosclerosis (hardening of the arteries), unfavourable ratios of high density lipoprotein cholesterol and low density lipoprotein cholesterol, insulin resistance and a tendency to central obesity.

Secondly, they use data showing that more egalitarian societies have better overall health: among developed countries, it is the most egalitarian that have the highest life expectancy, not the richest. They argue that this is because more egalitarian societies are more cohesive, as seen, for example, in higher levels of trust between people. Japan, which has the longest life expectancy in the world, has a much narrower income gap between the most and least affluent in society than many other developed societies. In 2001, households in the top fifth had 36% of the country's income and those in the bottom fifth had 11%. Equivalent figures for the USA and the UK, where health inequalities are much larger, were 46% and 5%, and 43% and 7%, respectively (Marmot 2004: 182). Moreover, Marmot argues that the low crime rates, high standards of educational performance and consensual pattern of industrial relations in Japan indicate a high degree of social cohesion. By contrast, it is argued that in Britain the level of social cohesion within communities has diminished over time and is reflected in widening differences in health between areas.

Both Marmot and Wilkinson make it clear that the competitive ethos or 'status syndrome', which impacts negatively upon health, is a macro or societal level phenomenon. As Wilkinson (2005: 203) puts it, government policies of countries such as the USA and the UK 'have showed little regard for social justice and often weakened the position of vulnerable sections of society'. They argue that in order to improve health we need to improve levels of social cooperation and trust. Thus Wilkinson claims that, 'it is only by improving the quality of social relations that we can make further improvements in the real quality of our lives' (2005: 314); this, of course, includes our health.

Researchers who support this overall explanation often propose social capital as the pathway by which income inequality is related to health (e.g. Marmot 2004). They propose that higher levels of social capital such as civic trust and social participation are associated with those more egalitarian communities or societies that have less health inequalities. Wilkinson (2005) claims that only by improving the *quality* of social relations can further improvements be made to the quality of people's lives. In his view, it is not simply a matter of reducing social divisions that promote stigma, violence, stress and intolerance, but of reducing the status competition that fuels the pressure to consume. Marmot (2004) stresses that 'action needs to be taken in improving opportunities for control and engagement for all', not only by governments, but also by individuals. From this point of view a key aspect of health care work, especially for community based nurses, is to develop community based support networks and to encourage people's participation in them (Chapter 2).

A number of criticisms have been levied against this overall thesis. The main criticism is that stressing the 'psycho-social pathways' which link socioeconomic status to health ignores absolute material deprivation, which is seen as the root cause of both health inequalities and relative psycho-social deprivation. In Coburn's view (2000: 137), it is not so much that income inequality produces lower cohesion and trust, leading to poor health, but that the neo-liberal market economy produces *both* higher income inequality and lower social cohesion. He concludes that where competition and individualism are valued above all, it is not surprising that we have seen a decline in community and trust between people. Lynch *et al.* (2001) broadly concur with this view, stressing that 'the structural, political–economic processes that generate inequality exist before their effects are experienced at the individual level'. Bartley (2004: 125–6) questions the emphasis that is placed on peoples' *perceptions* of their relative status: 'there is something rather depressing about this idea that not being a "top dog" in some kind of fixed hierarchy could be so psychologically catastrophic as to have an effect on life expectancy itself. (. . .) Do people really die of envy?'

Addressing socio-economic inequalities

Strategies to reduce socio-economic health inequalities must work alongside strategies that aim to improve the overall health of the population. However, there are no simple solutions to reducing socio-economic health inequalities because these are caused by factors operating at different levels. In terms of the 'layers of influence model' (Figure 3.2), strategies must address pathways from the 'outside in' (the social environment influencing the individual) alongside pathways from the 'inside out' (the individual influencing their personal social environment).

At the *societal level*, increasing prosperity and general standards of living have led to increased levels of health, increasing life expectancy and, probably, increasing years of healthy life expectancy in old age (Chapter 6). However, the gap between the top and bottom social strata has increased. If Marmot (2004) and Wilkinson (1996, 2005) are correct in their argument that, whatever their income, everyone tends to be healthier in a more egalitarian society, the implication for social policy is clear. A redistribution of wealth to create a more egalitarian and cohesive society will reduce health inequalities by improving the health of the worse off. Creating more socio-economic equality will not only reduce healthy inequalities but also improve the health of the nation generally.

Pierson (2002) identifies two broad societal-level strategies, those aimed at improving social cohesion and those aimed at improving social justice. The first attempts to integrate deprived people into UK society by providing similar opportunities for all members of the society in terms of education and access to work. The second aims to bring the disadvantaged up to the same level as the advantaged through a range of 'social engineering' activities such as special social security and other benefits and removing other barriers to access. He suggests that equal opportunity and anti-discrimination policies can have positive effects on reducing socio-economic health inequalities. In particular he identifies:

- maximising income and welfare rights for the disadvantaged;
- strengthening social networks for excluded people;

- building partnerships between helping agencies and those being helped;
- participation of those excluded from wider society in decision making;
- drawing the excluded into the mainstream by better understanding of their needs and wants.

Since 2002 taxation policy and increased benefits for those on lower incomes have reduced income inequalities in the UK (Shaw *et al.* 2005). The introduction of a minimum wage and winter fuel allowances for older people and improving social housing in deprived areas are other government strategies that should partially redress health inequalities.

At the *community* level one strand of government policy has been to improve access to health services through setting targets for health providers and the re-organisation of health services (Chapter 11; Department of Health 2005, 2006). Another strategy is to target communities with high levels of deprivation and associated ill health, and to recognise that health inequalities cannot be tackled by the NHS alone (Chapter 11). Local Strategic Partnerships are developing between health and local government, schools and social services in order to turn national targets into local action. Policies involve not only initiatives to improve the social environment in which people live (e.g. improved local recreational facilities, local facilities to help people stop smoking), but also stress the actions that individuals can take to improve their own lives (e.g. by actually taking advantage of local recreational facilities and enrolling on smoking cessation programmes).

Set in 2001, the targets included: to reduce by at least 10% the gap between the fifth of health authority areas with the lowest life expectancy at birth and the population as a whole; and to reduce by at least 10% the gap in infant mortality between manual occupational groups and the rest of the population. However, government targets and initiatives have been criticised as narrow, unambitious and piecemeal (Wanless 2003). Actions taken to reduce the *social* inequalities that produce *health* inequalities have been deemed ineffective as the gaps between the top and bottom social strata continue to widen (Department of Health 2005), leading Shaw *et al.* (2005) to argue that stronger redistributive policies are needed.

A third strand of government health policy has been the long-standing focus upon *individual health behaviours*. Health promotion activities, such as media campaigns publicising the risks of excessive alcohol intake and unhealthy eating, and health improvement initiatives targeting specifically identified vulnerable groups are at the centre of this approach. The aim here is to persuade individuals to take responsibility for their own health, to avoid health-damaging behaviour and to enhance their health by eating and drinking sensibly and taking regular exercise. This is sometimes reinforced by socio-environmental strategies to prevent unhealthy behaviours, for example by banning smoking in pubs, clubs and restaurants and making it illegal to drive without wearing a seat belt (Chapter 2).

However, it is important that strategies targeted at individuals work alongside strategies that aim to reduce socio-economic health inequalities at the community and societal levels. Take smoking as an example, health promotion strategies which focus on individual health behaviours are typically taken up more readily by those with better personal and local resources, i.e. those in higher socio-economic groups. Thus even though there has been an overall reduction in cigarette smoking in Britain, as we saw earlier there has been a widening socio-economic gap in smoking (Shaw and Smith 2005). Similarly, the 'better off' may take advantage of improvements in local areas, such as renovated housing and better shops selling fresh food produce. For these reasons, health improvement initiatives need to be targeted at specifically identified vulnerable groups.

Nurses and other health care providers will have a role to play in implementing national, regional and local policies to tackle health inequalities. In particular, the work of primary health services (PHS) has been broadened considerably to include not only service delivery (i.e. the effective diagnosis and treatment of individuals and their specific health problems), but also improving the general health of the wider local population, through health promotion and disease prevention activities. Miers (2003) discusses how nurses working in various settings have contributed to the amelioration of socio-economic health inequalities.

Summary

This chapter has reviewed the current evidence on socio-economic inequalities in health and examined the major explanations for these. The long history of health inequalities in Britain underscores their resilience, while more recent research shows that they are increasing. There is now a general acceptance in research and policy circles that health inequalities are socially caused, and that the major determinant is socio-economic inequality within society. Research on the biological, temporal and psycho-social pathways between socio-economic status and health are beginning to provide a better understanding of the relationships between socio-economic inequalities and health inequalities. At a societal level, strategies to address these health inequalities involve attempts to reduce socio-economic inequality and to improve social cohesion and social justice. At the community level, strategies focus on improving access to health care in disadvantaged communities, and at the level of individual behaviour they focus around health promotion and disease prevention activities. Nurses are increasingly expected to take a lead role in community and individual level attempts to reduce socio-economic health inequalities.

References

Acheson Report (1998) *Independent Inquiry into Inequalities in Health*. The Stationery Office, London.

Babb, P., Martin, J. and Haezewindt, P. eds (2004) *Focus on Social Inequalities*. Stationery Office, London.

Bajekal, M., Osborne, V., Yar, M. and Meltzer, H. eds (2006) *Focus on Health*. Office of National Statistics/Palgrave Macmillan. National Statistics website: www.statistics.gov.uk

Barker, D.J.P. (1998) *Mothers, Babies and Disease in Later Life*, 2nd edition. Churchill Livingstone, Edinburgh.

Bartley, M. (2004) *Health Inequalities*. Polity Press, Cambridge.

Blaxter, M. (2000) Rethinking social structure and health, in. S. Williams, J. Gabe and M. Calnan (eds) *Health, Medicine and Society*. Routledge, London.

Blaxter, M. (2004) *Health*. Polity Press, Cambridge.

Coburn, D. (2000) Income inequality, social cohesion and the health status of populations: the role of neo-liberalism. *Social Science and Medicine*, 51, 135–46.

Curtis, S. (2004) *Health and Inequality. Geographical Perspectives*. Sage, London.

Davey Smith, G., Dorling, D. and Shaw, M. eds (2001) *Poverty, Inequality and Health in Britain 1800–2000: A Reader*. Policy Press, Bristol.

Department of Health (2005) *Tackling Health Inequalities: Status Report on the Programme for Action*. Department of Health, London.

Department of Health (2006) *Our Health, Our Care, Our Say: A New Direction for Community Services*. HMSO, Norwich.

Doran, T., Drever, F. and Whitehead, M. (2004) Is there a north–south divide in social class inequalities in health in Great Britain? Cross sectional study using data from the 2001 census. *British Medical Journal*, 328, 1043–5.

Kuh, D., Hardy, R., Langenberg, C., Richards, M. and Wadsworth, M. (2002) Mortality in adults aged 26–54 years related to socioeconomic conditions in childhood and adulthood: post war birth cohort study. *British Medical Journal*, 325, 1076–80.

Lynch, J.W., Davey Smith, G., Kaplan, G. and House, S.J. (2001) Income inequality and mortality: importance to health of individual income, psychosocial environment, or material conditions. *British Medical Journal*, 320, 1200–4.

Marmot, M. (2004) *Status Syndrome. How your Social Standing Directly Affects your Health*. Bloomsbury, London.

Miers, M. (2003) *Class, Inequalities and Nursing Practice*. Palgrave Macmillan, Basingstoke.

Mohan, J., Barnard, S., Jones, K. and Twigg, J. (2004) *Social Capital, Place and Health: Creating, Validating and Applying Small-area Indicators in the Modelling of Health Outcomes*. Health Development Agency, London.

Petrou, S., Kupek, E., Hockley, C. and Goldacre, M. (2006) Social class inequalities in childhood mortality and morbidity in an English population. *Paediatric and Perinatal Epidemiology*, 20, 12–23.

Pierson, J. (2002) *Tackling Social Exclusion*. Routledge, London.

Shaw, M. and Davey Smith, G. (2005) Health inequalities and New Labour: how the promises compare with real progress. *British Medical Journal*, 330, 1016–21.

Townsend, P., Davidson, N. and Whitehead, M. (1988) *Inequalities in Health*. Penguin, London.

Wadsworth, M. (1999) Early life, in M. Marmot and R.G. Wilkinson eds *Social Determinants of Health*. Oxford University Press. Oxford.

Wanless, D. (2003) *Securing Good Health for the Whole Population. Population Health Trends*. HM Treasury, HMSO. Website: www.hm-treasury.gov.uk

Wilkinson, R. (1996) *Unhealthy Societies. The Afflictions of Inequality*. Routledge, London.

Wilkinson, R. (2005) *The Impact of Inequality. How to Make Sick Societies Healthier.* Routledge, London.

Williams, G. (2003) The determinants of health: structure, context and agency. *Sociology of Health and Illness*, 25, 131–54.

Further reading

Bartley, M. (2004) *Health Inequalities.* Polity Press, Cambridge.

A comprehensive introduction to the theories, concepts and methods used in health inequalities research.

Marmot, M. (2004) *Status Syndrome. How your Social Standing Directly Affects your Health.* Bloomsbury, London.

An accessible analysis of the relationship between social status and health in affluent contemporary societies by one of the leading researchers in this area.

Chapter 4

Ethnicity and health

Ethnicity and 'race' play a significant part in shaping the patterns of health and illness in the UK. Ethnic divisions and inequalities have a significant impact on health services and patients' experience of them, although they must be seen alongside the impact of other social divisions such as social class. Ethnicity is not restricted to minority groups supposedly at the margins of society, because everyone in the contemporary UK has an ethnic identity. For instance the 'racial' or ethnic group the nurse belongs to, or is *perceived* to belong to by the patient, might carry a particular set of meanings for the patient, or affect the nursing relationship in various ways. This chapter will:

- define concepts of 'race' and ethnicity;
- provide an overview of the main minority ethnic groups in the UK;
- examine ethnic variations in health;
- review explanations for ethnic variations in health;
- summarise the implications for health services and health care.

Race and ethnicity

Race

Historically, the term 'race' was used to draw distinctions between different groups of human beings that were based on *presumed* physical differences. Actual physical or biological differences are relatively superficial, but race has become a highly important *social* distinction because of the persistence of powerful beliefs or myths about the intrinsic nature of different 'races', such as intelligence or skills.

Racial characteristics cannot be used to explain differences between people but, in everyday life, racial stereotyping leads to assumptions being made about people's behaviour. For people with racist prejudices, the difference between 'black' and 'white' skin signifies deeper differences that derive from beliefs about differences in behaviour and, possibly, the innate superiority of one 'race' over another. Prejudice and discrimination can also arise in relations between ethnic groups. While ethnicity and race are overlapping social categories, ethnicity refers to the ways that social groups can be distinguished from one another according to their cultures and ways of life.

Ethnicity

Ethnicity can be defined as 'a socially constructed difference used to refer to people who see themselves as having a common ancestry, often linked to a geographical territory, and perhaps sharing a language, religion and other social customs' (Dyson 2005: 20). One the main limitation of studies of the health of ethnic groups is the difficulty and variation in operationalising such a definition. This can be seen in the different terms used in research, and hence in this chapter, to describe minority ethnic groups.

The UK has strong elements of a shared culture, marked, for instance, by the use of English as a common language. However, the UK also contains a number of indigenous cultures and two official languages (English and Welsh). There are marked cultural differences, as well as a shared British identity, among English, Irish, Scottish and Welsh groups. In addition there are minority ethnic groups such as the Jewish community, various European minorities (for instance Italian and Polish communities), and African, African-Caribbean and Asian minority communities. Included in the latter are people who are migrants, or who are the descendants of migrants, from Bangladesh, Pakistan and India – for instance Sikhs from northern India, or Gujerati-speaking people from western India. However, an ethnic group cannot be summed up simply as a community with a single, distinctive culture. There are three main reasons for this.

First, 'culture' is itself a complex and constantly changing mix of attitudes and beliefs, uses of language and accent, and cultural practices relating to dress, food, marriage, birth, health, illness and death. Cultures are never static – for instance, the outlook and attitudes of Bengali teenagers in east London today are very different from those of their migrant parents or grandparents. There is no single Bengali or Bangladeshi identity in Britain, and this point can be extended to all other minority ethnic communities.

Secondly, ethnicity is more than culture. Ethnic identity includes a people's sense of shared history and origins, and of a common destiny. Thus there can be a political dimension to ethnicity. Some ethnic groups develop political and religious organisations to defend or promote their interests, and in some countries there are ethnic political parties. In some respects belonging to an ethnic group that is highly conscious of its identity and distinctiveness can provide the kind of social solidarity, support and meaning in life that is beneficial for health (Chapter 2). In other respects belonging to a minority community in a rapidly changing society can cause tensions. Some individuals are torn between the moral codes and social expectations of their ethnic community or family group and the apparent freedoms of the larger society. This might have negative consequences for health, as illustrated, for instance, by above-average rates of mental health problems in some ethnic groups.

Thirdly, ethnicity can also be seen as 'more than culture' in the sense that it represents a set of structural influences affecting the standard of living and material circumstances in which individuals and groups live (Nazroo 2001). In some ways this reflects the importance of the social class positions of people in minority communities and the social and economic context in which they exist. Some ethnic minorities (such as the Bangladeshi community) include disproportionately high numbers of economically or socially disadvantaged people, while others (such as the Indian community) do not. However, the structural aspects of ethnicity represent more than the indirect impact of the class structure. Different minority communities are concentrated in different neighbourhoods or urban areas, and the environmental effects of living in each of these locations could explain some of the ethnic variations in health and illness rates that have been observed (Nazroo 2001).

Ethnic identity is influenced by internal and external definitions of ethnicity. Karlsen (2004) identified three dimensions of ethnic identity:

- *Multiculturalism* for the majority white population focuses upon ethnic integration. For ethnic minorities, it concerns the 'promotion' of ethnic difference through adherence to beliefs and practices traditional within their group and by exploring their feelings and attitudes towards multiculturalism.
- *Racialisation* is where an ethnic affiliation becomes politicised as a result of perceived racism (e.g. some Moslem identities following the 7 July 2005 bombings).
- *Community participation* is associated with the development and sustenance of ethnic identity through the self-presentation as a member of a particular ethnic group, the preservation of their culture and way of life, acculturation and the internalisation of external categories.

Karlsen concludes that the processes of ethnic affiliation are similar across minority and majority groups, but that 'ethnic identity could mean different things to people from different ethnic groups' (Karlsen 2004: 126).

Ethnicity, social inequality and discrimination

Racial and ethnic divisions and social inequalities in contemporary Britain occur because different ethnic groups have different social status, power and economic resources. Different concepts of *minority* status are a key to understanding this point. Some ethnic groups, for example the Jewish or Italian communities in Britain, might be in a minority, but are not particularly disadvantaged or discriminated against. In these cases, the majority generally accepts the right of the minority to maintain a degree of cultural difference. However, the values and beliefs of some minority ethnic communities are in conflict with dominant values, which may foster hostility, discrimination and intolerance on both sides. The status or identity of a minority ethnic community is not static but may change over time so that it is no longer labelled an 'immigrant' minority.

Discrimination against members of minority ethnic groups takes different forms. A basic distinction is between *direct* 'racial' or ethnic discrimination and *indirect* or institutional discrimination. Direct discrimination occurs when individuals act on their prejudices or beliefs to affect the welfare or opportunities of others. Indirect discrimination refers to a pattern of discrimination that arises at the organisational level. Disadvantage to a particular 'racial' or ethnic group may stem from the established working practices and culture of an organisation, even though these may be unintended and unrecognised.

It has been claimed that problems of institutional or indirect racism can be found in all the major institutions of contemporary British society, including the National Health Service (NHS). These can be difficult to deal with because this form of discrimination exists when the organisation treats everyone alike and *appears* to be fair. Paradoxically, treating everyone alike and 'not wanting to discriminate' can lead to a failure to recognise entrenched problems of racialised inequality. In preventive health care, for example, a local strategy on cervical screening that treated all women alike might miss important differences in the values and attitudes of different ethnic communities. Also, some health problems are more common in minority ethnic communities than in the majority population, while others are less common. These differences need to be recognised if the NHS is to provide an equal service to all sections of our culturally and ethnically diverse society.

Minority ethnic communities in Britain

The ethnic composition of the UK population is becoming increasingly diverse (Connolly and White 2006). The 1991 national population census included a question about 'ethnic' identity for the first time. The main categories used in this and the 2001 census and other official statistics are not ethnic groups in the sense defined above. The census refers to 'ethnic groups', but the official categories that householders were asked to choose between, when completing the census, are a mixture of *'racial'* categories (black or white) and *nationalities* or geographical regions (African, Bangladeshi, Chinese, Indian, Pakistani). 'Indian', for example, is not an ethnic group because the country India is populated by a host of different ethnic communities. Another problem with census definitions of 'race' and ethnicity is that the 'white' category (comprising 92% of the population in the 2001 census) is not subdivided into ethnic or national sub-groups. This implies that being white is an unproblematic, 'non-ethnic' majority status. Being 'ethnic', on the other hand, seems to be seen as a property of being black or Asian, and in a minority. There are also the problems that the terms used to categorise ethnic groups are not consistent, and that official statistics significantly under-represent the numbers of ethnic minorities in the UK (Chapter 1).

Most members of minority ethnic groups in the UK belong to communities with origins in Caribbean and African countries, the Indian subcontinent and Hong Kong/South China. There are also significant ethnic minorities with roots in Europe (e.g. the Irish community) and in other parts of the world. In the 2001 census, nearly 8% of the UK population were defined as members of minority ethnic groups (Table 4.1). The two main broad categories were

Table 4.1 UK population by ethnic group, 2001.

	Total population (%)	Non-white population (%)
White	92.1	
Mixed	1.2	14.6
Asian or Asian British		
Indian	1.8	22.7
Pakistani	1.3	16.1
Bangladeshi	0.5	6.1
Other Asian	0.4	5.3
All Asian or Asian British	4.0	50.3
Black or Black British		
Black Caribbean	1.0	12.2
Black African	0.8	10.5
Other Black	0.2	2.1
All Black or Black British	2.0	24.8
Chinese	0.4	5.3
Other ethnic groups	0.4	5.0
All minority ethnic populations	7.9	100

Source: UK population census, 2001. National Statistics website: www.statistics.gov.uk. Crown copyright material is reproduced with the permission of the Controller of HMSO.

'Asian or Asian British' 4% and 'Black or Black British' 2%. These are often referred to as black and minority ethnic groups.

Black and minority ethnic group members are mainly concentrated in a few (less affluent) areas in England, mainly London (45%), and the West (13%) and East Midlands (6%), with smaller proportions in the South-East (8%), North-West (8%), and Yorkshire and Humber (7%) (Connolly and White 2006). Minority ethnic groups in contemporary Britain have a younger age structure, with less than 5% of people over the age of 65, compared with about 17% in the population as a whole. They also have higher birth rates than the national average. These demographic characteristics affect both their demand for and use of health services. Minority ethnic group women tend to be poorer, less educated and less healthy than other women in the population. Both men and women from minority ethnic groups are under-represented in higher status occupational categories.

Data from the 2001 census show that more than half of the 4.3 million growth of the UK population between the 1991 and 2001 censuses was the result of immigration (2.2 million). There were nearly 500,000 immigrants from Ireland, over 446,000 from India and nearly 321,000 from Pakistan.

As official definitions of ethnicity are somewhat misleading, it is often more helpful to recognise the ethnic differences between communities that are acknowledged by the communities themselves, as well by outsiders. Box 4.1 identifies the largest minority ethnic groups in contemporary Britain based upon religious, cultural, community and language differences that mark out ethnic identity. It is important to stress that it is not a comprehensive list. Important groups, such as white European minority communities other than

> **Box 4.1 The largest ethnic minority groups in the UK**
>
> - **Irish** Forming the UK's single largest ethnic minority of about a million people, this community is comprised of people who migrated to settle in the UK from the Republic of Ireland and Northern Ireland, and their descendants.
> - **African Caribbeans** Those who have migrated from countries in the Caribbean, and their descendants.
> - **Black Africans** People who migrated from African countries (chiefly in West Africa) and their descendants.
> - **Indian Sikhs** People who have migrated from the northern Indian state of Punjab, and their descendants, who speak Punjabi and follow the Sikh religion.
> - **Indian Gujeratis** Mainly people who migrated from the western Indian state of Gujerat, and their descendants, who speak Gujerati and who are mainly either Hindus or Muslims.
> - **Pakistani Muslims** Almost all Pakistanis (and Bangladeshis) follow the religion of Islam. This community includes people and their descendants from various parts of Pakistan, including the northern state of Mirpur and the Pakistani region of Punjab (bordering on Indian Punjab).
> - **Bangladeshi Muslims** Migrants and their descendants from coastal areas and from Sylhet, an inland area of Bangladesh.
> - **'African' Asians** Migrants or refugees and their descendants, who had been living in various East African countries (e.g. Kenya, Uganda, Tanzania) before settling in the UK. This is a mixed group, in terms of religion and languages, and includes Sikhs, Hindus and Muslims.

the Irish, are missing. There is to date little substantial research on health and illness in these communities. The health experiences of 'new' or recent migrants who have arrived as refugees or asylum seekers (e.g. Albanians) or of other small minority communities (e.g. Somalis) are also little researched.

Health and illness in minority ethnic communities

The UK's ethnic diversity in terms of culture, standards of living and experience of 'racial' disadvantage is reflected in ethnic diversity in patterns of health and illness. There is no simple 'racial' divide in health, with the white majority being in a uniformly better off position in respect of rates of illness or mortality. Nor do all Black and Asian people share similar rates of illness or experience of health services. However, some clear patterns of health and illness in minority ethnic communities, compared with the white majority, have been identified in recent research. These can be summarised as follows:

- risks of poorer health and higher death rates are greater in most, but not all, minority ethnic communities;
- Indian and African-Asian communities have similar, and in some respects better, levels of health compared to the white majority;

- Bangladeshi and Pakistani men and women and black Caribbean women are more likely to report bad or very bad health than the general population;
- most ethnic minorities have *lower* rates of disease and mortality than the white population with regard to respiratory problems, lung cancer and breast cancer;
- in Asian groups the rates for diabetes and coronary heart disease are significantly higher than in the white majority;
- in black groups the rates for hypertension, stroke and diabetes are significantly higher than in the white majority.

These patterns underline the point that the relationship between ethnicity and health is a complex and changing one.

The rest of this section will consider the prevalence of long-standing illness, common conditions related to the circulatory system, diabetes and mental illness among minority ethnic groups, and two conditions found primarily within minority ethnic communities – tuberculosis and sickle-cell disorders. Davey Smith *et al.* (2003) consider a different set of comparisons.

The Health Survey for England (HSE) is an annual survey of self-reported health of adults and children living in private households. The 2004 HSE focused on the largest ethnic groups in England and is the most comprehensive source of information about the health of minority ethnic groups in the UK (Sproston and Mindell 2006).

Table 4.2 shows the prevalence of self-reported long-standing illness and limiting long-standing illness within minority ethnic groups. It shows that both increase with age among adults for all minority ethnic groups and for the general population. It also shows that there is considerable variation between minority ethnic groups, some with higher rates than the general population and others with lower rates. The prevalence of longstanding illness among men ranged from 22% for Chinese and 24% for black Africans to almost half (47%) of Irish men; it was also high for black Caribbean women (44%). The prevalence of long-standing illness was similar to that of the general population for black Caribbean and Irish children and lower than this among children in all other minority ethnic groups. Indian boys and those in the general population were more likely to have long-standing illness than girls but for all other minority ethnic groups this was similar for boys and girls.

Heart disease

It is well documented that men and women in South Asian communities have high rates of mortality from coronary heart disease (CHD) compared to the national average. The difference between their death rates and that of the general population is increasing. Taken as a whole, people who have migrated from the Indian subcontinent to the UK are more than half as likely again to die of CHD than people in the majority population. For black groups, rates are much lower than the national average, by about half for men and two-thirds for women.

Table 4.2 The prevalence of long-standing illness and limiting long-standing illness within minority ethnic groups in England, 2004 (%).

	Black Caribbean	Black African	Indian	Pakistani	Bangladeshi	Chinese	Irish	General population
Men (boys)*								
Long-standing illness	39 (21)	24 (11)	37 (18)	35 (18)	30 (14)	22 (17)	47 (23)	43 (24)
Limiting long-standing illness	24 (7)	10 (5)	23 (6)	20 (7)	24 (5)	9 (10)	26 (7)	23 (8)
Women (girls)*								
Long-standing illness	44 (22)	24 (7)	30 (9)	41 (13)	31 (10)	24 (13)	44 (17)	47 (20)
Limiting long-standing illness	28 (8)	15 (2)	19 (3)	30 (6)	21 (3)	10 (3)	23 (4)	27 (7)

*Men and women aged 16 and over; boys and girls aged 15 and younger.

Source: Sproston, K. and Mindell, J. (2006) *The Health of Minority Ethnic Groups*, Vol. 1. The Information Centre, Leeds (tables 2.5 and 12.1).

Balarajan (1995) found the proportion of excess CHD deaths to be 73% among Bangladeshis, 61% among Pakistanis and 53% among Indians. These death rates exceeded the rate for England and Wales, already high by international standards. Nazroo's landmark large-scale survey subsequently qualified this picture. He points out that while risk of contracting heart disease appears to be significantly higher among South Asians, compared to the white majority, 'this greater risk applied only to the Pakistani/Bangladeshi group' (Nazroo 1997: 132). Indian and African-Asian respondents were found to have the same risk of heart disease as whites. Harding (2003) examined the mortality of a large cohort of migrants from India to England and Wales over the period 1971–2000. She found that the mortality rates of these migrants increased over the period of their residence, regardless of the socio-economic status of the migrants. Mortality from cardiovascular disease was the main element within this increase, accounting for more than half of all deaths. She also found that cancer mortality increased with length of residence.

The HSE 2004 (Sproston and Mindell 2006) found differences *between* minority ethnic groups in terms of self-reported angina, heart attacks, hypertension and stoke (Table 4.3). For all minority ethnic groups and the general population, women had a lower prevalence of angina and heart attacks than men. Prevalence of these conditions was lowest among those aged 16–34, and increased with age in both sexes for all ethnic groups and the general population, with the highest rates for those aged 55 and above. Prevalence of these conditions was highest among the Pakistani and Indian minority ethnic groups and lowest for the black African and Chinese minority ethnic groups.

As far as heart disease is concerned, inequalities in the incomes, material resources and occupations of people in the different minorities are of key importance in understanding the observed variations. Nazroo (1997) concluded that social class differences could explain many 'ethnic' differences in heart disease. According to him, once socio-economic status is taken into account the risk of diagnosed heart disease as compared to whites drops for all South Asian communities, and falls to insignificant levels for the Pakistani/Bangladeshi group.

Hypertension and stroke

Hypertension (high blood pressure) is a significant risk factor in causing stroke, or haemorrhage in the brain. Table 4.3 shows that rates of hypertension vary significantly across ethnic groups and between men and women. Its prevalence is highest for black Caribbean men and women, and lowest for Bangladeshi men, Chinese women and Pakistani women. As with heart disease, the prevalence of stroke is higher among those aged 55 or over. Among men, black Caribbeans had the highest reported prevalence; among women, the highest rates were for the Bangladeshi and Pakistani groups.

Caution is necessary in epidemiological evidence about hypertension because raised blood pressure may not be noticed until the patient is examined or treated for something else. However, research on hypertension and

Table 4.3 Prevalence of common conditions related to the circulatory system among minority ethnic adults aged 55 and over in England, 2004 (%).

	Black Caribbean	Black African	Indian	Pakistani	Bangladeshi	Chinese	Irish	General population (2003)
Men								
Angina	3.4	0.7	4.9	6.9	3.1	1.6	4.0	4.8
Heart attack	3.2	–	3.9	4.1	2.9	0.3	3.0	3.8
Hypertension	38.4	25.1	32.6	19.9	15.9	20.2	36.4	31.7
Stroke	3.4	–	1.1	1.8	1.8	0.7	4.5	2.4
Women								
Angina	1.5	0.5	3.2	2.5	2.0	1.2	2.5	3.4
Heart attack	1.4	–	1.0	1.1	0.6	–	0.8	1.7
Hypertension	31.7	19.3	17.6	14.8	18.6	16.2	29.5	29.0
Stroke	1.8	1.2	1.2	1.06	1.8	0.4	2.7	2.2

Source: Sproston, K. and Mindell, J. (2006) *The Health of Minority Ethnic Groups*, vol. 1. The Information Centre, Leeds (tables 3.1 and 7.3).

the occurrence of strokes in different ethnic groups has produced consistent findings. Balarajan (1995), for instance, pointed to an excess of deaths from stroke among older African-Caribbeans (aged 65–74) that was 50% higher than the norm in England and Wales. He also showed that deaths from stroke were even higher in the Bangladeshi community (twice the England and Wales rate), significantly above in the Indian community, and slightly above the rate in the Pakistani community.

Although the risk of death from stroke is high in some Asian communities, the danger of hypertension has frequently been referred to in health research as an African-Caribbean problem. For example, Balarajan (2001: 236) points out that 'African Caribbeans around the globe are known to suffer disproportionately from hypertensive disease and stroke'. International studies of hypertension in African-American and African-Caribbean populations seemed to confirm a 'racial' difference, with black communities experiencing a significantly higher rate of hypertension than whites in all age groups. Medical research therefore began to conclude that genetic factors were strongly linked to a predisposition towards hypertension in all people of black African descent. However, research, including careful comparison of rural and urban communities in Africa, has shown that rates of hypertension and stroke are not uniformly high in all black communities (McKeigue 2001). Where they are particularly high, notably in relatively disadvantaged black communities in the USA, they seem to be closely associated with adverse environmental factors. McKeigue suggests that poverty, unhealthy high-calorie diets and obesity play a key role in causing significantly higher rates of these health problems.

Diabetes

The prevalence of diabetes in the UK is increasing, linked to the rapid increase in obesity. It is at least five times more prevalent among African-Caribbean and Asian communities. The majority of cases are type 2 (maturity onset) diabetes. The HSE (Sproston and Mindell 2006) found that the prevalence of doctor-diagnosed diabetes increases markedly with age (true prevalence may be higher). It is more common among men than women in all age groups, with the exception of Pakistani women aged 55 and over. Except for Indian men and Irish women it is rare among those aged 16–34. It is unclear whether rates of untreated diabetes vary between ethnic groups.

Research in the 1980s showed a significantly high rate of diabetes among black and South Asian minority ethnic immigrants to the UK. More recent studies, including both the immigrant generation and their UK-born descendants (Nazroo 1997, Health Education Authority 2000), have confirmed that, as with hypertension and stroke, the incidence of diabetes in most African-Caribbean and Asian populations remained at a significantly higher level in the succeeding, UK-born generations. For example, Nazroo (1997) showed that Pakistani and Bangladeshi communities experienced over five times the rate of diabetes found in the white population (8.9% compared to 1.7%, standardised for age and gender). The rates of diabetes in the African-Caribbean group were found to be over three times higher (5.3%), and in the Indian and African-Asian communities to be just under three times higher (4.7%), than in the white population. The Chinese group had the lowest rate among the minorities surveyed (3.0%), although this was still appreciably higher than in the white majority.

These ethnic differences in rates of diabetes remained significant even when socio-economic status was controlled for. In other words, diabetes rates are still significantly higher in middle class or better off sections of minority communities, as well as in poorer or less advantaged sections, when equivalent comparisons are made with the white majority. For this reason, some researchers have suggested that genetic factors could play an important part in causing relatively high rates of diabetes in black and Asian groups (Chandola 2001). However, it is not entirely clear how genetic differences alone could account for increased susceptibility to insulin intolerance and diabetes in these groups. Environmental and dietary factors also play an important part in explaining a marked global rise in diabetes in recent years. Complex interactions between genetic inheritance, changing diets and other environmental changes are most likely to explain the observed ethnic differences in this serious and growing health problem.

Tuberculosis

The rising incidence of this disease in the UK and the USA is a cause for concern. The appearance of resistant strains means that tuberculosis (TB) cannot be controlled as easily as it was in the past. In the UK disproportionate emphasis was initially placed on a higher rate of tuberculosis in migrants' home countries to explain the higher rate in minority ethnic communities. In fact, the incidence of tuberculosis was found to be low in some countries of origin, notably the Caribbean states. Further, in the twenty-first century, a growing proportion of black and Asian British people have been born in the UK. Thus, although some TB may be 'imported' to the UK by members of minority ethnic groups visiting their relatives in other countries, most of those who contract tuberculosis in the UK do so as a result of their living conditions in the society. As some minority ethnic communities, particularly the Pakistani and Bangladeshi minorities, experience a disproportionate amount of social disadvantage, medical researchers suggest that health inequalities in diseases such as tuberculosis are largely a result of poverty, poor diet and housing, and unemployment (Bhopal 2001: 28).

Sickle-cell disorders

The example of tuberculosis illustrates the important link between illness and living conditions (Chapter 3). However, there are several kinds of disease in which this link is not significant and which can only be explained by genetic differences between ethnic groups. Inherited conditions such as sickle-cell disorders are not entirely unknown in the majority population, but they are much more closely associated with specific minority communities.

Sickle-cell disorders are inherited disorders of haemoglobin in the red blood cells. The most common forms are *sickle-cell anaemia* (usually the most severe form) and *thalassaemia beta* (of which there is both a severe and a mild form). As many as 1 in 4 West Africans and 1 in 10 African-Caribbeans carry the sickle-cell trait. Thalassaemia is carried by 1 in 7 Cypriots (and is also found in other eastern Mediterranean populations), 1 in 10 Pakistanis and 1 in 30 Chinese (Dyson 2005). Carriers do not suffer from the painful and dangerous effects of these blood disorders, even in a mild form. Its presence as a trait has been associated with resistance to malaria – hence its geographical distribution in world regions where malaria is, or was, common. When both parents are carriers, there is a 1 in 4 chance that their children will experience illness as a result of a sickle-cell disorder.

The record of the NHS in providing help and information, genetic counselling and treatment for sickle-cell disorders has been patchy and inadequate. Dyson's study of screening and counselling for sickle cell/thalassaemia (Dyson 2005) provides a good account of the difficulties of providing a service based on ethnic screening.

Mental health

Whether minority ethnic groups have poorer mental health than the majority population is a question surrounded by controversy. This is partly because of the difficulties of obtaining reliable statistics of its prevalence and because mental illness itself is difficult to define (Chapter 8). It is also the case that responses to illness are affected to some degree by cultural values and social stereotypes, and this is particularly the case with mental illness. Psychiatric diagnoses have a record of unreliability, and the extent of some forms of mental illness in minority communities may have been over-estimated (perhaps greatly) by medical research.

Psychoses

Higher incidence rates for treated psychosis have been reported for minority ethnic groups, especially among black groups, than for the white population (Karlsen *et al.* 2005). Most of the research in this area has focused upon African-Caribbeans, finding higher rates of psychosis (usually schizophrenia) in this group than for the general UK population or in the Caribbean (Sharpley *et al.* 2001). For example, Sproston and Nazroo (2002) found that African-Caribbean and African people were much more likely than whites to be admitted to hospital with a first diagnosis of schizophrenia or other psychotic illnesses. Younger men experienced particularly high rates of hospitalisation.

In their review of pathways to psychiatric treatment, Morgan *et al.* (2004) reported that for African-Caribbeans there were high rates of police involvement and low rates of GP referral. There was also evidence that they are less likely to be referred to specialist services, experience longer periods of untreated psychosis, and have less family involvement in getting to care. They conclude that 'in general African-Caribbeans appear to follow more coercive and complex routes to psychiatric care' (Morgan *et al.* 2004: 742).

Morgan *et al.* (2004) examined two types of explanation for the significantly higher rates of psychosis among African-Caribbeans. Early research focused upon *patient characteristics* and *racial stereotyping* by psychiatrists and others in the referral process, and concluded that:

(1) African-Caribbeans were more severely disturbed at presentation;
(2) African-Caribbeans used more 'externalised idioms of distress', thus creating the appearance of more severe mental disturbance; and
(3) racial stereotyping led psychiatrists and others to see them as disturbed and threatening.

This third explanation led some researchers and commentators to conclude that racism was deeply seated in British psychiatry and in British society. Karlsen *et al.* (2005) suggested that experiences of racial harassment, workplace discrimination and perceptions of inherent racism in British society, are significantly associated with the prevalence of common mental disorders (CMDs; see below) and the risk of psychosis among the six largest minority ethnic groups in England. Other researchers have drawn upon a range of *social and cultural* explanations, such as social isolation (living alone, lower family involvement), the effects of living in deprived and disadvantaged neighbourhoods and the stigmatisation of mental illness among African-Caribbean groups (Sharpley *et al.* 2001, Karlsen *et al.* 2005).

Common mental disorders

There are concerns that some mental health problems among minority ethnic groups, and the distress they cause, are being missed by researchers and by health service providers. One of the main weaknesses of early research on ethnic variations in mental illness was that much of it was based on surveys of treatment or admission to hospital. This made interpretation of results difficult, as a wide variety of reasons other than mental illness itself could explain why higher numbers of people from certain ethnic groups were receiving institutional treatment, as we have seen in the preceding discussion.

The EMPIRIC study was a large-scale survey of the six largest ethnic groups (white, Irish, Indian, Pakistani, black Caribbean and Bangladeshi) living in England during 2000–2002 (Sproston and Nazroo 2002). This provides more reliable findings on the prevalence of mental health problems in different ethnic groups using evidence based on mental illness rates in the community, rather than on treatment or hospitalisation rates. This found relatively minor differences between ethnic groups (including the white majority) in terms of a set of common mental disorders (CMDs) such as anxiety, low mood and irritability. No ethnic group stood out as being particularly susceptible to CMDs, although there were differences between the experience of men and women in various ethnic groups. The most economically disadvantaged community (Bangladeshi) was found to experience the lowest rates of a range of CMDs.

A follow-up study (Weich *et al.* 2004) found no differences between the black Caribbean and white samples. For other groups there were only modest variations between them, with some variation by age and sex. Compared to white men, and controlling for socio-economic status, the prevalence of CMDs was significantly higher among Irish and Pakistani men aged 35–54. There were also higher rates of CMDs among Indian and Pakistani women aged 55–74 than among white women of the same age. Among Bangladeshi women who were interviewed in their own language (but not among those interviewed in English) there were lower rates of CMDs than among white women. The very low prevalence of CMDs among these Bangladeshi women contrasted strongly with their high levels of deprivation, which would have suggested high levels of CMDs.

The results reported in these (and other) surveys suggest that there is no clear link between ethnic group, material disadvantage and CMDs. This contrasts with ethnic inequalities in heart disease and the other physical health problems, discussed earlier, which do seem to reflect underlying patterns of class inequality and economic disadvantage in minority ethnic groups. It seems that differences in social support and integration (Chapter 2) may mediate the effects of economic disadvantage and racial discrimination in producing ethnic differences in rates of CMDs. Sproston and Nazroo (2002) suggest that social support and 'community social capital' can offset the effects of social deprivation, protecting some groups, for example the Bangladeshi community, from a higher rate of mental health problems. African-Caribbean communities, although supportive and a source of identity and help, are more likely to include single adult households than would be the case in most South Asian communities and, as noted above, this might have increased their vulnerability to the psychological effects of deprivation and social disadvantage.

As with psychosis, cultural misunderstanding, stereotyping and racism among health practitioners may be an important factor in the genesis, treatment and management of CMDs within minority ethnic groups, and probably affect their uptake of services negatively (Mclean *et al.* 2003). However, it seems unlikely that this is the main explanation for the pattern of ethnic variation.

Explaining ethnic variations in health and illness

The previous section has indicated a number of explanations for ethnic differences in health and suggested that there is no single explanation for them (see also Davey Smith *et al.* 2003). This section considers the main explanations.

Artefact

It is possible that the processes of data generation and analysis may create apparent health differences between ethnic groups that are not real. For example, the apparently higher prevalence of schizophrenia among young African-Caribbean men seems to reflect a greater chance of diagnosis. However, while there are particular artefactual effects, such as this, that may be significant, these are thought to be limited (Davey Smith *et al.* 2003).

Genetic explanations

Inherited blood disorders, such as sickle-cell disorders in certain minority communities, clearly do have a genetic cause. However, genetic explanations seem to have limited explanatory power because the incidence of most of the health conditions discussed seem to vary both *within* and *between* ethnic groups. While this may partly reflect inconsistency in the definition of ethnic groupings, there would no significant differences in disease rates within ethnic groups if genetic factors mainly determined rates of disease. Although ethnic differences in diabetes seem to have a genetic component, environmental factors, particularly changes in diet, seem to be strongly implicated in both a general rise in rates of diabetes and increases in the African-Caribbean community.

Migration and social selection

The migrant background of black, Asian, Irish and other minority communities in the UK provides another set of explanations for ethnic variations in health. Migration is an important factor in the establishment of ethnic communities and a sense of ethnic identity, and can be seen as having both positive and negative health effects.

First, migrants are a self-selected, healthier, group. Their health tends to be better than that of the populations from which they have come and they bring a certain advantage in health and life expectancy with them. This seems to be confirmed by a number of studies of migrant death rates. For example, in the 1950s and 1960s, mortality rates among migrant men in social classes IV and V were *lower* than among their white counterparts in the same social classes and age groups. Balarajan (1995) found that deaths from breast cancer were less than half the rate among women migrants from the Indian subcontinent, compared with the average in Britain, and were fewer in all the minority groups.

One of the criticisms of earlier studies of ethnicity and health is that too much emphasis was put upon mortality statistics of migrants and not enough on illness rates. It is possible for an minority ethnic group's *death* rate to be lower than average and for their rates of *illness*, at least for certain diseases, to be higher than the norm.

Negative aspects of migration, such as loss of support, stress and psychological problems of adjustment, may negatively affect migrants' health. As the migrant generations in the UK have aged, they have experienced relatively high rates of heart disease, hypertension, diabetes and other health problems.

However, when the health of migrant Asian and black people is compared with that of non-migrants in the same communities, in most cases migrants are found to have better physical and mental health (Nazroo 2001). These findings suggest that the shock, stress and disruption of migration cannot have had a very significant effect on migrants' health. It also appears that the 'health advantage' of the migrant generation has not been transmitted in any significant way to the second and third generations of minority ethnic groups in contemporary Britain (Davey Smith *et al.* 2003).

Socio-economic status differences

Many of the ethnic variations in health and illness can be explained by examining the impact of socio-economic status or social class on the comparisons being made. One clear example of this is that in many analyses health differences between minority ethnic groups and the indigenous white majority reduce, sometimes substantially, when socio-economic status is controlled for. For example, Nazroo (2003) reports that it is 'reasonably clear' that the socio-economic patterning of the health of ethnic groups exists in both the UK and the USA, reflected by the diversity across ethnic groups and a socio-economic gradient of health with ethnic groups. However, within each socio-economic category members of ethnic minorities have smaller incomes than whites. In the UK, whites have twice the income of Pakistani and Bangladeshi ethnic groups (the two poorest groups).

Comprehensive surveys of ethnic minority health (e.g. Nazroo 1997, Health Education Authority 2000) consistently show that socio-economic status is centrally important when making comparisons between ethnic groups. However, socio-economic status does not explain every variation in health between ethnic groups. As will be recalled, exceptions include the distribution of diabetes, which is significantly higher in minority black and Asian groups irrespective of socio-economic status. Another exception is the low rate of common mental problems in the economically disadvantaged Bangladeshi community.

Explanations based on socio-economic status also have their limitations when comparisons of health *within* ethnic groups, as opposed to *between* ethnic groups, are being made. For example, Chandola (2001) concluded there was little evidence of a class gradient in health within the relatively disadvantaged Pakistani and Bangladeshi communities. In the Indian community, on the other hand, a significant increase in social mobility since the 1980s and a widening social divide resulted in widening health inequalities. In the African-Caribbean community, there seems to be a mixed picture. According to Nazroo (2001), poorer people in the African-Caribbean community generally had poorer health, indicating a class gradient, although there were some exceptions, such as a higher rate of mental illness for those in non-manual occupations, compared with manual workers.

Of all the explanations considered, socio-economic status has perhaps the greatest explanatory power. However, establishing how exactly socio-economic effects influence ethnic patterns of health and illness can be complex (Davey Smith *et al.* 2003, Nazroo 2003). Minority ethnic groups are generally associated with lower socio-economic status and, thus, would be expected to have poorer than average health. Yet, some ethnic differences in health remain even when socio-economic position is controlled.

Cultural explanations

Cultural and lifestyle factors such as differences in smoking, diet and taking exercise have been closely associated with differences in health, particularly by governments in their public health and health promotion policies (Chapters 2 and 3). Evidence to support this explanation for ethnic health differences can be found in the significantly lower rates of respiratory disease and lung cancer found in South Asian communities, compared to both the black Caribbean community and the white majority, attributed mainly to the very low rates of smoking among South Asian women (Nazroo 2001). Another example is the low rate of common mental problems in the Bangladeshi community. These examples suggest that some cultural values and social habits have an enhancing impact on health.

There is, however, little evidence that other cultural or lifestyle differences between ethnic groups are very significant. Reviewing the evidence on unhealthy diets, lack of exercise and resistance to using medical services, Chandola (2001) concludes that it would be incorrect to attribute poorer health in South Asian or black communities to such health damaging behaviours. These are unlikely to have any more effect in these communities than in the white majority. Also, if cultural factors such as dietary habits are common to an ethnic group, they cannot explain significant differences *within* ethnic groups in rates of serious illness.

While cultural factors may play a role, focusing on cultural explanations for ethnic health inequalities at the expense of other factors can result in 'blaming the victim' for their own poorer health and in downplaying the structural and environmental causes of illness.

Racism and racial discrimination

Racial discrimination is thought to undermine the health of minority ethnic groups in various ways. Racial discrimination can be *indirect* or institutional, subtly affecting people's opportunities in education, employment, housing and other aspects of life that determine standards of living. Thus the health of some minority ethnic groups could be adversely affected because rates of illness are closely connected to inequalities in standard of living. The *direct*, personal, impact of racism could have a wide range of psychological effects, including anxiety and other mental health problems, and physical effects of stress such as high blood pressure. Nazroo (2003) argues that 'experiences of and awareness of racism appear to be central to the lives of minority ethnic people, and there is growing evidence that these contribute to ethnic inequalities in health'.

The impact on health of racism seems to vary. If discrimination affects everyone perceived to be 'black' or 'Asian' in approximately the same ways and to the same degree, we would expect to see approximately the same outcomes across the minority groups. But, as Chandola (2001) reminds us, there are significant differences in both illness and death rates between Indian men on one hand, and Bangladeshi and Pakistani men on the other. Significant differences in standard of living *within* ethnic groups, suggest that for various reasons, including social class position, some sections within minority ethnic communities can protect themselves better against the effects of racial discrimination on their health. The protective effect of belonging to an ethnic group is not solely dependent on economic and social position.

A more persuasive case has been made for the negative impact of racism and discrimination upon mental health (Karlsen *et al*. 2005). Thus, understanding the relationship between racism and health may be particularly relevant to understanding ethnic variations in psychosis and CMDs. Low rates of anxiety in the Indian community and of CMDs in the Bangladeshi community suggest that strong social support could be a factor mitigating the effects of racism on mental health.

Layers of influence

Research into socio-economic inequalities in health now accepts that it is important to examine the interaction between a range of macro and micro level factors that influenced health and illness (Chapter 3). It seems highly likely that the same can be said for any examination of ethnic differences in health, but there has been little application of this approach, and data on the lifecourse are noticeably absent.

Nazroo (2003) suggests two ways in which conditions can influence the health of ethnic minorities over the lifecourse. First, early exposure can 'set adverse biological processes in train', secondly, health disadvantages can accumulate over time (see Chapter 3). He then considers the impact of migration across generations. Finally, he argues that racial harassment and discrimination are related to ethnic inequalities in health. He concludes that further research is needed to examine the 'individual embodiment of social risks', psychological and social stress and how these lead to disease, and the 'centrality of racism'.

Health services and health care

Although medicine and health care have their limitations in terms of reducing mortality and contributing to positive improvements in health (Chapters 2 and 3), health services are of central importance in the management and treatment of illnesses. How they perform these functions in minority ethnic communities is therefore important. However, there is little information about the use of health services by minority ethnic groups in the UK, apart from that in the HSE, 1999. This reported that:

- South Asian and black Caribbean men were more likely to have consulted a GP than the general population. Among women, rates were significantly higher for South Asian and Irish women.
- Consultation rates for psychological distress (a CMD) were significantly higher for Irish men and lower for Chinese men and women and Bangladeshi women.
- Regular dental attendance was significantly low for men and women in all minority ethnic groups.
- Rates of inpatient, outpatient and day patient hospital attendance were similar to those of the general population for all groups except Chinese men and women, who had lower rates.
- The use of prescribed medicine was higher than for the general population for South Asian men and lower for Chinese men. Bangladeshi and Pakistani women had relatively high use and Chinese women had low use.

There seem to be both positive and negative aspects to the experience of health services among minority ethnic groups.

Positive aspects

Unlike social services, the NHS is a well-understood and well-used service among all the minority ethnic communities, and there are no significant problems of under-registration or exclusion from health services. This applies to use of hospital services as well as to GP or family doctor services.

As with the white majority, almost everyone in black, Asian and other minority ethnic communities is registered with a GP. Nazroo (1997) found that African-Caribbean men were the only group with lower registration rates (96%) than the general population. Rates of GP consultations are higher in most minority ethnic groups than in the white population. When health status is taken into account, black and Asian patients see their GPs more frequently than white patients. For example, Nazroo's (1997) survey showed that 35% of white respondents had talked to their GP about their health in the past month, compared with 41–50% of Indian, African-Caribbean, Bangladeshi and Pakistani respondents. Only African-Asians (32%) reported a lower rate of GP consultations. Minority ethnic patients, compared to whites, are also more likely to visit their GPs more than once each month.

Summarising a number of surveys on use of inpatient hospital services, Nazroo (1997) shows that patients from minority ethnic groups are as likely to be admitted to hospital as whites, taking reported illnesses into account. Younger minority patients are less likely to be admitted to hospital than is the norm in the white population, but rates of admission among older South Asian and African-Caribbean patients are similar to, or greater than, admissions of white patients in the same age group.

Negative aspects

The pattern of use of NHS services may be an indicator of a heavier burden of illness in minority ethnic communities. There is little evidence that patients from these groups 'over use' health services or facilities, compared to the white population. Where use of health services is more frequent than the national average, this seems to reflect medical need.

The use of preventative services, e.g. screening for cervical cancer, is lower than the national average among minority ethnic communities, and black and Asian patients are significantly less likely than white patients to receive follow-up services, or to be referred promptly to a consultant if they have a serious illness such as heart disease (Nazroo 1997). Many GPs are unwilling to work in the socially disadvantaged or inner city areas where most minority ethnic communities live. GP practices used by patients from minority ethnic groups are not as likely to have good facilities as practices in better-off areas. Also, physical access to the doctor's surgery has been found to be more of a problem for minority ethnic patients than for people in the white majority (Balarajan 2001).

A significant number of South Asian patients report communication problems with their GPs, mainly as a result of language differences. These difficulties mainly affect older patients and women, rather than younger patients and men. As many as half of Bangladeshi and Pakistani women are likely to have difficulty in communicating in English, and these proportions will be even higher among older women in these communities. Although there are now considerable numbers of South Asian GPs working in the NHS, this does not always mean that doctor and patient will be matched in terms of the Asian languages they can speak. There might also be considerable cultural and socio-economic status differences between Asian patients and Asian doctors.

The existence of language barriers between doctors and patients is not necessarily a criticism of the NHS, as factors that lie outside the control of the health service have helped to maintain these barriers (e.g. limited policies on teaching English to adults; cultural and linguistic preferences in different communities). However, communication problems may partly explain why Asian patients visit their GPs more frequently than white patients. If the doctor has not been well understood in the first consultation, this increases the chances of the patient having to return for further advice and treatment (Sproston and Nazroo 2002). Efforts to improve communication between family doctors and minority ethnic patients have been patchy (Health Education Authority 2000) and have been hindered by the general shortage of GPs.

Although the NHS has an ethnically and racially diverse workforce, there is evidence of direct and indirect racism (as discussed above), as well as a lack of understanding of the significance of ethnic and cultural differences. Evidence of indirect discrimination can be observed in the failure of the NHS to reach out sufficiently vigorously to the various minority communities. For instance, take-up of some preventive services is low, especially in Asian communities (Balarajan 2001).

Patients from minority ethnic groups do not expect to be given special medical or nursing care. Rather, their concerns are that the specific cultural practices of their community or requirements of their religious beliefs – in short, their ethnic identity – are understood by nurses and other health care staff. It is in this respect that a sociological understanding of the patient's cultural background and identity can be helpful to nurses. Where the care relationship involves cultural or ethnic difference, a shared understanding of these aspects of nursing cannot be taken for granted. There is a strong case, therefore, for maintaining an element of cultural awareness in the education and training of nurses. This is likely to be as valuable as training in awareness of racial discrimination.

Complementary and alternative medicine

The HSE 2004 (Sproston and Mindell 2006) found that among the general population women (33%) were more likely to have used complementary and alternative medicine (CAM) in the previous 12 months than men (21%). They found a wide range of usage among minority ethnic groups. Chinese women (47%) and men (30%) were most likely to have used CAM (acupuncture, Chinese medicine) in the previous 12 months and Bangladeshi men (6%) and women (4%) were least likely to have used it.

Summary

The relationships between ethnicity and health are complex, and sometimes contradictory. Rates of mortality and morbidity between and within ethnic groups do not consistently favour the white majority and, in some respects, health in minority ethnic communities is better. No single factor – genetic, migration, cultural, socio-economic or 'racial' discrimination – can explain the variations in health between ethnic groups. These are best seen as the outcome of a range of interacting causes. While access to health services is not generally a problem for minority ethnic groups, there are barriers to effective communication between some minority ethnic group patients and health service practitioners, and shortcomings in health services in areas such as follow-up treatment, preventive services and mental health care. It is important to recognise the importance of ethnic diversity for the provision of effective and comprehensive health care for all UK citizens.

References

Balarajan, R. (1995) Ethnicity and variations in the nation's health. *Health Trends*, 27, 114–19.

Balarajan, R. (2001) Challenges and policy implications of ethnic diversity and health, in H. Macbeth and P. Shetty (eds) *Health and Ethnicity*. Taylor and Francis, London, 233–42.

Bhopal, R. (2001) Ethnicity and race as epidemiological variables, in H. Macbeth and P. Shetty (eds) *Health and Ethnicity*. Taylor and Francis, London, 21–40.

Chandola, T. (2001) Ethnic and class differences in health in relation to British South Asians: using the new National Statistics Classification. *Social Science and Medicine*, 52, 1285–96.

Connolly, H. and White, A. (2006) The different experiences of the United Kingdom's ethnic and religious populations. *Social Trends*, 36, 1–8.

Davey Smith, G. Chaturvedi, N., Harding, S., *et al.* (2003) Ethnic inequalities in health: a review of UK epidemiological evidence, in S. Davey Smith (ed.) *Health Inequalities. Lifecourse Approaches*. Policy Press, Bristol, 271–309.

Dyson, S. (2005) *Ethnicity and Screening for Sickle Cell/Thalassaemia*. Elsevier Churchill Livingstone, Edinburgh.

Harding, S. (2003) Mortality of migrants from the Indian subcontinent to England and Wales: effect of duration of residence. *Epidemiology*, 14, 287–92.

Health Education Authority (2000) *Black and Ethnic Minority Groups in England: the Second Health and Lifestyles Survey*. Health Education Authority, London.

Karlsen, S. (2004) 'Black like Beckham'? Moving beyond definitions of ethnicity based on skin colour and ancestry. *Ethnicity and Health*, 9, 107–37.

Karlsen, S., Nazroo, J., McKenzie, K., *et al.* (2005) Racism, psychosis and common mental disorder among ethnic minority groups in England. *Psychological Medicine*, 35, 1795–803.

McKeigue, P. (2001) Approaches to investigating the genetic basis of ethnic differences in disease risk, in H. Macbeth and P. Shetty (eds), *Health and Ethnicity*. Taylor and Francis, London, 113–32.

Mclean, C., Campbell, C. and Cornish, F. (2003) African-Caribbean interactions with mental health services in the UK: experiences and expectations of exclusion as (re)productive of health inequalities. *Social Science and Medicine*, 52, 657–69.

Morgan, C., Mallett, R., Hutchinson, G. and Leffe, J. (2004) Negative pathways to psychiatric care and ethnicity: the bridge between social science and psychiatry. *Social Science and Medicine*, 58, 739–52.

Nazroo, J. (1997) *The Health of Britain's Ethnic Minorities*. Policy Studies Institute, London.

Nazroo, J. (2001) *Ethnicity, Class and Health*. Policy Studies Institute, London.

Nazroo, J. (2003) The structuring of ethnic inequalities in health: economic position, racial discrimination, and racism. *American Journal of Public Health*, 93, 277–84.

Sharpley, M.S., Hutchinson, G., Murray, R.M. and McKenzie, K. (2001) Understanding the excess of psychosis among the African-Caribbean population in England: Review of current hypotheses. *British Journal of Psychiatry*, 178, s60–s68.

Sproston, K. and Mindell, J. eds (2006) *The Health of Minority Ethnic Groups*, Vol. 1. The Information Centre, Leeds.

Sproston, K. and Nazroo, J. eds (2002) *Ethnic Minority Psychiatric Illness Rates in the Community (EMPIRIC)*. The Stationery Office, Norwich.

Weich, S., Nazroo, J., Sproston, K., *et al.* (2004) Common mental disorders and ethnicity in England: the EMPIRIC Study. *Psychological Medicine*, 34, 1543–51.

Further reading

Nazroo, J. (2001) *Ethnicity, Class and Health*. Policy Studies Institute, London.
Examines evidence of ethnic inequalities in health from two UK national surveys of physical and mental health and the explanations for these.

Nazroo, J.Y. and Williams, D.R. (2006) The social determination of ethnic/racial inequalities in health, in M. Marmot and R.G. Wilkinson (eds) *Social Determinants of Health*, 2nd edition. Oxford University Press, Oxford, 238–66. *Discusses the debate about the contribution of social and economic factors, particularly socio-economic inequalities, to the health of ethnic minorities using data from the UK and USA.*

Chapter 5

Gender differences in health

Research on gender differences in health in the UK and similar societies suggests that while women tend to have more illness throughout their lives, men die at younger ages. However, this oversimplifies the complex relationships between gender and health. Gender differences in health are the result of the complex interactions between biological and social factors, and as the social positions of men and women have changed over time so have patterns of morbidity and mortality. This chapter will:

- examine gender differences in mortality and morbidity;
- discuss the main explanations for gender differences in health;
- consider the implications of recent changes in health and gender roles.

Gender patterns in mortality

In contemporary Britain the marked female advantage in life expectancy is accepted as a 'fact of life'. However, this has not always been the case and it may not hold true in the future. Modern records began in the mid-eighteenth century when life tables were provided separately for men and women. Reconstructed data from the early seventeenth century onwards suggest that male and female mortality in most European countries differed very little and, if anything, there was a slight male advantage during the seventeenth and eighteenth centuries. The now familiar female advantage began towards the end of the nineteenth century and was well established by the early 1900s, although before 1930 girls and women at younger ages (about 10–30) were still more likely to die than boys and men (Gjonca et al. 2005).

The historical movement towards female advantage in life expectancy was related to changes in women's social circumstances. Death from childbirth was quite common up until the early twentieth century, although it was not the main cause of death for women; they were far more likely to die from 'killer diseases' like tuberculosis, scarlet fever, typhus and typhoid fever. Although men were afflicted by the same diseases, women's lives were harder than men's and they were less resistant to infection (Gjonca et al. 2005).

Grinding agricultural work, chronic exhaustion from maintaining the family, anaemia and malnutrition particularly took their toll.

Rapid urbanisation and industrialisation freed many women from the health damaging effects of rural life. The health problems that industrialisation and urbanisation brought in their wake affected men as much as women. From the late 1800s British women began to outlive men at all ages. Death rates began to fall significantly. By the early 1900s men could expect to live into their late 40s and women early 50s; by mid-century this had risen to mid-60s for men and early 70s for women; and by the start of the twenty-first century, to mid to late 70s for men and early 80s for women.

This consideration of history shows that gender differences in mortality are by no means fixed: while men had the slight advantage in the past, it is women who have the advantage today. This suggests that differences in mortality are unlikely to be a simple product of the biological differences between men and women. Rather, they are likely to result from the interaction of the different biological vulnerabilities of men and women and the different circumstances of their lives in different historical periods.

Explaining gender differences in mortality

Biology

It has been suggested that men die sooner because they are more biologically vulnerable. Support for 'male vulnerability' comes from studies of the male fetus, which is at greater risk of *in-utero* complications. Premature birth, still-birth, cerebral palsy and congenital malformations of the genitalia and limbs are more common in male infants. Sudden infant death syndrome, although uncommon, is also more likely to affect boys than girls (Office of National Statistics 2005). Moreover, at the time of birth boys are, on average, developmentally some 4–6 weeks behind girls. The chance of surviving the first year of life is also lower for boys. This suggests that girls may be born with a biological advantage.

Further support for 'female robustness' comes from studies of health in later life. For example, coronary heart disease (CHD) is a leading cause of death for both men and women, but it typically affects women at older ages. This later onset may be due to the protective effect of high levels of the female sex-hormone oestrogen and the subsequent post-menopausal drop in oestrogen levels.

The biological body does not exist in isolation, but develops in interaction with the social environment. However, until recently there was a marked tendency for research on the social and biological influences upon women's and men's health to proceed on the basis that differences in men's and women's health are either purely social or purely biological. This fails to appreciate that although underlying genetic, hormonal and metabolic differences exist, they can be modified by social processes. For example, any female biological advantage in the first weeks of life can be quickly overridden by social preferences for baby boys that confer health advantages, such as more food and closer attention to health problems. This is especially notable in some developing countries. Similarly, while oestrogen may protect women from CHD, the secretion of oestrogen by the ovaries is itself influenced by the social environment, particularly the kinds of lifestyles that women lead. Cigarette smoking, which in itself is a risk factor for CHD, appears to reduce women's secretion of oestrogen (and is also associated with an early menopause). Likewise, stress is thought to adversely affect ovarian function.

A final example of how biology is embedded in social experience is the propensity for men to engage in activities that carry a high risk of serious injury or death, such as dangerous sports or physical fighting, which may be associated with high levels of the androgen testosterone. However, it is also important to recognise that in most Western countries competition, physical aggression and risky behaviours are more actively encouraged among males than among females. Moreover, increases in levels of testosterone may be further stimulated by the anticipation of competition and risk that such encouragement brings (Courtenay 2002). These examples suggest that it is the *interaction* of biological and social factors that is important for gender and health.

Social factors

Gender is an important social division between people in modern patriarchal societies such as Britain. Patriarchy is a system of male dominance which operates by creating a strong gender divide, attributing certain 'natural' biological and psychological characteristics to men and others to women. For example, women are physically weak, men are physically strong; women are naturally caring, men are naturally aggressive; men are competitive, women are co-operative/supportive. These characteristics are often drawn together under the umbrella terms of 'femininity' and 'masculinity'. While feminists have strongly challenged female gender role expectations for decades, and the new discipline of men's studies is now questioning male gender role expectations, the concept of gender roles has had a very strong influence upon explanations of the health and health behaviours of men and women.

The conventional wisdom is that the gender roles and behaviours in contemporary Western society predispose men to early death and, conversely, prolong the lives of women. Traditional male gender roles and norms of masculinity appear to encourage behaviours that pose serious risks to health and increase the likelihood of an early death. Major accidents are far more common amongst men, as are fatal workplace injuries, principally because men predominate in high risk industries such as agriculture and construction. Young men (16–24 years old) have a substantially higher risk of work-related injury than older men (HSE 2002). Men are far more likely than women to experience risks to health and early death from the hazardous consumption of alcohol and illegal drugs, which are among the major risks for suicide, now the most common cause of death among young men in Britain (Chapter 8). This has been linked to men's relative inability to express emotions and their tendency to externalise problems, often through physical aggression towards themselves and others.

Just as male gender roles lead to the risk of an early death, female gender roles traditionally have been less likely to expose them to dangerous environments and less likely to lead girls and women to engage in risky behaviours that damage their health. Gender expectations mean that women are much less likely to drink alcohol at hazardous levels, to take illegal drugs or to risk their lives through reckless driving and dangerous sports. While women are undoubtedly exposed to an array of health risks at work, these are less likely to be the kinds of hazards that lead to death from accident or catastrophic injury. Women's longevity may thus be related to their more positive health-related behaviour.

Health-related behaviours are themselves part of building a particular gender identity. For women, attention to health and the body helps to define femininity (e.g. through managing diet in relation to body size). There is evidence that women may be more likely to follow healthy diets than men, although they are also at greater risk of eating disorders such as anorexia nervosa and obesity (Chapter 8). For some men, excessive drinking and aggressive driving may be an integral part of their identity as 'real men'. However, the consumption of alcohol and drugs and engaging in risky leisure activities are increasing among younger women in twenty-first century Britain.

Use of health services

It is possible that women's greater use of health services may help to explain their longer life expectancy. It has been suggested that women make greater use of health services because they are more likely to recognise symptoms of illness and to seek medical help for health problems at an earlier stage than are men. This may be because women are more attuned to bodily changes (for example, the menstrual cycle, pregnancy) and it is more acceptable for them to ask for help.

The difference in the use of services is most clear-cut with respect to medical general practice. In 2004, 16% of women and 11% of men reported consulting a general practitioner (GP) during the 2 weeks prior to interview. Women's higher use of GP services is related to reproductive health (visits for birth control or pregnancy), as indicated by the fact that the largest gender difference is found among the 16–44 age group, where women were twice as likely (16%) as men (8%) to have seen their GP (General Household Survey 2004). Taking visits for reproductive health out of the equation reduces but does not erase the gender difference in GP visits. Gender differences in the use of other health services, such as preventative screening and hospitals, are less clear-cut and harder to interpret.

While women's earlier and more frequent use of GP services may contribute positively to their health, there is also some evidence that gender bias in medical consultations may counteract this. For example, women are less likely to be routinely tested for cardiovascular symptoms and are more likely to suffer unrecognised heart attacks than men. Studies show that women who go to their doctor with severe symptoms are not as likely as men with lesser symptoms to be given a coronary arteriogram, catheterisation or bypass surgery (Shaw *et al.* 2004).

It has been argued that men are less likely than women to recognise or seek help for illness because independence and stoicism in the face of pain are defining features of masculinity (Banks 2001). Illness and injury are often seen as a kind of weakness to be overcome rather than given in to, for example 'rising above pain' and continuing to play contact sports when injured. This has led to the suggestion that if men were to heed health education messages and made greater use of health services this would improve their life expectancy.

Responses to the threats of reproductive cancers provide a good example of gendered differences in the use of health services. Women have been strongly encouraged to check themselves for the signs of breast cancer, the leading cause of cancer death for women, and to take up screening, with a 76% uptake in 2001 (Office of National Statistics 2002). In contrast, far less attention has been given to educating men to recognise the signs of prostate cancer, the third most common cause of cancer death for men, and testicular cancer, which has a rising incidence. There is an extensive lack of knowledge about these diseases among men. For example, a MORI poll in 2001 found that 60% of men could not correctly identify the early signs of prostate cancer. However, it is very difficult to make direct comparisons because timings have been different (the national breast screening programme began in 1988, there is currently no national programme for prostate or testicular cancer) and women aged 50–70 are routinely invited for breast cancer screening, whereas men need to be proactive in seeking prostate and testicular screening. Research from the USA indicates that uptake rates for prostate cancer screening are similar to female-specific programmes when they were first introduced, suggesting that there may be a time-lag effect in their uptake (Evans *et al.* 2005).

In summary, gender expectations and behaviours seem to be important in explaining the different life spans of men and women. Masculinity encourages behaviour that makes men vulnerable to early death, while femininity may support behaviour that protects women from early death and promotes longevity. Masculinity and femininity seem to affect health-seeking behaviour in opposite ways, although it is impossible to assess the specific contribution that gender differences in the use of health services makes to longevity.

The narrowing gap in gender mortality

The previous section has shown that gender differences in mortality are strongly related to gender roles and behaviours. For the whole of the twentieth century women outlived men (Table 5.1), an advantage that continues into the present century. Table 5.1 shows that even though both male and female life expectancy are still improving, men appear to have made swifter gains

Table 5.1 Life expectancy and healthy life expectancy at birth in the UK.

	1961	1971	1981	1986	1991	1996	2001	2003	Overall gain (1961 to 2003)
Male	67.8	69.1	70.8	71.9	73.2	74.2	75.7	76.2	8.4
Female	73.6	75.3	76.8	77.7	78.7	79.4	80.4	80.5	6.9
Gap	5.8	6.2	6.0	5.8	5.5	5.2	4.7	4.3	

Source: derived from *Social Trends 35* (2005), table 7.1. National Statistics website: www.statistics.gov.uk. Crown copyright material is reproduced with the permission of the Controller of HMSO.

since the 1980s than women. This is expressed as 'years of life gained'. The average 'years of life gained' by men over the period was 8.4 years, while for women it was 6.9 years. The projected figures for those born between 1999 and 2021 are 3.5 and 2.8 years for men and women, respectively. Thus, although the life expectancy of the UK population continues to grow, men are now making faster gains than women. This is mainly because middle-aged and older men (roughly ages 55–70) are living longer. If the difference in life expectancy between men and women continues to reduce at this rate, then in 100 years' time men will be living as long as women.

Explanations based on gender roles suggest that for men these gains might best be explained by changes in gender roles and behaviours that advantage men's health and disadvantage women's health. Such changes are thought to be the convergence of gender behaviours in which 'men have become more like women', and 'women have become more like men'. Many men are cutting back on harmful health behaviours while women are taking them up, and many men are now taking actions to protect and improve their health (Vallin *et al.* 2001). Given the complex relationship between health status and the circumstances of people's lives, it is difficult to make direct links between most of these broad changes and the declining gender gap in all-cause mortality. However, the examination of deaths from lung cancer, heart disease and skin cancer illustrates how changing gender-related attitudes and behaviour and changes in gender patterns of mortality are linked.

Lung cancer and smoking

Shifts in gender patterns of smoking have played a major role in the narrowing mortality gap between men and women. This can be appreciated by looking at changing patterns of deaths from lung cancer. Lung cancer has been the major cancer death for men since the 1940s (although male deaths from prostate cancer are increasing, they remain appreciably lower than those due to lung cancer) (Griffiths and Brock 2003). For women, breast cancer was significantly higher than lung cancer until it peaked in the late 1980s and lung cancer caught up, to the point that they are now about the same. Male deaths from lung cancer have always been and remain higher than female deaths.

The timing of peaks and troughs in incidence (the number of new cases within a time period) and mortality over time is quite different for men and women. For men, both incidence and mortality increased enormously from the early 1900s to reach a plateau in the early 1970s, after which they have declined. In contrast, for women, both incidence and mortality increased up to the end of the 1980s. Since then both have remained fairly stable, rather than fallen.

Lung cancer is closely associated with cigarette smoking. Figure 5.1 shows the trends in cigarette smoking for men and women in Britain between 1974 and 2002. Two points are important. First, the decline in smoking has been more marked amongst men than amongst women. Over 50% of men smoked in 1974, dropping to about 28% by 2002. For women, the drop is less evident: from about 40% in 1978 to 24% in 2002. Secondly, from the 1990s there has been very little difference in the percentage of men and women who smoked. The prevalence of smoking is highest among those aged 20–34, and it is younger women in particular who are taking up smoking.

Smoking among younger women appears to be part and parcel of the movement of women out of the private sphere of the home into the public sphere of paid employment and all that accompanies this, such as greater personal spending power and leisure time. The global tobacco industry uses positive images of glamour and emancipation to market cigarettes to women, but women's increased smoking is likely to be influenced by their socio-economic circumstances as well as such new found 'freedoms'. There is clear evidence that female smoking is associated with disadvantage. For example, as we saw in Chapter 2, there are associations between educational disadvantage and early and single motherhood and smoking, with the latter being a way of coping with poor and stressful lives (Graham *et al.* 2006).

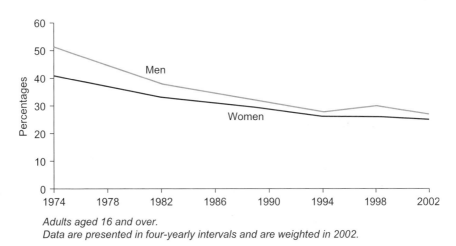

Adults aged 16 and over.
Data are presented in four-yearly intervals and are weighted in 2002.

Figure 5.1 The prevalence of smoking among adults 1974–2002.
Source: Bajekal *et al.* (2006) *Focus on Health*, Figure 4.1. National Statistics website: www.statistics.gov.uk. Crown copyright material is reproduced with the permission of the Controller of HMSO.

The incidence of lung cancer increases with increasing age, reflecting the time lag of about 20 years between taking up smoking and the onset of the disease. Men at the highest risk of lung cancer were born in the 1890s, while women at highest risk were born in the 1920s, when gender proscriptions against women's smoking began to lessen. This time-lag effect in lung cancer deaths is likely to be an important contributor to the narrowing gender gap in overall mortality which, as Figure 5.1 shows, began in the late 1970s/early 1980s. By this time women born in the 1920s would be around 60 years old and already subject to the negative health effects of smoking. Male smoking rates and lung cancer deaths were already declining by this time, especially amongst men in middle to older ages (ages 55–70), the male age cohort that has 'gained' most years of life in recent years.

Heart disease

Diseases of the heart or blood vessels [angina, heart attacks (CHD) and stroke] are associated with a complex set of lifestyle factors including: smoking, diet (linked to obesity and diabetes), low levels of physical activity, excessive alcohol consumption and stress. There is a definite association between the increased prevalence of cigarette smoking and CHD mortality, although it is difficult to identify its specific effects precisely given the constellation of risk factors for CHD. Unal *et al.* (2004) conclude that 60% of the CHD mortality decrease in Britain between 1981 and 2000 (for men and women combined) was attributable to reductions in major risk factors, principally smoking. However, CHD has historically been seen as a male disease and until recently very little attention has been given to CHD amongst women.

Heart disease is the leading cause of death for men and women in the UK. Death rates for heart disease have declined significantly since the 1970s for both men and women. Although they still remain higher for men, the decline has been more rapid amongst men than amongst women. However, for CHD, the decline in the death rate has been slower for younger ages, especially for women: the death rate for those aged between 35 and 44 fell by 35% for men and 32% for women between 1992 and 2002 (Petersen *et al.* 2005). It is thus highly likely that the gender differences in the decline in CHD mortality are associated with the age and gender differences in smoking patterns discussed earlier.

Unal *et al.* (2004) were unable to quantify the effect of alcohol consumption beyond the recommended daily rate, but this is also likely to be important in terms of gender differences. The picture is complex. The World Health Organisation (WHO 2002) estimates that the impact of alcohol consumption by women in developed countries is generally positive – if no alcohol was consumed there would be a 3% increase in CHD and a 16% increase in stroke. But excessive consumption, especially 'binge drinking', which is indirectly associated with CHD, has increased markedly over recent years in the UK. Men are more likely to drink to excess and to 'binge' drink than women in every age group, but the percentage consuming more than the recommended weekly level has remained more or less stable since the mid-1990s for men, but increased by over 50% for women (Petersen *et al.* 2005). Differences in heavy drinking are most similar at ages 16–24 (males: 32%; females: 24%) (Bajekal *et al.* 2006). Smoking and excessive alcohol consumption are only two amongst the set of factors associated with CHD mortality, but although diet, stress and level of physical activity also play a role it is extremely difficult to ascertain how these factors may have varied by gender over time and therefore their contribution to the decreasing gender gap in life expectancy.

Unal *et al.* (2004) suggested that 40% of the overall decrease in CHD was associated with changes in medical treatments, especially for acute myocardial infarctions, and surgical treatments. Since CHD in women has been 'underdiagnosed, under-treated and under-researched' (Mikhail 2005) it is highly possible that treatment biases that favour men may be inhibiting greater overall mortality improvements in women. For example, Shaw *et al.* (2004) found that women were less likely to be given coronary artery bypass grafting and percutaneous transluminal coronary angioplasty than men in England between 1991 and 1999. They report that, since these procedures were also less likely in older persons (and heart disease increases after the menopause), women are doubly disadvantaged because they generally experience CHD at older ages than men.

So far we have sought to explain the narrowing gap in life expectancy by reference to major causes of death that have been associated with particular improvements in life expectancy for men. Many other factors are also likely to play a role, even though it is not possible to assess their overall contribution fully. These may include a reduction in fatal workplace accidents for men following the decline in blue-collar industry; a decline in male fatal road-traffic accidents, alongside increased risk of death on the roads for women with more women drivers; and, possibly, increased health awareness amongst men (discussed below). Yet we need to offset these trends by rises in violent deaths and suicides amongst men since the early 1970s (although it should be noted that male suicide rates have been declining recently, Chapter 8) as well as the increase in some causes of death, such as prostate cancer. Skin cancer provides an good illustration of changes that appear to be disadvantaging men.

Skin cancer

Although it represented just 3% of all UK cancers in 2005, the incidence of skin cancer has doubled in the past 20 years and it has seen the largest increase in incidence of all cancers in the UK over the past 10 years, and is now the second highest in the world. Incidence rates have always been higher for women than for men (by about 4 : 3), but over the past 20 years have increased more swiftly for men (by 26%) than for women (by 20%). Although women are more likely to suffer from skin cancer, mortality has always been higher for men, and this too is increasing. Age-standardised death rates show a continual rise for males from an average of 1.2 per 100,000 in the early 1970s to

2.7 per 100,000 by the early twenty-first century. Age-standardised death rates for females averaged about 1.3 per 100,000 in the early 1970s, levelled off in the 1990s, and reached an average of 2.0 per 100,000 in the early twenty-first century. At the start of the twenty-first century the gap between men's and women's incidence of skin cancer is the narrowest for 25 years (Cancer Research UK 2006).

In the majority of cases skin cancer is caused by exposure to the sun's ultraviolet radiation (although better female survival rates may be due to thinner lesions in women). Changing male attitudes may have influenced this rapid rise in skin cancer amongst men. In particular, body image is now much more important to men, especially young men, than it was in the past and 'getting a tan' is part of this. However, men are much less likely than women to see sun exposure as a serious risk to their health and less likely to heed 'sun-safe' messages (Mintel Consumer Goods Intelligence 2004). They are less aware, or more cavalier, about health risks of sun exposure than women. Women are far more likely to take action to protect themselves by the use of sunscreens and protective clothing, and far less likely to get sunburnt than men (Office of National Statistics 2002).

Trend data suggest very little change in the use of suncream amongst men and women in recent years. In 2004, 48% of men and 63% of women aged 15 and over reported having used suncream in the past 12 months. For both men and women, use is highest in the 25–54 age range. Men under the age of 20 are especially resistant to its use (Mintel Consumer Goods Intelligence 2004). In 2002, 79% of women and 57% of men thought that taking precautions against over-exposure to the sun was very important, but a tenth of men thought that it was not important (Office of National Statistics 2002).

In this section we have seen that although women in the UK live on average 4–5 years longer than men the differential between them has been decreasing since the early 1980s. This narrowing gap in life expectancy is largely due to improvements in the major causes of death for men over this period, although less swift improvements for women also play a role. While it is difficult to identify the reasons for these changes precisely, gender-related changes in cigarette smoking are recognised to be very important. Finally, it is important to appreciate that not all recent changes in mortality advantage men because there are also trends for specific causes of death that favour women.

Morbidity: are women really sicker?

Although women live longer than men in Britain and other developed societies, researchers traditionally have argued that they are sicker throughout their lives. Broadly speaking, while men tend to suffer from serious illnesses that cause death at earlier ages, women live longer and experience more chronic, but not necessarily life-threatening, illness and disability. Thus women's 'extra 5 years' of life are typically not spent in good health. In terms of years spent free from disability or chronic illness, women's advantage reduces to just 2–3 years (Chapter 6).

Self-reported illness

The most readily available sources of information about morbidity are the measures of self-reported illness collected in the General Household Survey (GHS) shown in Table 5.2. The table shows that for all ages combined, females reported only slightly higher rates than males, with the exception of long-standing illness. However, a consideration of specific age groups shows varying gender patterns. For example, older women (65+) report much higher levels of 'restricted activity' than older men. For most conditions leading to a long-standing (chronic) illness there are no statistically significant differences between men and women. The main exception is musculoskeletal conditions (with rates of 52 and 85 per 1000 for men and women, respectively). The much larger proportion of older women suffering from arthritis and rheumatism mainly explains this (men 136, women 223 per 1000). Age-related gender differences also emerge for chronic respiratory problems, where men aged 65 and over report twice the levels of bronchitis and emphysema than women (General Household Survey 2004).

The overall picture these data present is of similar broad self-assessments of health for men and women, but also of age differences for specific categories, some favouring men, others favouring women. This national picture is supported by research on local and regional populations.

Table 5.2 Self-reported sickness: by type of complaint, gender and age, Great Britain 2004 (%).

	Long-standing illness	Limiting long-standing illness	Restricted activity*
Male			
0–4	15	4	10
5–15	19	8	10
16–44	20	10	8
45–64	43	26	15
65–74	57	33	16
75+	63	43	20
All	33	17	12
Female			
0–4	11	4	11
5–15	15	7	7
16–44	22	12	12
45–64	42	24	18
65–74	55	33	20
74+	63	48	26
All	32	19	14

*This refers to whether respondents had cut down on their normal activities in the 2 weeks prior to interview.
Source: General Household Survey 2004, table 7.2. National Statistics website: www.statistics.gov.uk.
Crown copyright material is reproduced with the permission of the Controller of HMSO.

Common mental disorders

There are also gender differences for common mental disorders. Women tend to report higher levels of mental distress than men, with higher levels of neurotic disorders (depression and anxiety, panic, obsessions and compulsions which cause distress and problems with daily activities) (Chapter 8). In 2000, the National Psychiatric Morbidity Survey of people living in private households (Office of National Statistics 2001) assessed 19% of women and 14% of men between the ages of 16 and 74 as having a neurotic disorder. The gender difference is largely due to higher rates of 'mixed anxiety and depressive disorder' among women (women 11%, men 7%). Women appear to experience more severe symptoms (18%) than men (12%).

One in 10 young people between the ages of 5 and 18 had a clinically recognisable mental disorder in Britain in 2004. Prevalence of 'any disorder' is higher in boys at ages 5–10 (boys 10%, girls 5%) and 11–16 (boys 13%, girls 10%). This is partly, but by no means wholly, explained by higher rates of 'conduct disorder' amongst boys (Office of National Statistics 2004).

Men and women may express psychological problems in different ways. While women under stress tend to become anxious and depressed, men under stress are more likely to drink heavily, take drugs or become physically and sexually abusive (Busfield 2000). These kinds of behaviours have often been left out of health statistics, contributing to the impression that they are a form of deviance, rather than an expression of mental ill health, and distorting the gender picture of mental health. Other problems may also be hidden. The incidence of self-harming is significantly higher amongst girls and young women than amongst boys and young men (Chapter 8). However, self-harming may be more likely to be concealed in boys, appearing as the result of attacks, accidents or fights (Mental Health Foundation 2006).

The evidence presented above suggests that gender differences in overall levels of morbidity are mainly attributable to higher levels of female morbidity for minor symptoms and some kinds of mental disorders. The gender differences in long-standing illness do not represent higher *overall levels* of sickness among women, but vary by condition. Thus it is important not to assume that women experience higher morbidity levels for *all* conditions. Further, although there may be aspects of women's lives in general that predispose them to higher levels of illness, and aspects of men's lives that predispose them to lower levels of illness, it is important not to be not blinded to similarities across gender and to differences within men and within women, for example differences by age (Chapter 6) and social class (Chapter 3).

Explaining gender patterns in morbidity

One difficulty in interpreting gender patterns in morbidity is that research on gender and health has traditionally emphasised women's higher morbidity and has been inhibited by the failure even to think about men's health in terms of gender, since gender traditionally has been synonymous with *women's* health. It is only since the late 1990s that men's health has been given any sustained attention. Even when men's health was brought into the picture, there was a tendency, which continues today, for researchers to make assumptions about the aspects of men's and women's lives that are important for their health *prior* to conducting their research. For example, conditions of paid work have been assumed to be important for men, while juggling home and work, caring for the family and supporting others have been assumed to be important for women. In making these assumptions, research has placed men and women into traditional gender roles and experiences, regardless of whether this was in fact the case. Moreover, it was assumed that it was the *differences* between men and women that were important rather than any *similarities*, so the latter were overlooked or disregarded.

Another difficulty is in determining how far the similarities and differences that are reported are accurate reflections of men's and women's health status. One concern is that rather than reflecting real health differences in sickness between them they may simply be artefacts, that is a reflection of the ways that men, women and health professionals think about and act upon their health. Two apparently competing explanations have been put forward.

The first explanation is that women's higher morbidity is real and a product of their poorer social circumstances. One way to test for this is to consider the health status of men and women in similar circumstances. Using a sub-sample of 20–60-year-olds from the Health Survey for England, Bartley (2004) found clear evidence that women experienced higher minor levels of psychological morbidity despite being in similar household and work situations to men, but there was no statistically significant difference in their self-rated general health. Moreover, an analysis of specific health conditions revealed few clear differences between men and women. Even where rates are higher in women the differences are often small and not statistically significant. The analysis did show that men have higher rates of heart and circulatory disease – as we would expect in light of age-related differences in their prevalence, discussed earlier.

The second explanation is that the health statistics simply reflect the propensity for women to *over-report* ill health and for men to *under-report* ill health. This could occur in self-reports, the main source of national data in Britain, and also in the assessments that others, such as health practitioners, make about the health of men and women. In its simplest and strongest form, this explanation argues that men (especially young men) are less likely than women to recognise illness or seek help for it, because independence and stoicism in the face of pain are defining features of their masculine identity, and this deflates their ill-health statistics. In contrast, the feminine 'caring role' makes women more attentive to bodily discomforts, more willing to seek help and more willing to adopt the 'sick role', resulting in the inflation of women's ill-health statistics. The implication is that self-reported measures such as 'restricted activity' due to illness (as in Table 5.2) may be as much about gender-related behaviours in response to illness, as about levels of severity.

Men and women are likely to think and behave differently in relation to health and illness, but in ways that are far more complicated than this explanation would predict. A recent study of help-seeking amongst a cross-section of men in Scotland (O'Brien *et al.* 2005) found widespread endorsement, especially amongst younger men and among healthier men, of the proposal that seeking help was a threat to their masculine identities. Yet some of the men in the sample embraced help-seeking when it would serve to *preserve* rather than threaten their masculinity (e.g. enabling them to keep working) or to *restore* valued aspects of masculinity such as sexual performance. This suggests that traditional notions of masculinity can also be associated with enhanced health-seeking amongst men. It is also important not to assume that women are always eager to seek help. For example, Free *et al.* (2002) found that some young women saw the use of emergency contraception as a 'failure' which generated embarrassment, a fear of what others might think, and a reluctance to seek help.

Health provision

Gender assumptions can also influence individual health practitioners, who may be more likely to diagnose some conditions in men and others in women, especially when the presenting symptoms are unclear. Indeed, it is precisely the milder forms of 'nebulous' illness, such as minor physical symptoms and neuroses, which permit greater discretion in terms of their perception, reporting of symptoms and their diagnoses, that show a female excess. This adds weight to the argument that the reported female excess morbidity is an artefact for at least some conditions, especially mild mental disorders.

Under-diagnosis can also occur. Arber *et al.* (2006) looked at how four patient characteristics – age, gender, social class and race – influenced decisions about CHD by primary care doctors in the UK and USA. The doctors viewed a video-vignette of scripted consultations with actors presenting with seven signs and symptoms strongly suggestive of CHD. Apart from the character-istics of the actor-patient the tapes were identical. They found no influence of social class or race, and no evidence of general ageism in doctors' behaviour. However, women were asked fewer questions, received fewer examinations, fewer diagnostic tests, and were prescribed the least medication for CHD. They also found evidence of 'gendered ageism' in that women in midlife were asked the fewest questions and prescribed least medication.

Irritable bowel syndrome (IBS) provides a good illustration of the interplay between the biological and social causation of disease and the gendered inter-pretation of symptoms by practitioners (Payne 2004). IBS affects between 20 and 40% of UK population, and has a much higher incidence amongst women. Biological risks are thought to be related to the reproductive system, especi-ally hormonal factors, given that women appear to be more susceptible during particular phases of the reproductive cycle. IBS is associated with stress and anxiety in both male and female sufferers, but women with the condition are more likely to report feelings of severe anxiety, depression, tiredness, crying and sleep loss. As reported above, depression and anxiety are generally higher in women than in men. Payne therefore concludes that 'there may be common causes of stress, poor mental health, and IBS that reflect gender relations' (Payne 2004: 22). Thus the higher incidence of IBS amongst women may result from a combination of biological factors and the stressful circumstances of their lives.

However, Payne also found that health practitioners might interpret the symptoms of IBS through the 'lens' of gender. IBS is often described as a 'diagnosis of exclusion', meaning that it is only determined when all other conditions have been ruled out. It is typical of nebulous conditions which are attributed to psychological causes, and women are especially vulnerable to being diagnosed in this way. IBS is therefore not only a useful illustration of the combined influence of the biological and the social, it also raises the question of how far gender differences are a *real* product of men and women's social circumstances and how far are they are a *construct* of gender stereotypes.

Much of the debate about whether gender patterns of morbidity are real or artefactual has been driven by concern about the possible inflation of women's ill health. If women are being inappropriately labelled as sick, then this creates the impression that they are vulnerable, weak and incapable. This in turn could lead to their exclusion from social positions, such as well-paid but demanding jobs, which benefit health through improved self-esteem and high financial rewards. The reverse is also true, if men's ill-health is under-reported and generally neglected, then their health problems are likely to be denied, leading to unnecessary suffering as they 'solider on' regardless (Men's Health Forum 2002). These negative consequences of gendered responses to illness for men have often been neglected because attention has typically been directed at the apparently higher levels of morbidity amongst women.

Gender, health and social change

Gender patterns of health and illness are highly sensitive to social change in the lives of men and women over time (Annandale 2003). For example, the narrowing gender gap in life expectancy is related to changes in circumstances (such as kinds of employment) and behaviour (such as smoking) that began several decades ago and are now affecting men and women in middle and older age. More recent changes in lifestyles and health-related behaviours of males and females, especially among younger age groups, are influencing contemporary patterns of sickness (e.g. increasing obesity). These changes result from fundamental changes within British society (Chapter 10), especially in the socio-economic, educational, employment, domestic and leisure circumstances of women and men.

The most important factors leading to changing gender roles and behaviours are employment and education. In Britain traditional areas of male employment such as heavy industry and manufacturing have been in decline since the second half of the twentieth century. This has been accompanied by a rise in the female-dominated service sector. As women's economic activity rates have risen, the rates for men have declined and there is now an almost equal gender balance in the workforce. Women's increased participation and their movement into the higher echelons of the workforce has no doubt been facilitated by their increased educational achievement. In 1974/5 girls and boys left school with more or less the same educational qualifications; by 2005, girls' achievements were significantly outstripping boys (Equal Opportunities Commission 2006).

Changes in working patterns have had *direct effects* upon mortality through reductions in male deaths from work-related accidents, although it should also be noted that higher male unemployment is associated with social exclusion and depression (Lindsay 2003). For women, paid work is strongly associated with improved health and longevity (Klumb and Lampert 2004). The *indirect effects* upon health and morbidity through gender-related changes in lifestyle associated with changing education levels and patterns of employment are just as important.

There used to be a very strong association between the kind of work that people did and the lifestyles that they led. The new service economy is changing this by breaking down barriers between consumption and lifestyles of what were once clearly defined and tightly bound social groups (Chapter 10). Consumerism allows the expression of lifestyles and identities that are no longer tied so directly to social class and gender (Charles 2002). The boundary between work and home, once firmly entrenched for men as they kept their work and home life separate, is blurring as home and the family become the centre of consumption. Conversely, women, once largely confined to the 'housewife' role, are experiencing the separation of home and work through their paid employment in a working life outside the family.

This is not to say that men and women are necessarily becoming *equal*. For example, although the earnings gap has reduced considerably over the past 30 years, from 29% in 1975 to 17% in 2005, women still earn less per hour than men. Moreover, part-time work attracts lower pay than full-time work, and women are far more likely than men to work part-time (42% of women and 9% of men worked part-time in 2005) (Equal Opportunities Commission 2006). Nor is it the case that the attitudes and behaviours of men and women are becoming *the same*. Rather, gender expectations are now less fixed and both men and women can engage in behaviour previously confined to the other gender, although it is important to appreciate that this varies by age.

The rising incidence of skin cancer amongst men, discussed earlier, provides an example of the result of the interaction of 'new' and 'old' forms of masculinity. The 'new' expectations of the desirable/healthy looking tanned body, previously a female preoccupation, work alongside 'old' feelings of invulnerability, which lead young men to ignore the need to protect themselves from sun. For young women the benefits to health from their 'new' social and economic independence, linked to better educational qualifications and entry into the labour force, may be cancelled out by opportunities to engage in dangerous behaviours usually associated with earlier death for men. The substantial major increase in young women's consumption of alcohol, a direct contributor to death from liver disease and accidental death, and a major contributor to CHD, breast cancer and upper digestive cancers, is a good example of this.

Recognising that there are *similarities* between men and women as well as differences, leads us to appreciate that men and women are not homogeneous groups. There are also *differences within* genders and it is more appropriate to refer to masculinities and femininities in the plural, than to masculinity and femininity in the singular. For example, sociologists have suggested that it is one form of masculinity, the 'traditional' ('macho') form of masculinity, often called hyper-masculinity, which is particularly negative for men's health (Courtenay 2002).

Age is a particularly important marker of differences within men and within women. The convergence of gender roles, experiences and behaviours is more likely among younger men and women. Young women's lives have become a dominant metaphor for social change and the touchstone for society's problems (McRobbie 2000). Much has been made of the dangers to health from women's liberation. For example, a recent article in the *British Medical Journal* concluded that 'the historic gap between men and women's life expectancy could vanish as more and more women accustom themselves to the work hard–play hard culture of modern Britain' (Brettingham 2005: 656). While young women do need to heed the message that cigarette smoking and binge drinking are a danger to health, it is important not to dwell on these behaviours (as the media tends to do) to the exclusion of the very real gains to women's health from their growing economic self-sufficiency and personal autonomy. Above all, it is important to appreciate that the relationship between the lives of men and women today and their health is highly complex and it has become increasingly difficult, and hence inadvisable, to draw simple one-to-one associations between a person's gender and their health.

Implications for nursing practice

In contrast to some other countries, such as Canada which has adopted gender mainstreaming policies, most UK health policy has been gender-blind. However, the new 'gender duty', which comes into force in April 2007 as part of the Department of Trade and Industry's Equality Bill, will require NHS Trusts and health authorities to identify gender equality goals and to make clear the action they will take to implement them. It is expected that NHS services will be required to carry out equality impact assessments to determine whether policies have a disproportionate effect on women or men, to set equality goals and outcomes, and to publish equality action plans and to collect gender disaggregated statistics.

The new duty will require NHS staff to 'mainstream' gender into their practice and to take into account whether men and women have different health needs. In much the same way that nurses and other staff have been encouraged to develop race awareness, they will now be required to become gender aware (Doyal *et al.* 2003). Nurses will need, for example, to be able to recognise that men and women may present symptoms such as those of heart disease and mental illness differently, and to be able to take this into account in diagnosing and treating illness. It may be advisable to tailor rehabilitation programmes after illness such as stroke, or preventative services such as smoking cessation programmes, to the different expectations and needs of men and women.

The new gender duty will require nurses above all to be 'gender sensitive'. Gender sensitive health care is not easy to achieve. It involves recognising that gender matters. For example in the context of biological or sex-linked diseases, where patients hold highly gendered beliefs, or act in gendered ways in relation to their health. But it also requires nurses (and other staff) to be aware that people do not always behave in gender-stereotypical ways and that, as we have seen, gender roles and gender expectations are in flux. Therefore, nurses will need to be alert to the possible significance of gender while also appreciating that there is no simple one-to-one association between being male or female and a specific set of gender attitudes and behaviours in relation to health.

Summary

This chapter has argued that gendered patterns of mortality and ill health in contemporary Britain are more complex and less clear-cut than is often presented. For mortality, the gap in life expectancy between men and women persists but appears to be very slowly narrowing. For morbidity, gender differences are small or non-existent when considering general measures of morbidity for all ages together, but some differences are seen for specific conditions at particular ages. It is unclear whether the reported patterns of morbidity have always been more similar than they seemed, since differences reported in the past may have been an artefact of the kinds of questions that were asked and/or the failure to report similarities. However, it does seem that gender patterns of death and ill health are becoming more similar in contemporary Britain. For young people in particular, gender identity is likely to be negotiated in ways that open men and women up to experiences that both protect and undermine their health in complex, and perhaps competing, ways. This does not mean that gender is less relevant for health and illness, but that it may no longer operate in such a clear-cut way.

References

Annandale, E. (2003) Health, illness and the politics of gender, in S. Williams, G. Bendelow and L. Birke (eds) *Debating Biology: Sociological Perspectives on Health, Medicine and Society*. Routledge, London.

Arber, S., McKinlay, J., Adams, A., *et al.* (2006) Patient characteristics and inequalities in doctors' diagnosis and management strategies relating to CHD: a video-simulation experiment. *Social Science and Medicine*, 62, 103–15.

Bajekal, M., Osborne, V., Yar, M. and Meltzer, H. eds (2006) *Focus on Health*. National Statistics/Palgrave Macmillan. Available at www.statistics.org (accessed June 2006).

Banks, I. (2001) No man's land: men, illness and help seeking. *British Medical Journal*, 323, 1058–1060.

Bartley, M. (2004) *Health Inequality.* Polity Press, Cambridge, 135–48.

Brettingham, M. (2005) Men's life expectancy is catching up with women's. *British Medical Journal*, 331, 656.

Busfield, J. (2000) *Health and Health Care in Modern Britain.* Oxford University Press, Oxford.

Cancer Research UK (2006) Available at http://info.cancerresearchuk.org/cancerstats/types/melanoma/mortality (accessed May 2006).

Charles, N. (2002) *Gender in Modern Britain.* Oxford University Press, Oxford.

Courtenay, W. (2002) A global perspective on the field of men's health: An editorial. *International Journal of Men's Health*, 1, 1–14.

Doyal, L., Payne, S. and Cameron, A. (2003) *Promoting Gender Equality in Health.* Equal Opportunities Commission, Research and Resources Unit, Manchester. Available at http://www.eoc.org.uk/PDF/promoting_gender_equality_in_health.pdf (accessed May 2006).

Equal Opportunities Commission (2006) *Facts about Women and Men in Great Britain.* EOC, London.

Evans, R., Brotherstone, H., Miles, A. and Wardle, J. (2005) Gender differences in early detection of cancer. *Journal of Men's Health and Gender*, 2(2), 209–17.

Free, C., Lee, R. and Ogden, J.Y. (2002) Women's accounts of factors influencing their use of non-emergency contraception: in-depth interview study. *British Medical Journal*, 325, 1393–8.

General Household Survey 2004. Available at www.statistics.gov.uk

Gjonca, A., Tomassini, B.T. and Smallwood, S. (2005) Sex differences in mortality, a comparison of the United Kingdom and other developed countries. *Health Statistics Quarterly*, 26, 6–16.

Graham, H., Frances, B., Inskip, H., *et al.* (2006) Socioeconomic lifecourse influences on women's smoking status in early adulthood. *Journal of Epidemiology and Community Health*, 60, 228–33.

Griffiths, C. and Brock, A. (2003) Twentieth century mortality trends in England and Wales. *Health Statistics Quarterly*, 18, 5–17.

HSE (Health and Safety Executive) (2002) *Levels of Trends in Workplace Injury: reported Injuries and the Labour Force Survey.* Stationery Office, London.

Klumb, P.L. and Lampert, T. (2004) Women, work and well-being 1950–2000: a review and methodological critique. *Social Science and Medicine*, 58(6), 1007–24.

Lindsay, C. (2003) A century of labour market change: 1900 to 2000. *Labour Market Trends*, March, 133–44.

McRobbie, A. (2000) *Feminism and Youth Culture*, 2nd edition. Macmillan, London.

Men's Health Forum (2002) *Soldier it! Young Men and Suicide.* Men's Health Forum, London.

Mental Health Foundation (2006) *Truth Hurts. Report of National Inquiry into Self-harm amongst Young People.* Mental Health Foundation, London.

Mikhail, G. (2005) Editorial. Coronary heart disease in women. *British Medical Journal*, 331, 467–8.

Mintel Consumer Goods Intelligence (2004) *Suncare Preparations – UK – December 2004.* Mintel Group.

O'Brien, R., Hunt, K. and Hart, G. (2005) 'It's caveman stuff, but that is to a certain extent how guys still operate': men's account of masculinity and help seeking. *Social Science and Medicine*, 61, 503–16.

Office of National Statistics (2001) *Psychiatric Morbidity among Adults, 2000.* Stationery Office, London.

Office of National Statistics (2002) *Social Trends* 32. Stationery Office, London.

Office of National Statistics (2004) *Survey of the Mental Health of Children and Young People in Britain 2004.* Stationary Office, London.

Office of National Statistics (2005) *Social Trends 35.* Stationary Office, London.

Payne, S. (2004) Sex, gender, and irritable bowel syndrome: making connections. *Gender Medicine,* 1(1), 18–28.

Petersen, S., Peto, V., Scarborough, P. and Rayner, M. (2005) *Coronary Heart Disease Statistics 2005 edn.* British Heart Foundation, London.

Shaw, M., Maxwell, R., Rees, K., *et al.* (2004) Gender and equity in the provision of coronary revascularisation in England in the 1990s: is it getting better? *Social Science and Medicine,* 59(12), 2499–507.

Unal, B., Critchley, J.A. and Capewell, S. (2004) Explaining the decline in coronary heart disease mortality in England and Wales between 1981 and 2000. *Circulation,* 9 March, 1101–7.

Vallin, J., Mesle, F. and Valkonen, T. (2001) *Trends in Mortality and Differential Mortality.* Council of Europe Publishing, Strasbourg.

WHO (2002) *The World Health Report 2002. Reducing Risks, Promoting Healthy Life.* WHO, Geneva.

Further reading

Annandale, E. and Hunt, K. (2000) Gender inequalities in health: research at the crossroads, in E. Annandale and K. Hunt (eds) *Gender Inequalities in Health.* Open University Press, Buckingham.
A useful and widely cited review of the current status of research on gender inequalities in health with particular references to theoretical and methodological issues.

Payne, S. (2006) *The Health of Men and Women.* Polity Press, Cambridge.
An excellent up-to-date review of data, theory and explanations about differences in men's and women's health in the UK.

Chapter 6

Health and disease in old age

The relationship between health and ageing, and in particular the health of older people, is an important issue not only in the world of health services but also in the wider public arena. Appreciating this relationship requires an understanding of the links between biological and social aspects of ageing. Despite the continuously increasing length of life in our society, negative depictions of old age as a time of increasing illness and dependency often distort the ways in which ageing and old people are discussed in the mass media and in health and social policy debates. This chapter examines the relationships between health, illness and old age and the implications of Britain's 'ageing society' for both older people and health services. It will:

- define and discuss the concept of an 'ageing society';
- discuss the biological and social aspects of ageing;
- describe the social position of old people in contemporary Britain;
- discuss patterns of health and illness among older people;
- discuss health care for older people.

Older people and the ageing of society

It is important not to see 'old people' as a homogeneous group as there is great diversity among the 'elderly' population of contemporary Britain. One reason for this is that pre-existing differences, such as those described in Chapters 3 and 4, continue into old age. Another reason is that the category 'old people' covers an age range of some 40 years, and people aged 65 can expect to live for another 25–30 years. We would not expect a 25-year-old and a 50-year-old to be 'the same', neither should we expect a 65-year-old and a 90-year-old to be the same.

While the process of ageing clearly describes biological changes, sociologists have shown that it also reflects changes in social status, reflected by a variety of indicators such as retirement from work, receipt of pension, reaching an arbitrary chronological age, and the loss of independence due to chronic ill health. Taking this approach to old age suggests that it is a variable social status, entry to which depends upon a number of factors in addition to chronological age.

An ageing society is one in which the *proportion*, rather than the sheer number, of older people in the population is increasing relative to the proportions of young and middle-aged people. Declining birth and infant mortality rates are the main cause of an ageing society. In twentieth-century Britain the birth rate gradually declined (despite the mid-century 'baby boom') and the lower percentage of children and young people in the population at the end of the century meant that the proportion of older people in the population had increased. The trend towards living longer is the other, less significant, aspect of an ageing society. Men who had reached the age of 60 towards the end of the twentieth century could expect, on average, to live for another 15.6 years, only two more years than men aged 60 at the beginning of the century. The rise in women's later life expectancy during the twentieth century was more marked. Women aged 60 at the end of the century could, on average, expect to live for more than another 20 years, compared to only 13 more years for women aged 60 in 1901. Life expectancy at birth in 2001–2003 was 76 for males and 81 for females (Soule *et al.* 2005).

Throughout the twentieth century the numbers of people over the age of 65 and as a proportion of the total population of the UK have increased continuously, although more slowly since 1971. The 2001 census found that for the first time people over the age of 60 (21%) exceeded children under the age of 16 (20%) as a proportion of the UK population. Just over 7% of the population were aged 75 or over (the 'old old') and there was a big increase in the number of the 'oldest old', aged 85 or over (1.1 million), who made up 1.9% of the population (as compared to 0.4% in 1951). In this age group women outnumbered men in the ratio 5 : 2. For all minority ethnic groups the proportion of elderly people was 4%.

A much more rapid rise in the numbers of very old people is expected, becoming especially evident between 2030 and 2050 when the 'baby boom' cohort of the 1960s reaches very old age: the 'oldest old' are expected to reach 9.1% of the population in 2031. It is expected that the proportion of people over retirement age will be about 25% of the total population by 2021 (Soule *et al.* 2005, Arber and Ginn 2006).

The projected rise in the numbers of over-85s particularly worries health service planners. Although they will still form only a small minority of the total population in the future, they are assumed to be a group that will continue to need a disproportionately high amount of expensive health care (see Figure 10.1, p. 214). However, a large proportion of such increased costs may be explained by the significantly larger proportion of deaths amongst the oldest old as compared to the rest of the population: regardless of age, health care costs are high in the few months before death (Arber and Ginn 2006). As we will discuss later, there is also a view that older people are becoming healthier than those in previous generations.

The ageing of British society and the prospect of rising numbers of older people are often portrayed in the mass media as threats to the viability of the pensions and welfare system and as an intolerable future burden on society (Mullan 2000). Public perceptions have tended to concentrate on the supposed problems caused by 'too many' older people. Instead of celebrating the rise in the numbers of long-living people as one of the great successes of rising standards of living and better health care, there have been gloomy predictions of the effects of the so-called 'demographic time bomb' on an already overstretched care system. In health care, concerns have focused upon whether the health services of the future will be able to cope with ever-growing numbers of frail and chronically ill people. However, although the numbers and proportion of older people in Britain will continue to rise, contrary to some alarmist media stories, the associated rise in pension and health care costs may be less than expected (Arber and Ginn 2006).

Understanding ageing and health in older people

Discussion about rates of illness and death in the older population focuses on a rather medicalised view of later life. However, ageing is not merely a process of biological change, it is also a process of social change. To understand the role of nursing and of health services in the lives of older people we must take into account both of these aspects of ageing.

The medical approach to ageing and health

The medical approach to ageing (Chapter 2) is widely used and understood by nurses and other health professionals, and the general public. It focuses upon the ageing individual, and views human ageing as a process of physiological and biological change. Ageing is seen as being determined by an in-built biological process (a 'biological clock') programmed by our genetic make-up that governs significant bodily changes from early development to maturity through to the decline and loss of functions in later life. Ageing means an inevitable loss of health, and represents a decline from optimum levels in youth. Life stages – infancy, childhood, puberty and adolescence, adulthood and maturity, and old age – are predetermined. Although individuals may vary in the chronological age at which they enter and leave each stage, normal development includes passage through all the stages. Human health, growth and development are strongly influenced by these stages and as individuals age they take on the characteristics of their biological age group, leaving behind the behaviour and interests of the earlier stages.

The 'medical model' focuses on the 'mechanical' processes of ageing. Different parts of the body such as knee and hip joints, the heart and liver, may age at different rates, much as different components in a car might fail sooner, or last longer, than expected. Thus, some of the negative aspects of physiological ageing are 'fixable', to a degree, by medical intervention. From this perspective old age comes to be seen as a form of disease or a complex of conditions that are treatable.

The social approach to ageing and health

The social approach to ageing emphasises the importance of social factors in shaping people's experiences of growing old. It suggests that the both the ageing process itself and how it is viewed in a society are shaped socio-economic conditions and cultural values throughout the lifecourse (Chapter 3). While ageing is a biological reality, it is influenced by social and economic factors. Both health and the average life span have improved very significantly in industrial societies since pre-industrial times, and life expectancy is greater in today's industrial developed economies than in most poorer countries. In contemporary Britain and similar societies what is regarded as the 'natural', biological life span has been revised upwards.

As people age they tend to carry their health experience and their identities with them, rather than changing fundamentally at each stage, as the medical model suggests. As each cohort ages, it is likely to experience social, cultural and economic influences that are specific to their historical time. Thus, future cohorts of older people are likely to be different in significant ways from those of today. For example, they might be more assertive and 'consumer minded' in their expectations of nursing and health care. Instead of seeing an older person's behaviour or health simply as a reflection of the physiological stage they have reached, it is important also to consider how the health of older individuals is influenced by the experiences of their age cohort (Chapter 3).

Health and illness in later life are influenced by the social roles older people adopt, as well as by the physiological or 'mechanical' failure of different parts of their bodies. The social model draws attention to the important links between social role, bodily functioning and self-conceptions (Chapter 7). For many older people in contemporary Britain, especially men from lower socio-economic classes, entry to old age has been/is signalled by retirement from paid work and the receipt of a pension. Social arrangements and negative social attitudes in interaction with reduced income and increasing chronic illness may make it harder for some old people to participate fully in the whole range of 'normal' life.

The social process of ageing may thus become marked by a progressive 'emptying out' of roles and activities and decreasing social integration within the wider community, and the loss of these may adversely affect self-conception and the sense of identity. This can have a detrimental effect on their morale, leading to lower performance of the immune system and physical illness. Conversely, valuing older people and recognising their worth can lead to better health, or at least to a more tolerable experience of illness. This has been found to be the case even with older people who have organic brain disorders such as Alzheimer's disease (Kitwood 1997).

The medical and social approaches to ageing are best seen as complementing or informing each other, rather than as being in conflict (Chapter 2). As the social approach acknowledges, chronological age ('clock time') does not reliably predicate the onset and progression of disease in old age or the ability to benefit from treatment. Nor does it correlate reliably with the social activities, interests and aptitudes of older people. Taking account of the social aspects of ageing can lead to a better understanding of elderly people, their health and illness and their capacity to benefit from health care. For example, physical decline and social aspects of ageing, such as the loss of meaningful or valued roles in work or family, may reinforce each other, creating a negative effect on morale and physical health. The impact of illness is mediated by social support (Chapter 2). Older people with supportive social networks are likely to be less adversely affected by the same level of illness or disability than those who are socially isolated. Old age is thus best seen as a biologically based category that has been socially shaped and patterned. By understanding this, nurses may avoid the dangers of stereotyping old people and 'elderly patients' as a single group. It is therefore important to look at the social contexts that influence older people's health and shape their experiences of ageing.

Older people in contemporary Britain

Previous chapters have shown that health, people's socio-economic status, income and material resources; their religious and cultural values and beliefs; their sex and ethnicity; and their family relationships shape their health, illness and health care. We therefore look at some of these factors with reference to older people.

Marital status

For older people marital status has important consequences for their living arrangements, financial status (especially for women), sources of social support, help and immediate care, and social isolation.

Entering old age, the great majority of older people are married and living with their spouse. However, as they become older this situation changes. Older men are much more likely to remain married than older women, while older women (especially aged 85+) are much more likely to be widowed. Men are therefore more likely to have a partner for companionship and support. In 2001 17% of men and 47% of women aged 65+ were widowed (Arber and Ginn 2006). Becoming widowed leads to the loss of the main source of company and support for older people. Living alone increases with age, especially among women; 80% of widowed people live on their own.

Place of residence

Where people live is a good indicator of their autonomy and social status and the 'social capital' (Chapter 3) they may be able to draw upon. In terms of *neighbourhoods*, older people living in deprived areas are at least twice as likely to experience poverty than those living elsewhere. They also are much more likely to be excluded from social participation. About half the expenditure of older people (65+) with severe deprivation goes on housing, fuel and food.

The great majority of older people (about two-thirds) own and live in their own home in the community. About 10% of older people living in the community are in sheltered housing, with a fifth of those aged 85 or over living in such accommodation. The majority of older men (about 70%) live with their spouse or partner, but less than 40% of women do so. This decreases with age for both men and women, with a third of men and over half of women aged 85 or over living alone. Older Asian people are more likely to live in multi-generation households and less likely to live alone than those from other ethnic groups. Older people over 85 and/or living alone are most likely to be receiving statutory and voluntary services such as home care, meals, community nursing and occupational therapy services.

Housing conditions have an important effect on health and quality of life. Like most households in Great Britain, in 2003/4 over 90% of older people had central heating and a refrigerator in their homes, and nearly all had a telephone (99%). However, those aged 85 or over were less likely to own washing machines (73%), microwaves (68%), or video recorders/players (54%). Having a car is an important factor in maintaining independence and social participation in contemporary Britain. About 80% of the 'young old' households have a car, although women, especially at the oldest ages, are more likely to lack access to a car and are thus more likely to be dependent upon public transport. Almost half of all those aged 85 or over were living in 'non-decent' housing, usually because of cold housing conditions. Living in such accommodation is likely to have an adverse affect upon the health of older people, especially in winter.

About 4% of older people live in residential or nursing care homes, although the proportion of those living in these settings rises sharply with age. In 2001 13.5% of those aged 85–89 and 16% of those aged 90, and over 16% of men and 28% of women were living in such homes. The larger proportions of women than men is related to women being less likely to have a spouse to care for them because they are widowed, and their higher level of disability. Like widows, people who never married are also more likely to live in communal establishments. Older people from minority ethnic groups are less likely to live in care homes than those from white and mixed ethnic groups.

Retirement, income and material resources

In the UK one of the most important markers of entry into old age has been retirement from paid work. This has been especially important for men, particularly those in manual and lower skilled white-collar employment. Barnes and Parry (2004) report that men are more likely to find retirement painful than women because they are more likely to have a strong attachment to their work. Women's continuing 'caring' roles provide greater continuity and 'pre-empt' the role changes and losses associated with retirement.

There is a strong link between retirement and income. In 2004 the employment rate for older men was substantially lower than in 1979 (when data began), while there has been a rise in the employment of older women, reflecting wider social changes (Chapter 5). Over a third of the people aged 50–69 who were forced to retire did so mainly because of health problems. Most people aged 65 or over will be primarily dependent upon a pension, and those with occupational pensions are likely to be better off than those depending upon a state pension.

Income, health and well-being are strongly associated. Income is crucial in affecting the quality of life of older people, and for maintaining their independence. Not only does an adequate income provide for the physical necessities of life such as housing, heating, food and clothing, but it is also essential in maintaining their social involvement with others, such as visiting family and friends and engaging in leisure activities. Income levels among older people vary greatly, and reflect earlier socio-economic differences. As we saw in Chapter 3, those with lower incomes have poorer health.

Income tends to fall in old age, although a substantial proportion of pensioners will have other sources of wealth. Looking at those on low income (less than 60% of the national median income), 21% of pensioners are on low income, compared to 14% of working age adults. Single pensioners are twice as likely to receive income support than those who are married. Single women are more likely to receive income support (21%) than single men (14%) and minority ethnic group members (29%) are more likely to receive income support than whites (19%) (Soule *et al.* 2005). While the more affluent older households are likely to be spending about a quarter of their income on food, heat, light and heating, the poorest households are likely to be spending about 70% of their income on these essentials (Vincent 1995).

Social participation and support

Although most older people maintain contact with friends and relatives on a regular basis, those who are in good general health are more likely to make frequent visits to them and to maintain contact with neighbours. Visiting others and contact with neighbours decreases with age. Frequent visits from others to older people are associated with poor general health.

Bajekal *et al.* (2004) found that there were clear differences between the older (and largest) four ethnic groups in Britain in terms of their social networks and participation. The white group ranked highest in terms of participation in formal networks (and material circumstances and health), the Indian and Caribbean groups were second and third and the Pakistani group ranked lowest. However, for the frequency of family contacts and perceived desirability of their neighbourhood these rankings were reversed.

Older people are both recipients and providers of care and social support. Older spouses will look after each other and with other family members provide most of the social care for older people living in the community. However, this declines sharply with increasing age. Not only do they provide care and support to each other, but many older people also provide support to their adult children, such as providing day care for grandchildren whose parents are working. For older people living in their own home, their spouse and families (especially daughters) are the main sources of practical and emotional support.

Chronic illness and disability in old age

Old age in contemporary Britain is associated with increasing levels of chronic illness and disability, and the increasing likelihood of death, usually from chronic illness (Chapter 9). The prevalence of a number of diseases – coronary heart disease, stroke, chronic obstructive pulmonary disease and diabetes – increases rapidly in the older age groups, and are more common among older men than older women.

Types of chronic illness and disability

Table 6.1 provides an overview of the main types of illness experienced by older people in Britain. By far the major causes of chronic illness are the circulatory system and the musculoskeletal system. The latter causes serious disabilities for about 10% of those living in private households and 65% of those in care homes (Health Survey for England 2000). Respiratory diseases are also a significant cause of disability. Only a small proportion of older people report long-standing illness resulting from neoplasms (cancers and benign growths).

In 2003 the death rate from cancer in England and Wales declined steeply from 36% of deaths for men and 56% for women aged 50–64 to half that rate among men over 85 (18%), and to an even lower rate among women (11%). For the other main causes of death in old age, circulatory diseases (mainly heart attack and stroke) are more common for men than women, and respiratory diseases are similar for men and women (Soule *et al.* 2005, table 5.4). Seymour *et al.* (2005) noted that dementia is an increasing and important cause of death for older people, but is infrequently recorded as the primary cause of death. Rates of mental illness increase with age and, as with younger adults (Chapter 5), mental illness is more common among women than among men.

Table 6.1 also shows that there are differences between older men and women in the sorts of illness that typically affect them. The most striking contrast is for arthritis – a major source of pain and disability for both older men and women – which is twice as prevalent for women. The table does not support the commonly held view that leading illnesses among older men tend to *decrease* with age while women's health problems tend to increase with age.

Limiting long-term illness

Table 5.2 (p. 103) shows that self-reported ill health increases with old age. In 2004, well over half of men and women aged over 65 reported a long-standing illness; over one-third reported a limiting long-standing illness (LLTI) and over

Table 6.1 Chronic sickness: rates per 1000 of older people reporting selected long-standing conditions, Great Britain 2004.

Condition	65–74 years old	75 years old and over	All ages
Musculoskeletal			
Arthritis and rheumatism			
Men	110	136	52
Women	194	223	85
Back problems			
Men	59	21	44
Women	37	26	36
Other bone and joint problems			
Men	43	65	37
Women	60	94	38
Heart and circulatory			
Hypertension			
Men	92	87	38
Women	119	107	48
Heart attack			
Men	84	83	23
Women	51	67	18
Stroke			
Men	17	54	8
Women	12	28	6
Respiratory			
Asthma			
Men	43	34	40
Women	57	49	48
Bronchitis and emphysema			
Men	34	28	8
Women	15	14	5
Endocrine and metabolic			
Men	110	116	47
Women	109	89	56
Digestive system			
Men	41	49	26
Women	47	58	32
Nervous system			
Men	28	42	28
Women	34	29	28
Neoplasms and benign growths			
Men and women	30	42	n.a.
Mental disorders			
Men and women	11	16	n.a.
Genito-urinary system			
Men and women	22	39	n.a.
Average number of conditions reported by those with a long-standing illness	1.7	1.8	

n.a., not applicable.

Source: General Household Survey 2004, tables 7.13, 7.14 and 7.15. National Statistics website: www.statistics.gov.uk. Crown copyright material is reproduced with the permission of the Controller of HMSO.

Table 6.2 Trends in limiting longstanding illness and restricted activity* among older men and women, 1975–2004 in Great Britain (percentages reporting).

Sex/age group	1975	1991	2004
Limiting long-standing illness			
Men 65–74	36	40	37
Women 65–74	39	34	33
Men 75 and over	44	46	43
Women 75 and over	49	51	48
Restricted activity			
Men 65–74	8	14	16
Women 65–74	12	18	20
Men 75 and over	12	16	20
Women 75 and over	13	21	26

* This refers to whether respondents had cut down on their normal activities in the 14 days before interview.
Source: General Household Survey 2004, table 7.2b. National Statistics website: www.statistics.gov.uk.
Crown copyright material is reproduced with the permission of the Controller of HMSO.

one-fifth reported that their activity was restricted. Those living in private households are much less likely to have an LLTI than those living in communal establishments (Bajekal *et al.* 2006).

There is no conclusive evidence that LLTI is becoming either markedly more or less common in older age groups. Comparing the years 1975, 1991 and 2004, Table 6.2 shows no clear pattern in the incidence of LLTI reported by older men and women over time. It is unclear why men aged 65–74 reported higher rates than women in 1991 and 2004. At ages 75+ the rate is consistently higher for women than for men, but the gap between them is decreasing. The rates for restricted activity increased sharply from 1975 to 1991 and again to 2004, with women having higher rates than men. One difficulty in assessing this evidence is that it is mainly based on 'snapshot' comparisons of surveys of older people in different years. As yet there are no results from longitudinal surveys of health in older people in Britain that track the same age cohort through time.

LLTI and restricted activity give only a general view of the extent of health and illness among older people. Another measure of the impact of illness in old age is the prevalence of serious disability. In 2000 the prevalence of serious disability among those aged 65 or over was 16%, with a sharp increase with age for those living in private households in England (Health Survey for England 2000). Serious disabilities were reported by 10% of those aged 65–79 and by 25% of those aged 85 or older. Over 70% of residents in care homes reported serious disability.

The most common disability was locomotor disability, reported by about 30% of those in private households and 75% of men and 81% of women in care homes. Disabilities negatively affecting personal care were much more common in care homes (men 58%, women 66%) than in private households (14%). While sight and hearing deteriorate with age, they are unlikely to involve severe disability for older people living in the community, although severe hearing disability in care homes was reported by 15% of men and 23% of women.

Serious functional disability affects only a minority of older people at any given time (Bernard 2000). While a considerable number are affected by LLTI, about 80% of men and women over the age of 85 are able to feed themselves, bathe themselves, get in and out of bed, and use the toilet without help. While these are relatively minimal requirements for the maintenance of independence and life satisfaction in old age, the great majority of the very old can still manage to meet them. Concentrating on the extent of illness and disability makes it easy to forget that at any point in time a large majority of older people are in relatively good health and are leading active lives.

Socio-economic status and ethnicity

Socio-economic status is very influential in determining patterns of health and illness (Chapter 3) and socio-economic health inequalities that exist at younger ages persist, and perhaps intensify, in old age. For example, in England and Wales in 2001 a greater proportion of people aged 60–64 from semi-routine or routine occupations reported LLTI than those from a managerial or professional background. At all ages above 60 those in the highest income group reported lower rates of LLTI than those in the lowest income group. Differences by occupation and income lessen after the age of 75, probably reflecting the greater survival of healthier old people (Soule *et al.* 2005).

Health differences between ethnic groups are less marked among those aged over 65 than at younger ages, but South Asian groups report higher levels of LLTI than the white majority and people of Chinese origin report a significantly lower level (Soule *et al.* 2005).

Healthy life expectancy

Although life expectancies have lengthened in wealthy modern societies such as the UK (see Table 5.1, p. 98) it is also important to consider how many of these extra years of life would be healthy years of life. This led to the development of the concept of 'healthy life expectancy', measured in terms of expected years spent in good health, free from LLTI or serious disability. Two interpretations developed. The pessimistic view was that people were living longer with poor health (i.e. the 'expansion' of morbidity) and, consequently, were making more demands upon health services. The alternative view was that morbidity was being 'compressed' into a relatively short period of time at the end of life because older people were becoming healthier. Thus, they would make fewer demands upon health services. Age Concern (1999) strongly supported this optimistic view, suggesting that preventive and rehabilitation strategies should work alongside clinical research and improved practice to achieve the compression of morbidity.

Subsequently, a pattern of increasing life expectancy in old age accompanied by the increased prevalence of less severe and disabling chronic diseases emerged in some countries. This led to a third interpretation, that there was a 'dynamic equilibrium' whereby the increase in chronic diseases in old age was counterbalanced by their lower levels of severity. During the 1980s and 1990s declining mortality among the 'oldest old' was accompanied by the increased prevalence of chronic diseases (and possibly an increased prevalence of disability), although these diseases led to severe disability less often than previously (Robine and Michel 2004).

Robine and Michel suggested that three patterns can be seen in 'low mortality' countries such as the UK:

- a regular increase in life expectancy at the age of 65 since 1970;
- stagnation in disability-free life expectancy, whatever the level;
- improvement in life expectancy free from severe disability.

They argue that how older people *perceive* their health is also a factor in healthy life expectancy, and that this can follow a different pattern from disability (i.e. people with disabilities may see themselves as in 'good health'). They also observe that the increasing numbers of the 'oldest old', as indicated by the increasing number of those over the age of 100, suggests that frailty should also be added to the presence of chronic diseases and functional capacity as an indicator of healthy life expectancy. Box 6.1 shows their proposed model of population ageing.

Comparisons of illness rates between people over 85 years and those in their sixties and early seventies show that rates are lower in the older group for some significant diseases (Mullan 2000). For example, various forms of cancer and heart disease peak in the 60–70 age group and become less common in later life. Developments in pharmacological and surgical treatment, such as techniques to reverse neurological impairment and to prevent strokes, are already beginning to have a positive impact on the effects of long-term illness in older people (Dalley 1998). Relatively inexpensive and routine surgical treatments that greatly improve mobility and sight appear to have particularly beneficial effects and reduce the dependency of older patients on further treatment or care services. Many elderly patients gain as much from surgery and medical treatment as younger patients, and recover just as well (Mullan

---

Box 6.1 A simplified picture of population ageing

(1) Increased survival of sick people and the expansion of morbidity.
(2) Control of chronic disease progression, resulting in increased years of life and the increase of functional limitation and disability.
(3) Improved health behaviours and health status of people entering old age, leading to the compression of morbidity.
(4) Emergence of very old and frail cohorts, with a new expansion of morbidity.

Adapted from Robine, J.-M. and Michel, J.-P. (2004) Looking forward to a general theory on population aging. *Journal of Gerontology: Medical Sciences*, 5A, 590–7.

2000). For example there is no age difference, in terms of post-operative illness or mortality, in outcomes following coronary bypass surgery or kidney transplantation. It is expected that improvements in health among the 'young old' are likely to reduce the total burden of illness in the elderly population as a whole, and will compensate for rising need among the growing group of people aged over 85.

The common perception of later life as a period of inexorable decline in health is thus open to question. Those who live into their eighties and nineties are the people who have been selected out as survivors, and a significant proportion are in relatively good health until a year or so before death.

In the UK, disability-free life expectancy increased for older men and women between 1980 and 1998. In 1980, life expectancy for men at age 65 was 4.3 years, of which 2.7 could be expected to be free from disability, and in 1988 these had increased to 5.3 and 4.2 years, respectively, meaning that the proportion of disability-free further life had increased from 61% to 79% (Soule *et al.* 2005: 40–1). The Parliamentary Office of Science and Technology (2006) reported the percentage of life spent in 'good' or 'fairly good' health in the UK was 88.5% for men and 85.6% for women in 2001. Table 6.3 shows different types of life expectancy for people at birth and at age 65 in 2001.

We should, however, be cautious about taking an overly optimistic view of health and ageing. First, as we have noted, the evidence about the nature, extent and consequences of chronic illness and disability among older people is still not clear. Robine and Michel (2004) suggest that the 'compression' and 'expansion' of morbidity can vary over time within a society as the nature of age cohorts change (Box 6.1). In contemporary Britain some old people experience healthy life well into old age, some live the latter period of their lives with distressing illness and disability, while for others there is a 'dynamic equilibrium' between the longer prevalence of a number of chronic conditions and low levels of severity.

Table 6.3 Life expectancy, healthy life expectancy and disability-free life expectancy at birth and age 65, Great Britain, 2001.

	Life expectancy	Healthy life expectancy*	Disability-free life expectancy#	Years with disability
Males				
At birth	75.7	66.8	60.4	15.7
At age 65	15.9	11.9	8.8	7.1
Females				
At birth	80.4	69.9	62.9	17.5
At age 65	19.0	14.0	10.3	8.7

* Good or fairly good health.
# No long-term illness, health problem or disability which limits daily activities or work.
Source: Health expectancies in the UK and its constituent countries, 2001. *Health Statistics Quarterly* (2006) 29: 18–25.

Secondly, the socio-economic inequalities in health discussed in Chapter 3 continue, and are exacerbated, in old age. A healthy old age and the compression of morbidity is most likely to be found among relatively affluent older people entering old age in good health; older people in poorer social groups are likely to experience increasing illness and disability throughout later life. Healthy old age for the latter therefore depends to some extent on the success of social and health policies in improving or maintaining health in the poorer sections of society, and addressing rising social and economic inequality.

Thirdly, there is no guarantee that succeeding generations of people who are now in their youth or young adulthood will continue the trend of continuous health improvement. Threats to children's and young people's health from increasing obesity, lack of exercise, smoking and drug use are causing concern. It is possible that in the future the onset of diabetes, heart disease, cancer and other serious illnesses will occur much earlier in the life course in significant numbers of people, rather than being compressed into later life.

A final reason to be cautious lies in the subjective nature of illness. Despite growing social divisions, material living standards and health have improved steadily in Britain over the past few decades. But while health might continue to improve in the future, there is a strong possibility that people's *expectations* of health in later life will continue to rise faster than actual improvements (Chapter 10). The present generation of older people seem to be prepared to put up with a certain amount of illness and accept some chronic conditions as an inevitable part of growing old. Future cohorts of older people may be much less likely to do so. It seems likely that the next generation of older people will report illness more frequently and expect more expensive and sophisticated treatments than those that are accepted today.

Health care and older people

Apart from babies and infants, people aged 65 and over make the highest use of health services within the UK. They occupy almost two-thirds of general and acute hospital beds, account for 50% of the recent growth in emergency admissions, and their care accounts for 43% of the total NHS budget, and 44% of the total Social Services budget (Commissions for Health Care, Audit and Inspection 2006) The use of health services is particularly high among people aged 75 and over. However, it is unclear how effective health and social care services are in protecting older people against ill health and in helping them to deal with their ill health. While some older people benefit significantly from health care interventions, for others deficiencies in their health care may compound their problems.

Use of services

A major consequence of the development of community care in the 1990s was to reduce the role of the NHS as a provider of long-term health care for older people and other groups significantly (Ham 2005: 96). The NHS now mainly concentrates on providing primary health services (through the GP service) and acute hospital based care.

Preventive health care

The potential benefits of a preventative approach and of widening older people's access to inexpensive but effective forms of treatment have long been recognised in British government health policies. For example, requiring GP practices to monitor the health of all patients over the age of 75 annually to improve preventive health care of older people.

The success and the impact of health promotion and preventive strategies on health and life expectancy for older people have been variable, and appear to be relatively weak. Preventive strategies have emphasised the individual and behavioural determinants of health to the neglect of material and environmental influences, although the latter are now receiving more attention (Chapter 3). Hypothermia illustrates how a social or economic perspective is vital to a fuller understanding of what an effective preventive strategy requires. Hypothermia (having a core body temperature of less than 35°C) is much more common in older than younger people, because in old age the human body has a decreased capacity to regulate temperature. Lack of heating in the bedroom, or low temperatures in the home generally, can easily lead to accidental hypothermia in older people. Despite the government's scheme of winter fuel payments to older people, the main cause of inadequate heating and insulation in the home is 'pensioner poverty'. In Sweden, which has much lower temperatures in winter than Britain, the occurrence of hypothermia is negligible because older people's standards of living and housing are high. Although there may be considerable benefits to a policy that helps to identify illnesses earlier and provides preventative and remedial treatment more effectively, raising the incomes of poorer old people well above the income support level is likely to be more effective than any preventive health care strategy.

Primary care

In 2003 about a quarter of men and women aged 65+ consulted a GP and 12% consulted a practice nurse in a 2-week period. Such consultations increase with age; for example, 28% of women aged 75 and over consulted a GP. People over the age of 65 make more visits to a GP over the course of year than any other age group, apart from infant boys. Consultations have risen over time – in 1972 14% of those aged 65–74 saw a GP, rising to 20% in 2003. This rise may be due to initiatives to improve the health of older people, such as free annual influenza immunisation (used by 72% of those eligible in 2004). While consultations have increased, the number of home visits by a GP has fallen (7% in 2003), reflecting the large overall reduction of home visits since the 1970s. Those aged 75 and over are much more likely to receive home visits (Soule *et al.* 2005). The use of community nursing by older people seems surprisingly low, with 2–5% of those aged 65–79, 10% of those aged 80–84 and 19% of those age 85 and over using this service in 2001/2 (Soule *et al.* 2005).

Secondary care

The use of hospital services by older people (65+) increases with age for both men and women, apart from inpatient admissions, which decrease. Older women are much more likely than older men to be admitted as a hospital inpatient and men aged 75 and over are more likely to attend as day patients. About a quarter of older people (65+) use hospital casualty and outpatient services in a year, with little difference between men and women. This level of use probably reflects their greater propensity to have an accident in the home, especially a fall, than younger people. The use of hospital services by older people increased significantly between 1981/2 and 2004.

Not only is the frequency of hospitalisation greater among older people, but their length of stay remains appreciably greater, despite strong attempts by hospitals to reduce this. For example, in 2004 the average number of nights stayed in hospital as an inpatient rose with age, from 4 nights for 16–44-year-olds to 13 nights for those aged 75 and over (General Household Survey 2004). Any reductions in use of inpatient services by older people have been achieved by reducing length of stay rather than the number of times older people are admitted to hospital, and by the increasing use of day care services for minor operations. It is likely that as medical techniques have improved and some interventions have become more effective, both demand and need for hospital care have increased faster than population growth in the group aged 75 and over.

Geriatric medicine plays a central role in the acute hospital care of older people. The development of its body of specialist knowledge and skills has brought benefits, especially in the field of rehabilitation, and may also prevent inappropriately aggressive forms of drug therapy or surgery for older patients. However, it has traditionally been seen as a low status specialty and geriatric medical teams and departments have, as a result, often been less able than higher status medical specialities to attract sufficient staff and resources to provide a satisfactory service.

By reinforcing the use of chronological age, rather than 'biological' age or medical need, to determine the services that are offered to older patients, geriatric medicine may sometimes play a role in diverting elderly patients from better and more prompt treatment. For example, older patients might be referred less quickly to specialists in the treatment of cancers and other life-threatening diseases. In a study of nurses' assessment and care of older people admitted to an acute medical unit (Latimer 2000) it seems that the role of geriatric medicine was restricted to social factors, especially how these might affect discharge. In their review and report of the care for older people in England, the Social Care Inspectorate, the Audit Commission and the Healthcare Commission (Commissions for Health care, Audit and Inspection 2006) failed to mention, let alone comment upon, the role of geriatric medicine.

Intermediate care

Intermediate care plays a potentially important role in enabling older people to maintain their independence by 'bridging' the gaps between care in the home and in hospitals, and is an integral part of government attempts to provide 'seamless care'. Its main goals are to prevent inappropriate hospital admissions, provide comprehensive assessment and provide supportive care over a short time, thus reducing long-term care. Most referrals to intermediate care come from GPs and are delivered in the community, and many of the services are nurse-led. Andrews *et al.* (2004) report great variation in older people's experience of nurse-led intermediate care and 'little evidence' of their participation in decisions about intermediate care. So far there is no clear evidence that intermediate care is reducing long-term care and the use of hospitals.

Co-ordination of care

There have been consistent concerns about the patchy nature of access of older people to primary care and hospital services and the referral and communication between these. In 2006 the 'Commissions review' found significant improvements in some areas such as stroke care, access to cardiac procedures, hip and knee replacements, and home support in England. However, there were also negative findings:

- in hospitals elderly people were being treated with a lack of dignity and respect;
- fragmentation and a lack of clear direction resulted in a lack of 'joined up' services;
- mental health services for older people were particularly poor due to the organisational division between working age and older adults 'resulting in an unfair system' for older people;
- chiropody services, a key service for preserving mobility and quality of life, were poor;
- there were unacceptable delays in accessing services for people with dementia;
- the needs and aspirations of older people were not considered;
- older people were not involved in the planning of services.

To be effective, health services for older people need to be coordinated not only with each other but also with social services that help to maintain the independence and quality of life of older people – both those who are ill and those caring for them. Spouses, who are themselves elderly and possibly with their own health problems, and other family members provide the majority of social care for older people. Over a third of the 1.4 million informal carers aged 65 and over provide 50 or more hours of unpaid care a week (Soule *et al.* 2005). The extent of non-family support from health and social services is unclear.

The 'Commissions review' (Commissions for Health care, Audit and Inspection 2006) found that better co-ordination was needed between local authorities and health services. In their study of the commissioning of care services for older people in England, Ware *et al.* (2003) found that although there was general satisfaction from users, many care managers had significant difficulty in finding sufficient care services to meet the assessed needs of their users and were concerned about the poor recording of unmet need. They concluded that the fragmentation of assessment and care management could lead to discontinuities in the care of older people and their carers.

It seems that the extent of local community services are increasingly being focused upon the intensive care of those defined as being in greatest need (Soule *et al.* 2005). This raises questions about how such need is identified, and whether targeting services at those most in need is detrimental to the support of other older people and their carers. Henwood (2001) reports that older people from ethnic minorities have greater difficulty in accessing support services and rely heavily upon voluntary agencies. The 'Commissions review' (2006) reported that health organisations and local authorities in England 'were not always effective in engaging with black and minority ethnic groups' (Commissions for Health care, Audit and Inspection 2006: 10).

Many older people in need of long-term health and personal care can no longer use NHS hospital or nursing home services and instead must use a combination of services provided by local authorities and the private and voluntary sectors. This is of key importance in comparing the use of health services by younger and older age groups because a considerable proportion of the care (including nursing care) provided to older people now lies outside the NHS. The wealth of older people and their adult children may profoundly influence access to such care.

Discrimination and rationing of care

In general, service use by older people, particularly those aged 75 and over, is appreciably greater than among young adults, although more so for in-hospital services than GP services. These patterns of health service use suggest that older people are not experiencing particular problems in terms of access to health care. In particular, despite difficulties in providing adequate GP services in some areas, most older patients are able to call a doctor to their home if they are physically unable to attend a surgery. While access to primary health care services is not particularly problematic, research on older people's experience of the *quality* of both GP and hospital services has raised important questions. As Bernard (2000: 14) puts it, 'high consultation rates do not necessarily . . . translate into satisfaction with either services or professional responses'.

The 'Commissions review' (2006) found that explicit age discrimination in the NHS and Social Services in England had declined since 2001, but that:

> . . . there is still evidence of ageism across all services. This ranges from patronising and thoughtless treatment from staff to the failure of some mainstream public services such as transport, to take the needs and aspirations of older people seriously. Many older people find it difficult to challenge ageist attitudes and their reluctance to complain can often mean that nothing changes (Commissions for Health care, Audit and Inspection 2006: 7).

A number of reasons for this may be suggested. Doctor and patient may agree that symptoms that would lead to a fuller examination of a younger person are simply to be expected and accepted as part of the inevitable decline of old age. Some older patients may be anxious that younger adults, including nurses and doctors, will inappropriately take charge of their lives, so it may seem 'safer' to agree with doctors who discount a treatable illness as simply a problem of old age rather than precipitating a series of unwanted medical investigations and changes in their life. However, many older people feel that doctors and other health practitioners have not listened to them and that they have not been given adequate explanations of their health problems or treatments (Bernard 2000).

There is other evidence that ageism may influence access to health services, and concerns are regularly expressed in the mass media about the unspoken use of age criteria in a wide range of medical treatments and in health services generally. A survey of senior health and social services managers in 2001 found that three-quarters of them believed that age discrimination existed in some form in services in their area (Levenson 2003). In particular, that access to some forms of treatment were based on age rather than clinical need, that cost ceilings for services for older people were lower than those for younger people, and that referral to residential care might be based upon cost rather than individual needs and preferences.

Summary

In contemporary Britain the number and proportion of older people will continue to increase, a prospect that alarms health policy makers because of the anticipated consequences for the costs of health care. However, there is disagreement about whether the ever-extending lives of older people will result in longer periods spent in illness and dependency or whether they will be spent in healthy old age. Becoming and being old in contemporary Britain is not a uniform experience but varies by generation, social class, ethnicity and gender. It is thus difficult to generalise about the relationships between health, illness and old age. It is, however, wrong to suggest that, at a given chronological age, every older person will be ill, frail and disabled, or have a well-defined range of health care needs. Nevertheless, older people will remain the largest users of health services for the foreseeable future. The effectiveness of these appears to be variable, and indirect and direct discrimination on the grounds of age are evident. While the health of older people is likely to continue to improve in the future, there is a strong possibility that older people's *expectations* of health in later life will rise faster than actual improvements (Chapter 10). The present generation of older people seem to be prepared to put up with a certain amount of illness and accept some chronic conditions as an inevitable part of growing old. However, future cohorts of older people may be much less likely to do so, and will expect more expensive and sophisticated treatments.

References

Age Concern (1999) *The Future of Health and Care of Older People: The Best is Yet to Come*. Age Concern England, London.

Andrews, J., Manthorpe, J. and Watson, R. (2004) Involving older people in intermediate care. *Journal of Advanced Nursing*, 46, 303–10.

Arber, S. and Ginn, J. (2006) Ageing and gender: diversity and change. *Social Trends 34*. Office of National Statistics, available at www.statistics.gov.uk (accessed April 2006).

Bajekal, M., Blane, D., Grewal, I., *et al.* (2004) Ethnic differences in influences on quality of life at older ages: a quantitative analysis. *Ageing and Society*, 24, 709–18.

Bajekal, M., Osborne, V., Yar, M. and Meltzer, H. (eds) (2006) *Focus on Health*. Office of National Statistics/Palgrave Macmillan. Available at www.statistics.org (accessed April 2006).

Barnes, H. and Parry, J. (2004) Renegotiating identity and relationships: men and women's adjustments to retirement. *Ageing and Society*, 24, 213–34.

Bernard, M. (2000) *Promoting Health in Old Age*. Open University Press, Buckingham.

Commissions for Health Care, Audit and Inspection (2006) *Living Well in Later Life. A review of progress against the National Service Framework for Older People*. Social Care Inspectorate, Audit Commission and Healthcare Commission. Available at www.healthcarecommission.org.uk (accessed June 2006).

Dalley, G. (1998) Health and social welfare policy, in M. Bernard and J. Phillips (eds) *The Social Policy of Old Age*. Centre for Policy on Ageing, London, 20–39.

General Household Survey (2004) Available at www.statistics.gov.uk

Ham, C. (2005) *Health Policy in Britain*, 5th edition. Palgrave Macmillan, Basingstoke.

Health Survey for England (2000) *The Health of Older People*. National Statistics. The Stationery Office, London.

Henwood, M. (2001) *Future Imperfect? Report on the Kings Fund Care and Support Inquiry*. The King's Fund, London.

Kitwood, T. (1997) *Dementia Reconsidered*. Open University Press, Buckingham.

Latimer, J. (2000) *The Conduct of Care*. Blackwell Science, Oxford.

Levenson, R. (2003) Institutional ageism. *Community Care*, 17–23 July, 42–3.

Mullan, P. (2000) *The Imaginary Time Bomb – Why an Ageing Population is not a Social Problem*. Tauris, London.

Parliamentary Office of Science and Technology (2006) Healthy life expectancy. *Postnote 257*. Available at www.parliament.uk/parliamentary_offices/post/pubs 2006.cmf

Robine, J.-M. and Michel, J.-P. (2004) Looking forward to a general theory on population aging. *Journal of Gerontology: Medical Sciences*, 59A, 590–7.

Seymour, J., Witherspoon, R., Gott, M., *et al.* (2005) *End-of-life care. Promoting comfort, choice and well-being for older people*. Policy Press, Bristol.

Soule, A., Babb, P., Evandrou, E., *et al.* (2005) *Focus on Older People*. Department of Work and Pensions/Palgrave Macmillan. Available at www.statistics.gov (accessed April 2006).

Vincent, J. (1995) *Inequality and Old Age*. UCL Press, London.

Ware, T., Matosevic, T., Hardy, B., *et al.* (2003) Commissioning care services for older people in England: the view from care managers, users and carers. *Ageing and Society*, 23, 411–28.

Further reading

Soule, A., Babb, P., Evandrou, E., *et al.* (2005) *Focus on Older People (2005)*. Department of Work and Pensions/Palgrave Macmillan. Available at www.statistics.gov (accessed April 2006).
Provides comprehensive coverage of the social position of older people in Great Britain and their health and illness.
Walker, A. (guest editor) (2004) Understanding quality of life in old age. *Ageing and Society*, 24 (Part 5).
An excellent introduction to the range of factors that inter-relate with health and illness in old age.

Part III

Illness and dying

Chapter 7

Chronic illness and physical disability

Introduction

In contemporary Britain the main burden of disease comes from long-term chronic illnesses. There are also many members of our society, especially among the elderly, who have long-standing physical disabilities. Most nursing work, both in hospitals and in the community, involves working with people who have chronic long-term conditions. These are typically made sense of and treated within the biomedical model of illness (Chapter 2) with varying degrees of success. Through the application of the biomedical model our ability to manage chronic long-term conditions has become more effective and the lives of sufferers extended and enhanced. However, to be ill is also to be in a socially altered condition and individual experiences of chronic illness and physical disability are shaped by wider social contexts. This chapter will:

- outline approaches to chronic illness and physical disability;
- discuss chronic illness and physical disability in contemporary Britain;
- examine factors affecting the experience of chronic illness and physical disability;
- discuss factors influencing adjustment to living with a long-term condition;
- discuss care and caring.

Approaches to chronic illness and disability

In contemporary Britain long-term conditions, including both chronic illnesses and physical disabilities, affect the lives of the majority of the population either directly or indirectly. They also constitute a huge burden on health and social services.

Chronic illnesses are long-term conditions from which there is no possibility of a complete return to the pre-morbid state enjoyed by the individual before they became unwell because the physical changes in the body are permanent. The long duration of the experience of the person who is chronically ill means that they develop a degree of expertise in their own treatment (Department of

Health 2001). It also means that because of their expertise, their involvement with their medical carers is different from that of people who experience short acute episodes of illness. With many acute episodes of illness the sufferer may expect to recover fully following medical intervention. In contrast, most chronic conditions are continuous but not necessarily stable and many worsen over time, and medical and nursing intervention, while alleviating symptoms, will not lead to full recovery. While some chronic illnesses may lead eventually to death or have life-threatening complications, it is important to remember that many chronic illnesses also have acute episodes.

Physical disabilities are sometimes associated with chronic illness but may also result from acute illness, accidents or congenital conditions. The definition of disability is highly contested. However, we can distinguish between two broad types of definitions, those that focus upon the individual and those that stress that disability is socially constructed (Priestley 2003). Over time there has been some rapprochement between proponents of these two approaches and, rather than seeing them as alternatives, it is more fruitful to see them as focusing upon different aspects of disability.

Individual approaches

The central aspect of individual approaches, such as the biomedical model (Chapter 2), is that they see illness and disability as located in the individual as a result of departures from the normal structure and functioning of the human body, which reduce and/or hinder functional capacity. For acute and chronic illnesses, physical departures from a biological norm are the focus of therapeutic intervention, the purpose of which is either to return the acutely ill person to normal or to ameliorate, in some way, the physical problems of the person with a chronic illness. Therapeutic actions based on this biological approach have been very effective in helping to manage chronic illnesses like diabetes, epilepsy, angina, and interventions like hip replacement surgery have helped many people regain and enjoy a good quality of life (Bunker 2001).

For people with physical disabilities, prosthesis and technical support like a wheelchair or other aids to living allow them to be more like able-bodied people in functional terms. However, because the disabled person finds it difficult to perform normal activities (e.g. walking, hearing) without assistance, it may be assumed that they have difficulty with social roles and obligations, such as going to work or having sexual relations. As Priestley (2003: 12) puts it, 'the kind of social disadvantages commonly associated with disability in modern societies [are] viewed largely as an individual problem caused by impairment'.

One of the paradoxes of modern medicine is that its very success in improving life expectancy in long-term chronic conditions creates ever increasing demands upon health services for continuing clinical care and/or technical support – some of it very expensive. Despite the medical successes that have done so much to improve the quality of life of so many people with chronic conditions and physical disabilities, individually oriented approaches have attracted criticism from proponents of social models of illness.

Social approaches

It is clear that the extent to which people with apparently similar physical impairments become disabled and dependent upon others varies according to a range of social factors, such as their age, gender and wealth. The central feature of social models of disability is that disability is not caused by physical impairments but is socially shaped and created. From this perspective disability is seen as 'a social problem caused by social processes' (Priestley 2003: 13).

Sociologists studying chronic illnesses emphasise the importance of understanding the *experience* of living with chronic illness, something which the biomedical model either does not focus on or treats as incidental. Across a number of chronic diseases common experiences ensue which, in social and psychological terms, are very similar. A variety of behaviours central to the experience have been identified, including:

- coping with symptoms and the way others respond to the symptoms;
- dealing with changes in relationships with family, friends and workmates;
- reorganising life expectations;
- adjusting to the physical limitations imposed by the illness;
- dealing with economic disadvantage;
- dealing with various degrees of discrimination.

Sociologists emphasise that these experiences are social and cannot be understood or predicted on the basis of the biological changes in the human body caused by the disease. Moreover, the problems attached to the care of people with chronic disease and physical disability are as much about social and psychological consequences as they are about the physical needs emphasised in the biomedical model (Bury 2001).

Since the 1980s disability activists have used a social approach to disability to challenge the exclusion of disabled people from social life, contributing to a range of anti-discriminatory legislation such as the Disability Discrimination Act of 1995. Disability activists argue that the focus upon physical impairments and the social and psychological problems associated with living with them not only misses the fundamentally oppressive social experiences of disability but, more importantly, hides the fact that 'society' *creates* disability. They argue that the institutions of society (e.g. schools, work organisations, the legal system) are based on the wants and needs of its able-bodied adult members and systematically discriminate against people who have disabilities. For example, Oliver (1996: 33) argued that '. . . it is society which disables physically impaired people. Disability is something imposed on top of our impairments by the way we are unnecessarily isolated and excluded from full participation in society'. Such writers argue that responses focusing only on therapeutic interventions, rehabilitation and care, even when driven by compassion, may not be beneficial for people with disabilities (Swain *et al.* 2003). At the extreme, it is argued that the negative consequences of having a disability can only be overcome by transforming society itself. However, while retaining the focus on the social sources of disability and social exclusion, many disability activists have now incorporated the work of sociologists and accept that physical disabilities do have consequences that changes to social arrangements cannot affect, such as blindness and being unable to drive (Barnes and Mercer 2003).

Chronic illness and physical disability in contemporary Britain

Estimates put the number of people in Great Britain with a chronic disease as between 17 and 25 million people, and those of adolescents and adults with the overlapping category of a disability (physical or mental) as between 11 and 36 million. Official statistics suggest that at the start of the twenty-first century some 17.5 million adults in the UK had a long-term condition and 10.8 million (18% of the population) had a limiting long-term illness (Bajekal *et al.* 2006). Box 7.1 lists the most common chronic and disabling conditions in Britain.

The number and severity of chronic and disabling conditions increases with age (Chapter 6). The principal exception to this is spinal injuries which occur mainly among young adults. Table 5.2 (p. 103) shows that there are significant variations in the pattern and distribution of chronic illness in adults by age, with over 60% of men and women aged 75 or over reporting they had a long-standing illness. The number of people who experience long-standing problems and come to be defined as disabled in some way is increasing with the ageing of the population and the greater number of people living beyond 75 (Chapter 6). Between two-thirds and three-quarters of these will have one or more long-standing illnesses and consequent disabilities; three times the rate for those aged 16–24 (Department of Health 2001)

Many elderly people remain fit and active until very late in their lives. However, chronic illness and physical disability are a reality for some people as they grow older. A typical progression might be to experience at first non-serious levels of reduced mobility, vision and hearing, which do not threaten autonomy and independence. Then these may deteriorate into a situation marked by multiple pathology and disability that, although restricting, do not compromise independence. A further decline in health and increasing disability may lead an elderly person to become dependent upon others (usually their partner and family) for help with basic activities of living if they are to remain in their own home. Finally, this situation may break down, perhaps as a result of an episode of acute illness or an accident (such as a fall that leads to hospitalisation) and the long-term loss of independence. The effects of these changes will be mediated by the social support older people receive. Those who are isolated are likely to be more adversely affected by the same level of sickness or disability than those with supportive networks (Chapter 2), and are more likely to be admitted to nursing homes or hospitals.

Chronic conditions are not restricted to adults but comprehensive recent information about their extent among children and adolescents is unavailable.

Box 7.1 Common long-term conditions in the UK

- **Arthritis** Rheumatoid and osteo-arthritis are major causes of disability in the UK, affecting about 8.9 million adults and 415,000 children. Arthritis is uncommon before the age of 40. Approximately half of arthritis sufferers are below and half above the age of 55. Above 65, women are twice as likely as men to report osteo-arthritis and rheumatism. For more information see www.arc.org.uk

- **Asthma** It is estimated that asthma affects 1 in 5 households in the UK, with over 5 million people, including over 1 million children, receiving treatment for it. It is the most common childhood disease, and its prevalence is rising. It affects approximately one-fifth of all teenagers. For more information see www.asthma.org.uk

- **Back pain** is thought to be the most commonly reported type of pain. It affects about 40% of adults, with 15% of sufferers in pain throughout the year. It is most prevalent among those aged 45–64, and is related to occupation, particularly manual work. Men are more likely to suffer back problems than women. For more information see www.dh.gov.uk

- **Blindness** In 2005 there were about 378,000 people registered as blind or partially sighted in the UK and about 2 million who defined themselves as having a sight problem. Most people who are blind lost their sight gradually as they became older. About 70% of those registered as blind or partially sighted are aged 75 or over. For more information see www.rnib.org.uk

- **Chronic obstructive pulmonary disease (COPD) Bronchitis** and **emphysema** are the main forms of COPD, which affects 1 person in 7 in the UK. The most common causes of COPD are smoking and, among men, occupational factors such as exposure to dust. COPD increases significantly with age, especially for men. It is uncommon among those under the age of 40 but affects about 10% of those aged 60–85. Above 75, men are twice as likely as women to report chronic respiratory problems. For more information see www.lunguk.org

- **Cancer** is commonly seen as a fatal disease. However, earlier detection and improved treatment mean that many cancers are becoming similar to other chronic conditions. It has been estimated that 1 in 3 Britons will eventually be diagnosed with cancer. For more information see http://info.cancerresearchuk.org

- **Coronary heart disease** affects about 2.4 million men and 875,000 women in the UK, mainly those over the age of 55. Its prevalence increases sharply with age and it is more common among men aged 45 and over. Men aged 65–74 have more than double the rate of CHD than those aged 55–64. Heart failure has been estimated to affect about half a million people annually. For more information see www.heartstats.org

- **Cystic fibrosis** is the most commonly inherited condition in the UK, affecting 2% of the white population. It mainly affects the lungs and digestive system. Although infants born with CF do not have a long life expectancy, this has increased considerably, to 30–40 years at the start of the twenty-first century. For more information see hcd2.bupa.c.uk/fact_sheets

- **Deafness** There are about 8.6 million deaf and hard of hearing people in the UK, about 673,000 of whom are severely or profoundly deaf; 20,000 children (0–15 years old) are moderately or severely deaf, about half of whom were born deaf. Deafness and loss of hearing increase with age, with 55% of those over 60 being hard of hearing. A higher proportion of men than women are hard of hearing. For more information see www.deafcouncil.org.uk

- **Diabetes** About 3% of the UK population have diabetes, although its prevalence in the UK is increasing, linked to the rapid increase in obesity. About 80% of diabetics are diagnosed in middle age or later, with the non-insulin dependent form. Insulin-dependent diabetes is most likely to appear in childhood. Diabetes is at least five times more prevalent among African-Caribbean and Asian communities. Diabetes increases the risk of cardiovascular disease, stroke, kidney problems and blindness. For more information see www.diabetes.org.uk

- **Epilepsy** is the most common serious neurological disorder, affecting about 2% of the UK population. It can affect people at any age and from any walk of life. Over half the children with epilepsy grow out of it and most people with epilepsy can take part in everyday life and half are free from seizures. For more information see www.erf.org.uk

- **Hypertension** About 30% of the UK population have hypertension, which is a major risk factor for heart attack and stroke. About one-fifth of all heart attacks and strokes are due to a history of hypertension. For more information see www.heartstats.org

- **Multiple sclerosis** is one of the most common diseases of the central nervous system. It is estimated to affect about 85,000 people in the UK. It is the most common disabling condition of the central nervous system affecting young adults (20–40 years old). MS affects women more than men, in the ratio 3 : 2. For more information see www.mssociety.org.uk

- **Sickle-cell diseases** are inherited blood disorders that affect a significant minority of people in South Asian and Cypriot communities (about 15,000 people in 2005). It is about twice as common as cystic fibrosis. For more information see sicklecellsociety.org.uk.

- **Strokes** are the largest single cause of severe disability in the UK. Over 80% of strokes occur in people aged 65 or older, with higher rates among men than women. In 2005 there were more than 250,000 people with disabilities caused by stroke in the UK. A quarter of men and one-fifth of women can expect to experience a stroke if they live to the age of 85. For more information see www.stroke.org.uk

Bone and Meltzer (1989) found that the most common types of disability among children were behavioural (affecting 2.5% of those aged 5–15 years), followed by disabilities in communication, locomotion and intellectual functioning. The rates in the behavioural disabilities declined after age 15. Limiting long-standing illnesses and restricted activities are much less common among children than adults and are slightly more common among boys than girls (Table 5.2, p. 103). The rates for these increase for adolescents, but remain lower than those for adults (Matheson and Summerfield 2000).

There are much higher volumes of both chronic illness and disability among the least advantaged. People from lower socio-economic strata as compared to those from middle and higher strata are more likely to experience chronic illness and disability, and are more likely to experience financial, domestic and work related difficulties (including unemployment) as a result of their condition (Chapter 3). There are also particular disabling chronic illnesses, such as diabetes in South Asians and sickle-cell disease in African-Caribbean and Cypriot groups (Chapter 6), which overlie this picture (Ahmad 2000). There are no significant gender differences in the overall reported prevalence of common long-term conditions; apart from musculoskeletal disorders where more rheumatoid and osteo-arthritis among older women results in a higher overall prevalence among women (Chapter 5).

Body and identity

While health care professionals focus on the sick or disabled individual, sociologists are interested in the effects of an illness or a disability upon people's relationships and attachments. The personal and social identities arising from these relationships are central to understanding the adjustment to chronic conditions (Millward and Kelly 2003, Kelly and Millward 2004).

Our sense of self or personal identity is the private subjective sense of who and what we are, while our social identity is the way other people publicly define and see us on the basis of our behaviour and appearance (Chapter 2). Just as the body may be thought of as providing a physical 'thread' of continuity through life, despite its constant changes, the sense of personal identity provides a socially shaped sense of continuity through the life course. For most of the time there is a near congruence between the roles and statuses to which we aspire and play, and our own sense of who we are and the way that others respond to us. For example, a person may think of herself as a good and caring nurse, and positive comments from her patients and colleagues would reinforce this self-conception. Our sense of who we are is normally relatively stable and enduring and only becomes an issue if our identity is mistaken by others, or some serious life event such as an illness causes us to question our place in the world and to rethink our sense of who and what we are. Changes in the appearance of the body and in its functioning resulting from chronic illness or physical disability may profoundly effect the way people think about themselves and their levels of self-esteem. For all chronic conditions the sense of personal identity will be affected because the condition can never be entirely ignored by the person, even if others do not know about it.

One of the ways in which personal identity, the body and 'society' mesh in chronic illness and physical disability is through the technologies that are used to assist with managing the restrictions on social life resulting from them. A range of technologies are now available that can facilitate:

- communication with others
- mobility
- physical safety
- control over one's body
- independence
- participation in work
- participation in the community.

In their qualitative study of people with disabilities Lupton and Seymour (2000) found that their respondents felt that their disabilities should not define their identities and that 'technologies were valued for allowing them to tame the disorderly aspects of their bodies and thus facilitate social integration' (Lupton and Seymour 2000: 1857). Technologies that were 'normalising' (especially computer technologies) integrated the user unobtrusively into social life and relationships and were highly valued. Conspicuous technologies (e.g. wheelchairs) that highlighted the disability, although beneficial, also served to 'separate out' their users and were perceived more negatively.

Chronic illness and physical disability involve not simply the loss or change of functions or roles; they also have the potential to change the very sense that people have of themselves. Not only does their body function differently, but their normal roles and activities will also be disrupted. Their inability to walk or to exert themselves as much as previously may prevent them from continuing highly valued activities, leading to the diminution of social contacts and attachments at work, in their leisure activities and within their home life. In the face of persistent and continuously debilitating symptoms, they may have to come to terms with the fact that they will not work again, that they will not be able to play energetically with their grandchildren, and that they will not be able to make love to their partner with the passion and frequency that they did before they were ill, thus leading to a changed sense of personal identity.

Strong feelings and emotions may be aroused as people try to come to terms with the loss of their previous abilities and social roles and struggle to maintain positive feelings of self-worth and personal identity. In a seminal paper, Charmaz (1983) suggests that the 'loss of self' is a fundamental form of suffering for chronically ill people; but this may not be the case for all people with chronic conditions. It is likely to vary over time, particularly in relation to variations in the impact of the chronic condition. For example, Lowton and Gabe (2003) found in their study of 31 adults with cystic fibrosis (who had been diagnosed as chronically ill since infancy) that the majority of them maintained a positive attitude and sense of well-being, and typically spoke of themselves as healthy. Because they had an active social life, did not require hospitalisation, or were in paid work, they could 'normalise' their symptoms by seeing them as affecting their lives in similar ways as the effects of minor illness on people without their disease whom they knew. However, this depended upon them being able to control their symptoms effectively, and several respondents found the disease distressing and, in four cases, 'all encompassing'. The critical factor here was the worsening progression of their physical condition (e.g. the onset of CF-related diabetes), leading to the loss of the roles and identities they had previously maintained.

Medical diagnosis and entry to the sick role (Chapter 2) play an important role in shaping the experience of chronic illness by creating an public identity that guides the actions and interpretations of oneself and others. Sometimes in chronic illness the sick role has a highly positive connotation, facilitating access to a range of potentially helpful resources. In particular, where the symptoms of the disease are ambiguous and take a long time to diagnose, e.g.

multiple sclerosis, the eventual diagnosis may be received with relief because of the certainty and legitimacy it provides. However, many physical disabilities are not caused by illness and many disabled people are not ill, so their role is not easily defined within the frameworks provided by the sick role for the management of illness. While there may be some benefits for sufferers of treating disability as if it were a sickness, there are also disadvantages. Requiring the disabled person to assume the sick role in order to gain access to a range of benefits and services may both restrict their autonomy and lead to dependency.

Experiencing chronic illness and physical disability

The experiences of people with chronic conditions can be very different, and it is important to recognise the varying extent of both of the intrusiveness of symptoms and/or impairment and their social consequences. A very large proportion of people with chronic conditions lead full and normal lives with the aid of medical technologies, support from health services and other carers, and their own resilience and ability to cope. It is important to remember that there are now effective remedies that facilitate a normal life, the most common being the correction of poor eyesight and hearing. Chronic conditions occur across a continuum running from virtual normality to high dependency and complete involvement in the sick role, with many chronic conditions moving towards the latter over time. Where a condition is located along the continuum is determined by the way that biological and social processes interact.

At the 'normal' end are treatable chronic conditions, such as cataracts and hypertension, that can be managed quite successfully, and where considerable disability can be alleviated. There are also a very wide range of conditions, such as diabetes, epilepsy and rheumatoid arthritis, where a combination of clinical intervention and self-management enables people to live with their condition in a predictable and satisfactory way for most, or some, of the time, and to engage in everyday activities such as work, leisure and sexual relations to varying degrees. To an external observer who does not know that there is an underlying disease, the person with a well-managed chronic condition appears to be living a completely normal life. To the person with the illness, on the other hand, a great deal of effort has to go into maintaining the appearance of normality. With these conditions a person may move in the direction of the sick role at some times and towards a virtually normal life at other times.

Heart disease and diseases of the circulatory system, respiratory illnesses, and cancers are not so readily amenable to restorative intervention, but varying degrees of successful management can be obtained for significant periods of time. With these diseases increasing limitations upon individuals and the requirements for more intensive support accumulate as the disease progresses. This may eventually lead to high levels of dependency and incapacity, as epitomised by patients receiving intensive ongoing clinical care, such as someone who is housebound with emphysema and dependent upon oxygen.

It is quite common for someone to progress towards the sick role end of the spectrum and for symptoms and impairments to become more disruptive and intrusive of social life with increasing age (Chapter 6).

Onset

The time of life when the chronic conditions or disabilities are acquired is important. There are three principal ways in which chronic illness or disability is acquired: at birth or in infancy, suddenly (perhaps as a result of an accident), or through the development of a chronic illness in later life (Table 7.1).

At birth

Some people are born with their disease or disabling condition, perhaps as a result of a genetic condition (e.g. cystic fibrosis) or due to a problem

Table 7.1 Three patterns of physical disability.

Type of onset	Age at onset	Typical conditions	Main typical problems and difficulties
At birth or infancy	0–5	Cystic fibrosis Spina bifida Down's syndrome	*For parents* Shock Loss of a 'normal child' Interpreting developmental delays *For children* Mastering normal developmental tasks Learning they are different Living a normal social life despite obstacles to education, work and sexual relations
Sudden and unexpected	Teenage and young adult	Paraplegia	Shock and loss Impact on identity and self-image Rehabilitation Reconstructing their lives despite difficulties for work, leisure and sexual relations
	Middle age	Coronary heart attack	Shock Changing pattern of work and family roles and responsibilities
	Old age	Stroke	Shock Rehabilitation Dependence upon others
Slow and gradually worsening	Middle and old age	Arthritis Respiratory diseases Parkinson's disease	Maintaining a balance between normal social activities and the demands and restrictions of the condition Increasing dependence upon others For some conditions, uncertainty over stability and deterioration of condition

preconceptually, during pregnancy or at birth (e.g. a neural tube defect leading to spina bifida). Infants may acquire a disability through infections; for example, deafness resulting from bacterial meningitis. The main initial problems associated with such disabling conditions concern the adjustment of the parents, whose reactions have been described in terms of coping with loss. Nurses and other health workers may also experience emotional reactions, and be particularly upset if an infant is impaired as a result of a technical failing during or shortly after delivery.

Problems for the individual with the disability acquired this way concern both the technical consequences of learning how to live with their illness and disability(s) and in learning and adjusting to the fact that they are different from other people. Experiences of early childhood and family life vary according to whether children are treated, and think of themselves, as 'normal' and 'no different' from others, which is linked to whether ongoing medical treatment or personal care is required (Grewal *et al.* 2006).

Transitions to independence are important (Grewal *et al.* 2006). Critical stages in coming to terms with their identity as a disabled person occur when the child first leaves the shelter of his family on entry to school, and again when leaving full-time education. This typically occurs at an earlier stage than for able-bodied children, is less likely to involve further or higher education, and often may not result in entry to full-time paid work. Finally, for those individuals who are severely disabled and living in their parental home, the death of their parents may lead to institutional care.

Sudden onset

The acquisition of a disability as a result of sudden trauma is most likely to occur among teenagers and young adults, frequently as a result of accidents or injury. The individual is likely to feel initially overwhelmed by the physiological aspects and consequences of their injury. In the longer term they are confronted with the dual problems of coping with their physical losses and the restrictions of their disabilities and coming to terms with the social disadvantages that result. Life plans and goals in sexual relations, parenthood and career may come into question or become impossible to achieve, thus posing major questions for identity and self-conception. The development of new self-conceptions incorporating their changed physical and social status is vital to successful adjustment.

Other relatively common causes of sudden disability are stroke and heart attack, conditions that mainly affect the middle aged and elderly. Although older people will experience problems of adjustment, they may have fewer difficulties than young people. This is because they may believe, or come to convince themselves, that they have achieved (or failed to achieve) their life plans and goals.

Gradual onset in later life

The development of chronic disease in middle and old age is the most common pattern of onset. This may be slow and insidious, with a gradual process of accommodation and adjustment to increasing levels of impairment and activity restriction. Greater disability as a result of the progression of a chronic illness may be one of the factors leading to retirement from paid work. At this stage of life, illness and disability may be more readily accepted as a normal part of ageing. However, there may be more social isolation, and people in old age may have less physical and financial resources to call upon in coping with their condition.

Visibility

The visibility and intrusiveness of a condition (e.g. facial burns, constant hand tremors) are important because people who are notably different in appearance or behaviour from normal expectations are most likely to be noticed by others. This may undermine the taken-for-granted assumptions which underpin everyday social encounters. Although chronic illness and disability are by no means inevitably stigmatising, people with highly visible impairments or disabilities are likely to experience stigmatisation (Chapter 2; Goffman 1990). Where the stigmatised condition is very visible or intrusive it may be difficult for people to escape the coercive power of attributed identities, or to have control in managing their interactions with others. At the extreme, a negative spiral of exclusion from meaningful interaction, self-withdrawal, and diminished self-esteem may result (Figure 7.1).

In a very visible condition, what many sufferers find very frustrating is the failure by others to recognise any aspect of their social identity other than their disability or the publicly visible aspect of their illness. This is because other people overlook the other aspects of the person (e.g. their humour, intellectual attainment) that make up their individuality and personal identity, and focus instead on the disability. For example, when meeting someone in a wheelchair for the first time the wheelchair may provoke ideas about dependency, and feelings of sympathy and possibly embarrassment. As the participants in Galvin's study (2005) reported, 'being patronised or pitied, singled out for unsolicited attention or treated as invisible, being stared at or reviled' (Galvin 2005: 397) because of a visible impairment has a demoralising negative impact upon personal identity.

The situation is different in the management of interpersonal relations where the chronic illness or disability is not immediately apparent. Here the disability or illness may only become apparent as interaction unfolds and as relationships develop. There are several examples reported in the literature. In the case of epilepsy, people who have that disease may conceal it because of their fear of the social consequences of the disclosure, such as the loss of a job or the loss of credibility, even though there is no evidence that they are being discriminated against (Jacoby 1994). As noted in Chapter 2, their sense of 'felt stigma' may cause them more anxiety and distress than the actual results of disclosure, and may have damaging consequences for their self-conception.

Another example is people who have had ileostomies following surgery for ulcerative colitis. When they are dressed, including in swimming costumes,

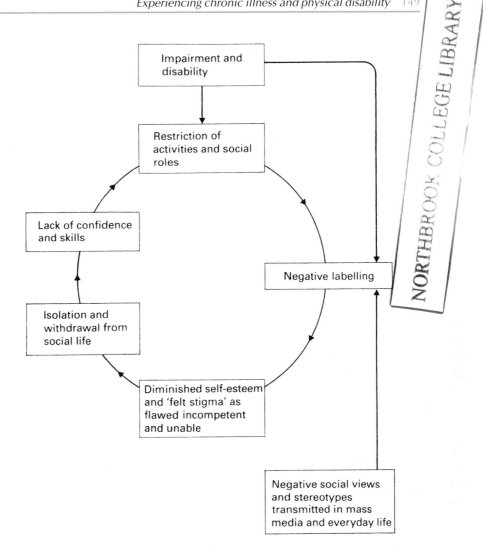

Figure 7.1 Feedback between stigmatisation, self-esteem and participation in social activities.

the ileostomy is neither visible nor obvious. However, when trying to buy life insurance, or applying for a new job, it will need to be disclosed. If they enter into a sexual relationship not only will it need to be disclosed, but the presence of the bag and its potential to get in the way during sexual intercourse will need to be actively managed not just by the person with the ileostomy but also by their new partner (Millward and Kelly 2003).

Unpredictability and disruption

Disruption and unpredictability are key characteristics of chronic illness or disability (Bury 1997, chapter 2). Disruption takes many forms, going well beyond the interruption to the normal round of everyday activities that is characteristic of any illness to some degree, and is an important determinant of where upon the continuum from independence to dependence a person is located.

Symptoms are one obvious source of disruption in chronic illness, and coping with a hostile social and physical environment is highly disruptive of ordinary living in the case of physical disability. In some chronic conditions (e.g. multiple sclerosis or rheumatoid arthritis) symptoms themselves can be highly unpredictable and the person may not know from day to day whether it will be a good or bad day, or whether their symptoms will be intrusive or manageable (Robinson 1988). For example, in arthritis the sufferers may not know until they wake up whether it is a day when they will be able to get about easily, or whether they will be wracked by pain. It may not be clear whether medication will bring relief or not. This unpredictability makes any kind of medium- to long-term planning very difficult. The simple things in life are not/no longer simple. This is highly disruptive of ordinary living.

Many, perhaps all, of the things that the person with the illness or disability wants and needs to do are made more difficult than they are for well or able-bodied people and require more effort. Getting up and washing for someone with a spinal cord injury is a major task. For someone with colitis, planning a simple journey is fraught with the danger of a sudden attack of diarrhoea. For someone with diabetes, choosing when and what to eat are major issues. For someone with emphysema, climbing a flight of stairs requires an enormous effort. Finding directions if someone is visually impaired, or listening to announcements at a railway station for the hearing impaired, are major problems. To be accomplished, these everyday tasks require hard work, or assistance, or both.

In addition, biomedical therapeutic interventions designed to help may actually add to the burden of difficulties and make things even more complicated. Taking combinations of medication, attending hospital, undergoing investigative procedures and reorganising home life to accommodate physical needs and equipment, are all disruptive phenomena flowing from the illness that add to the difficulties the person has to cope with and the effort to overcome them.

Economic and social effects

Chronic illness and physical disability have economic as well as social effects (Grewal *et al.* 2006). People who are chronically sick or disabled may be unable to work, or can participate in the labour market in only very limited ways and then often only in less well paid work. Yet it is more costly to be chronically ill or have a disability than to be in normal health. Direct costs may be incurred through the alteration of the home to accommodate disability, more frequent laundry, special dietary requirements, additional heating costs and the employment of additional help in the home. Indirect costs may also be significant as activity restriction may affect access to large (and cheaper) supermarkets and require the use of taxis. Not only may people with disabilities suffer loss of income through restriction or loss of paid employment, but their partner or other main 'lay carer' may have to give up their paid employment in order to look after them. Loss of income and the increased costs of being ill or disabled are unlikely to be adequately compensated by the range of financial arrangements available through the welfare state systems. These economic disadvantages are not simply an outcome of chronic illness or disability but may also reflect the social patterning of disadvantage (Chapter 3).

Adjusting to a chronic condition

Possibly the most important factor in the adjustment to chronic conditions is the nature and extent of *control* that is possible. This varies with the intrusiveness, stability, severity and disruptiveness of the condition, may change over time for a particular condition, and will vary between different long-term conditions. The self-management of diabetes provides a good illustration of the interplay of the various factors involved.

Campbell *et al.* (2003) identified a common pattern of response to, and self-management of, diabetes across different countries and health systems. The ability 'to attain a balanced life with diabetes' was 'strongly associated with "strategic non compliance", involving the monitoring and observation of symptoms and an ability to manipulate dietary and medical regimes as fully as possible, rather than limiting social and work activities in order to adhere rigidly to medical advice' (Campbell *et al.* 2003: 67). They found that a sense of well being and of control of their diabetes developed over time and was associated with six factors:

- experience of monitoring and observing one's body and its reactions;
- trust in one's own actions to manage diabetes;
- a less subservient and more questioning approach towards care providers;
- some knowledge of the mechanisms of diabetes;
- acknowledgement of the seriousness of diabetes;
- supportive care providers.

Campbell *et al.* (2003) suggested that rather than locating people within a particular category or trying to place them on a particular 'trajectory' it is better to recognise that they have to pass through critical stages and overcome certain obstacles before they can manage their diabetes effectively and achieve a degree of balance and control over it.

Kelly (1992) suggests that adjustment and coping can be considered at four levels:

- the technical and practical management of the condition;
- managing relationships with others;
- the management of thoughts and feelings (emotional coping); and
- interpreting and making sense of the condition.

In one form or another these constitute the routines that make life possible and shape the ways in which social and public identities will develop.

Technical tasks

The technical tasks of coping with chronic illness and disability involve both the learning and mastery of new skills (e.g. using an artificial limb, changing colostomy bags) and gaining useful information (e.g. about how to manage special diets). Some of these skills, such as taking medication or the self-administration of blood or urine tests, are additional to normal daily activities like dressing, eating and going to the toilet. For some people who are ill or disabled the latter may require considerable effort and/or help from others. In many conditions they have to be planned and organised in ways that can come to dominate the waking hours of the ill person and their lay carer(s).

Unless and until these technical tasks are managed successfully other aspects of life take second place. Physical aspects of the environment, such as ease of access to and within buildings and to transport, are significant here, as they enhance or restrict the lives of individuals who have a physical disability or chronic illness. Nurses can play an important role in providing information about, and access to, ways of improving their patients' physical environments.

Relating to others

Chronic illness and disability are not merely personal experiences, but are the result of shared experiences and interactions with other people, so another important task is that of relating to others. This may involve establishing new types of relationships with people (e.g. those involving greater dependency) and the renegotiation of existing relationships, especially within the household. These link very closely to the technical tasks described above, since the degree to which the technical difficulties posed by the condition are brought under control have a defining effect on the success or otherwise of the management of interpersonal matters. Household members and significant others may be involved directly in providing the technical tasks of managing the condition.

Managing thoughts and feelings

Strong feelings and emotions may be aroused as people try to come to terms with their loss of previous abilities and social roles. People with chronic illnesses and disabilities respond with the entire range of human emotions, including anger, resentment, good humour, fear, stoicism, anxiety and depression. Such feelings can, and do, have a significant impact on the relationships people have with others, and both the person with the condition and those they spend time with must somehow come to live with these emotions and feelings.

One response, especially following traumatic physical disability, is *denial*. This concept has come to embrace any kind of psychological response that seems to amount to failing to face up to the 'reality' of a situation. However, it must be acknowledged that denial, especially in the immediate aftermath of a trauma, can be a useful response that may allow other processes of adjustment to occur. Denial is only a problem if it persists and stops someone adjusting to their condition in the long run. *Anger* is another common response, often manifesting itself against the illness, oneself or others who are providing care. *Resignation*, giving up and submitting to an invalid status, letting the condition dominate one's life and becoming completely enveloped by the sick role and adopting an extreme form of dependency on others is another extreme psychological response.

It is important for health professionals not to see such psychological responses as inevitably pathological. Ordinary people facing extra-ordinary situations respond in extreme ways and their psychological suffering and emotional responses are likely to be highly charged. For the majority of chronically ill and physically disabled persons their emotional responses are well within the range of normal behaviour. To ignore such feelings or to view them as another form of illness – this time psychological – is unhelpful: a minority of persons will respond psychologically to their situation in ways that will require clinical help. Nurses may be able to help their patients and their lay carers to understand, discuss and manage their emotions by acknowledging that it is quite natural to respond from time to time with emotions such as anger or depression, and that the expression of such feelings may be psychologically healthy because they may be part of the healing process.

Making sense of the condition

The sick or disabled person will need to make sense of their condition before they can fully adjust to it. Until they can do this they may be unable to develop stable and predictable ways of managing their disability or illness. Language and story telling play an important role here. The language used to describe the illness and its symptoms is highly important in shaping the way that people make sense of their illness. Among the most powerful and useful languages is medicine, both with its explanations of cause, treatment and outcome and through its influence on wider lay understandings of illness.

The narratives (or stories) that people tell to others is another way of making sense of chronic illness and physical disability (Chapter 2). Bury (2001) suggests that there are three main types or levels of illness narrative. *Contingent narratives* are concerned with the origins and temporal development of the condition and its everyday effects upon the individual and others. *Moral narratives* address and sometimes attempt to shape the types of evaluative judgements that are made about people with a chronic illness and/or disability. Such narratives are essentially about changing identities and their location in social circumstance, addressing issues such as who or what is to blame and the presentation and maintenance of the person's social worth. *Core narratives* link the person's experiences with cultural meanings of illness and suffering and draw upon these shared understandings to cope with their condition, e.g. to distance oneself from the illness by using humour. These three narrative types perform different functions, and any story of illness or disability may include more than one of them. It is important for nurses to listen to the stories that their patients tell as this will help them to recognise important non-clinical social and psychological concerns, expectations and areas of help.

Care and caring

The experiences of chronic illness and physical disability are socially defined in interaction with other people. Chapter 2 discussed the crucial role of emotional, instrumental and informational social support in illness and disability, and observed that there may be some negative consequences for those providing social support. People with disabilities may challenge our ideas about what is 'normal' behaviour, possibly making us uncomfortable about the range of activities and capacities we take for granted. They may take longer over mundane tasks such as eating or dressing, may only be able to perform them with a lot of effort and in unusual ways, or require assistance with them. Not only do chronic illness and physical disability affect the individual's own activities and abilities but they may also limit the lives of other people by restricting their activities and requiring the reorganisation of their previous routines, roles and ways of viewing the world. In the short term, such disruption may be acceptable, but over the long term it is likely to create difficulties for 'lay carers' and others closely associated with people with disabilities.

Family and friends

Family and friends will have an intimate knowledge of the person and their condition and are the main providers of emotional and instrumental support. For example, many long-term conditions require the effective management of diet and the assimilation of this into family practices is important in promoting a sense of 'living a normal life' (Gregory 2005). They have insight into the experiences of people who are chronically ill or have a physical disability, because of their close association with them. The impact of chronic illness and disability upon family and friends can be profound, with their work and social life being disrupted by the needs of care and the restrictions on activity which arise from living with someone who has a disability. Close associates may themselves become stigmatised because of their relation to the ill or disabled person (Chapter 2; Goffman 1990). Although strong emotional strains may arise, for example as a result of the burden of care or the difficulties of giving non-disabled children in the family the care and attention they deserve, there is no evidence of higher than average marital break-up or difficulties.

Health and social care workers

Professional health and social care workers are another important source of help and support. They are in a position to shape the experience of chronic illness and disability through the instrumental help and informational support they provide, and by the way they define such illness and disability. Because of their central role in the care of people who have a chronic illness and/or disability in hospitals and the community, nurses play a particularly important role. In many cases their attitudes towards the chronic illness or disability (as well as to the person who has it) may be critical in shaping the response of their patients towards it.

Chronic illnesses may be difficult for nurses to deal with because their patients won't get better and some are likely to become progressively worse. In particular, they may experience difficulties when they are unable to provide adequate relief of symptoms. Another difficult situation is when they are required to give 'bad news', which may lead them to pretend that there is still uncertainty about the prognosis (even though they know the patient will get worse) or to disclose only some of the bad information initially, hoping that the patient will come to realise that all is not well. Nurses can provide both practical and emotional support which may enhance both the patient's coping skills and their sense of self-esteem.

The provision of information and advice can be very important. Nurses can answer many questions that patients and their lay carers have, about:

- the nature of their condition ('Will it get worse?', 'Why is the skin like that?');
- probable activity restrictions ('Will I be able to go back to work?', 'How long before we can resume sexual relations?');
- how to manage the condition ('When is the best time to do the injections?', 'I don't want to use my nebuliser too often.');
- where to find help and support ('Where can I get a better bed?', 'How do I get help at night?').

They may also be able to point out the unanticipated potential for activity which may remain ('You may find that you can continue with your gardening provided that directly you feel breathless you take deep breaths and don't become anxious.').

However, the different perspectives of patients and nurses give rise to a number of potential pitfalls. Nurses may be seen to be unresponsive to the wishes of patients and their carers because they apply their own (professionally based) judgements of need and value rather than those of the patient. Thus, they may mis-define or ignore what patients feel they need, while giving care and treatment that is perceived as inappropriate or unnecessary. What may be trivial to the nurse may be central to the patient, and vice versa. Nurses may fail to recognise the ability and knowledge that sick and disabled people and their families have about their condition and its consequences for everyday life.

Because of patients' long-term involvement with their condition, perhaps including their involvement with self-help groups or other activists, they accumulate a great deal of knowledge, experience and practical wisdom about it and how best to manage it. In the developed world the recognition of the expertise of people with long-term conditions has led to an attempt to harness their practical wisdom in the 'expert patient' movement (Department of

Health 2001, Bury *et al.* 2005). Yet despite the increasing acknowledgement of the important role of patient expertise and their participation in the management of their chronic illness, it can be difficult for doctors and nurses to see beyond the clinical problem to the person with wants and needs which are much broader than the biomedical imperatives of the illness or disability. Disability activists claim that the various health and welfare institutions of British society that are intended to help them are in fact sources of their handicap and oppression (e.g. Oliver 1996). Unless nurses (and other professionals) pay sufficient attention to the knowledge and abilities of people who have a chronic illness or disability they are in danger of underestimating their abilities and preventing them from being used.

Nurses, especially community nurses, may become caught up in problems associated with the frequent lack of co-ordination among care givers, and may even become caught in the crossfire of competition between different professional experts involved. Unless these various problems are avoided, the nurse may deliver non-responsive and even coercive advice, 'help' and care.

Alternative therapists

The common use of alternative therapists (i.e. those with non-medical training or qualifications) by chronically ill people may, in part, be related to the better communication and information they are often thought by the patient to provide (Sharma 1995). The main reason why people use alternative therapies is the perceived failure of medicine to deal with chronic conditions in a satisfactory way (Sharma 1995). Not only may modern medicine be unable to cure chronic disease, but it may also be unable to palliate symptoms such as chronic pain adequately. Further, many sufferers find their drug therapy undesirable or the medical regimes over-invasive. The impersonality and lack of adequate information characteristic of much modern medical and nursing practice (especially in hospitals) is in sharp contrast to the time, information and personal attention received from alternative therapists. Sharma suggests that patients feel empowered and informed by alternative therapists, with greater control over the choice of treatment.

Self-help organisations

The role of self-help organisations and informal contact with others in a similar situation cannot be underestimated. At the personal level, self-help groups can provide mutual help and support and may be particularly important in sustaining positive self-concepts in the face of negative experiences. They can provide invaluable psychological support, insight into the person's problems and difficulties, relevant and practical information and help, and a source of sociability. At the local level, they may be a valuable source of information about how to access services, and can also act as pressure groups to bring about improvements. At the national level, organisations such as

Diabetes UK and the Disability Alliance have played an important role in raising public awareness of issues and exerting political pressure. At all these levels involvement with others with similar experiences may empower individuals to take greater control of their lives. Access to self-help and other disease-specific organisations via the internet has provided an important additional source of information and support for people with chronic illnesses and disabilities that transcends the limitations of physical proximity.

Summary

In this chapter we have focused upon fundamentally important social aspects of chronic illness and physical disability that cannot be subsumed within the framework of the bio-medical model. Such chronic conditions are socially patterned, especially by age and socio-economic status, reflecting the inequalities in health manifested in society as a whole. Chronic conditions affect not simply bodily functioning and appearance but also self-conceptions, identities and social attachments and relationships with others. Their impact on these is influenced by the onset of the condition, its visibility and its salience for others, and its disruption of everyday life. Four key tasks were identified in coping with chronic conditions: the technical and practical management of the condition; managing relationships with others; emotional coping; and interpreting and making sense of the condition. Finally, other people, including nurses, have an important role in shaping the experience of chronic illness and disability.

References

Ahmad, W.I.U. (2000) *Ethnicity, Disability and Chronic Illness*. Open University Press, Buckingham.

Bajekal, M., Osborne, V., Yar, M. and Meltzer, H. eds (2006) *Focus on Health*. National Statistics/Palgrave Macmillan. Available at www.statistics.org (accessed June 2006).

Barnes, C. and Mercer, G. (2003) *Disability*. Blackwell, Oxford.

Bone, M. and Meltzer, H. (1989) *The Prevalence of Disability among Children*. Office of Population Censuses and Surveys. HMSO, London.

Bunker, J. (2001) Medicine matters after all, in B. Davey, A. Gray and C. Seale (eds) *Experiencing and Explaining Disease*. Open University, Buckingham.

Bury, M. (1997) *Health and Illness in a Changing Society*. Routledge, London, 110–40.

Bury, M. (2001) Illness narratives: fact or fiction? *Sociology of Health and Illness*, 23, 263–85.

Bury, M., Newbould, J. and Taylor, D. (2005) *A Rapid Review of the Current State of Knowledge Regarding Lay Led Self Management of Chronic Illness: Evidence Review*. National Institute for Health and Clinical Excellence, London. Available at www.nice.org.uk (accessed May 2006).

Campbell, R., Pound, P., Pope, C. *et al.* (2003) Evaluating meta-ethnography: a synthesis of qualitative research on lay experiences of diabetes and diabetes care. *Social Science and Medicine*, 56, 671–84.

Charmaz, K. (1983) Loss of self: A fundamental form of suffering of the chronically ill. *Sociology of Health and Illness*, 5, 168–95.

Department of Health (2001) *The Expert Patient: A New Approach to Chronic Disease Management for the 21st Century*. The Stationery Office, London.

Galvin, R. (2005) Researching the disabled identity: contextualising the identity transformations which accompany the onset of impairment. *Sociology of Health and Illness*, 27, 393–413.

Goffman, E. (1990) *Stigma: Notes on the Management of Spoiled Identity*. Penguin, Harmondsworth, Middx.

Gregory, S. (2005) Living with chronic illness in the family setting. *Sociology of Health and Illness*, 27, 372–92.

Grewal, S., Joy, S., Lewis, J., *et al.* (2006) *'Disabled for Life?' Attitudes Towards, and Experiences of, Disability in Britain*. DWP Research Report 173, Leeds.

Jacoby, A. (1994) Felt versus enacted stigma: A concept revisited. *Social Science and Medicine*, 38, 269–74.

Kelly, M.P. (1992) *Colitis*. Routledge, London.

Kelly, M.P. and Millward, L.M. (2004) Identity and illness, in D. Kelleher and G. Leavey (eds) *Identity and Health*. Routledge, London, 1–18.

Lowton, K. and Gabe, J. (2003) Life on a slippery slope: perceptions of health in adults with cystic fibrosis. *Sociology of Health and Illness*, 25, 289–319.

Lupton, D. and Seymour, W. (2000) Technology, selfhood and physical disability. *Social Science and Medicine*, 50, 1857–62.

Matheson, J. and Summerfield, C. (eds) (2000) *Social Focus on Young People*. The Stationery Office, London.

Millward, L.M. and Kelly, M.P. (2003) Incorporating the biological: Chronic illness, bodies, selves and the material world, in S.J. Williams, G.A. Bendelow and L. Birke (eds) *Debating Biology: Sociological Reflections on Health Medicine and Society*. Routledge, London.

Oliver, M. (1996) *Understanding Disability: From Theory to Practice*. Macmillan, Basingstoke.

Priestley, M. (2003) *Disability. A Life Course Approach*. Polity, Oxford.

Robinson, I. (1988) *Multiple Sclerosis*. Routledge, London.

Sharma, U. (1995) *Complementary medicine today. Practitioners and Patients*, revised edition. Routledge, London.

Swain J., French, S. and Cameron, C. eds (2003) *Controversial Issues in a Disabling Society*. Open University Press, Buckingham.

Further reading

Barnes, C. and Mercer, G. (2003) *Disability*. Blackwell, Oxford.
A useful and accessible introduction to the main elements of disability studies.

Bury, M. and Gabe, J. (eds) (2004) *The Sociology of Health and Illness: A Reader*, Part 4. Routledge, London.
A useful collection that contains some of the key sociological work in this area.

Chapter 8

Mental disorders

In any social situation there are expectations as to how people should normally behave and communicate. At one time those whose behaviour departed radically from social norms were variously labelled as 'idiots', 'lunatics' or sometimes as 'possessed' by demons or evil spirits. However, in modern societies such people are more likely to be seen as suffering from mental disorders and in need of care and treatment from specialist health professionals. To many people this trend is an indication of a more enlightened, humane and compassionate society. Others disagree, arguing that many mental disorders are not 'really' diseases and to label them as such may be counterproductive by further restricting the opportunities of the mentally disordered to lead comparatively normal lives and, sometimes, by legitimising an oppressive form of social control over them. This chapter will:

- compare different theoretical approaches to mental disorders
- examine suicidal behaviour and eating disorders
- look at changing patterns of care of the mentally disordered
- discuss the contested nature of the concept of mental illness and the relationship between psychiatric care and social control

Approaches to mental disorders

The term 'mental disorder' covers a wide and ill-defined area, but it is possible to distinguish between three overlapping populations. First, there are those suffering from impaired bodily function, such as people with learning disabilities or senile mental confusion. Secondly, there are people with behavioural problems, such as alcohol or drug abuse, who are often treated by health care professionals *as if* they had diseases. Thirdly, there are those who have what are called mental illnesses, such as schizophrenia, depression and anxiety states, where it is not clear if they are diseases or behavioural problems.

There are many different theoretical approaches to mental disorders, but a broad distinction can be made between biological, psychological and sociological perspectives (Table 8.1). Biological theories argue that all, or most, mental disorders are symptomatic of an underlying *bodily* malfunction and should be managed by medical treatments of one sort or another. Psychological theories suggest that some mental illnesses and behavioural disorders may be

Table 8.1 Models of mental illness.

	Medical	**Psychological**	**Social**
Definition/ diagnosis	Mental illnesses are diagnosed by doctors in terms of clearly defined criteria and are symptoms of underlying *bodily* disease	Mental illnesses are diagnosed by doctors or therapists. Precise diagnosis difficult. Mental illnesses are diseases of the *mind* which may, or may not, have an organic basis	Diagnosis of mental illness problematic. Often owes more to social factors than clinical evidence Behaviour 'labelled' as 'illness' may be response to difficult, or oppressive situation
Causes	Uncertain, but growing evidence of genetic predisposition and biochemical causes	Often caused by experiences in patients' past, especially in early childhood	Triggered by social circumstances that create stress, lower self-esteem and sense of control
Treatment	Medical, surgical and nursing care	Psychoanalysis to help reveal subconscious conflicts or cognitive disorder Behaviour modification	Individuals may require help and treatment in short run, but condition will not improve if changes are not also made in their life situation
Goal	To restore patient to health through treatment, or at least control symptoms and prevent condition getting worse	To give patient insight into origins of problems and help develop strategies for combating them	To help reduce rates of mental illness by revealing social influences

a product of personal experiences that distort thought processes and are thus 'diseases of the *mind*' rather than the body. Psychological theories do not necessarily reject biological influences or medical treatments, but argue that they should be accompanied, or substituted, by various therapies aimed at giving people more insight into the psychological sources of their mental distress or behavioural disorder. Sociological approaches focus on *relationships* between individual experiences of mental disorder and distress and wider patterns of social organisation. Sociologists are interested in the role of social influences in the *causes* of mental disorder, its *recognition* and the social organisation of treatment and care of the mentally disordered.

Biological approaches

Many mental disorders, such as Down's syndrome or Alzheimer's disease, are now known to have an organic basis. However, with mental illnesses, such as schizophrenia and depression, evidence of biological causation is less conclusive.

Some types of mental disorder tend to run in families, suggesting a genetic predisposition to the disease, but in practice it is difficult to isolate genetic influences from environmental ones. Biological research has also suggested that mental disorders may be the result of an imbalance of chemicals (called neurotransmitters) in the brain. For example, there is some evidence that schizophrenia may be the result of over-activity of a neurotransmitter called dopamine, while depression and self-harming behaviour have been linked to low levels of another neurotransmitter called serotonin. In this context, treatment involves trying to correct the imbalance with medication. However, there are difficulties with this biochemical approach. First, the results of research exploring the effects of treatment have been inconsistent. Secondly, it is difficult for researchers to be sure whether biochemical changes in the brain are a cause of mental disorder or a *consequence* of stressful life experiences. Thus it is also important to take into account the influence of external events in triggering mental illnesses.

Psychological approaches

Psychological theories attempt to locate the sources of some mental disorders, such as depression and anxiety, in patients' experiences. A number of theories have examined the relationship between the 'formative' experiences of early childhood – especially traumatic experiences – and mental disorder in later life.

Psychoanalytical theory, derived from the work of Freud, argues that there are crucial stages in the *emotional* development of the child, such as separation from the mother and the recognition of sexual identity. Unresolved conflicts at one or more of these crucial stages can remain in the person's *unconscious* mind and produce anxieties and neuroses in later life. Psychoanalytic therapy aims to help to provide insights into the childhood origins of the patient's present distress. While many feel they have benefited from such therapy, its clinical effectiveness remains unproven, as it is difficult to test objectively.

Cognitive psychology focuses on thought processes in the *conscious* mind and argues that there are distinct stages in the child's *intellectual* development as it comes to think rationally about itself and the world. From this perspective, it is argued that factors, such as traumatic childhood experiences, can impede this process and lead to distorted cognitive perceptions in later life. For example, the stage of cognitive development where the child starts to appreciate the effect of its actions on others may fail to materialise for various reasons, leading to a 'psychopathic' personality where acts of gross cruelty can be undertaken without any apparent remorse. In cognitive psychology thought processes are seen as causal influences in their own right and not mere reflections of biochemical changes or unconscious impulses. Cognitive-behavioural therapy, developed from the work of Beck (1991), focuses on the patient's 'irrational' or 'distorted' beliefs, testing them against reality, and trying to establish more rational perceptions and behaviour patterns.

Another psychological approach tries to locate the sources of mental disorder and its development in *social* relationships, particularly within families. In a classical study developing this 'family model', Laing and Esterson (1964) attempted to show that 'schizophrenic' behaviours were in fact unconscious 'strategies' to cope with unliveable family situations. From this point of view, the source of mental illness is the *interaction* between the patient and other family members. Schizophrenia is evidence of a disordered family rather than simply of a disordered individual. This approach has been widely criticised as unscientific and untestable, and for failing to explain why among people exposed to more or less similar experiences a few become schizophrenic while the majority do not. However, the 'family model' of mental illness has been influential and many practitioners treating mental disorders focus on families rather than individuals. More recent research in this area has explored the role of families in the *course* of mental illness rather than its cause (Hooley *et al.* 2005). A number of studies have suggested that the chances of relapse into mental illness amongst discharged patients is much more likely when they return to families with high levels of expressed emotion, such as hostility, criticism and over-concern. From this perspective, it is argued that rehabilitation programmes need to focus on patterns of interaction in families, particularly the management of expressed emotion.

Sociological approaches

Sociological theories focus on the social contexts from which mental disorders emerge and are recognised and treated. Two distinct sociological approaches can be identified. The first explores the extent to which recognised psychiatric conditions, such as anxiety or depression, are caused by social factors. The second is more concerned with the social reaction to mental disorders, and to mental illness in particular.

Social causes

Epidemiological research has shown that specific mental disorders, such as schizophrenia and depression, are not distributed randomly in populations but are consistently linked to socio-demographic variables, suggesting that mental disorders may also be caused, or triggered, by factors in the wider social environment. For example, in Britain, rates of recorded mental disorders for people from African-Caribbean groups and for some groups of Asians are higher than for the general population (Chapter 4). Women have higher rates of reported mental disorder than men, although men are slightly more vulnerable to schizophrenia (Chapter 5). Mental disorders have also been found to be related to social class and social disadvantage. For example, two recent studies in Britain, found the prevalence of mental disorder was positively correlated with social deprivation in England (Evans *et al.* 2004) and in Wales (Skapinakis *et al.* 2005).

Although socio-demographic factors are positively correlated with mental disorders, their causal impact is not clear. Researchers try to explain why factors, such as low social class, are associated with mental disorder, how they are linked to other factors and why particular individuals within these groups are more vulnerable than others. For example, in their influential work Brown and Harris (1989) identified stress factors that led to higher rates of depression amongst working class women compared to middle class women. Working class women were doubly disadvantaged. First, they were more likely to experience long-term major difficulties, such as poor housing, unemployment or the death of a family member. Secondly, they were more vulnerable to the effects of stress (Chapter 2) because of the greater prevalence of certain key 'vulnerability factors'. The presence of three or more dependent children at home, the loss of a mother before the age of 11, lack of paid employment and absence of a close confiding relationship, were all found to lower the women's self-esteem and leave them more vulnerable to the damaging effects of stressful life events. As these factors arose from *social* situations, Brown and Harris concluded that although depressive illness is a biological condition, its origins lie primarily in social factors.

Social reaction to mental disorders

While the sociological approach described above explores how social factors may contribute to the onset of mental disorder, other sociologists have adopted a more sceptical approach and questioned the diagnostic categories themselves, particularly in relationship to mental illness. They are interested in why some actions (but not others) are seen as symptoms of mental illness and why some individuals (but not others) are labelled as mentally ill. For example, as we saw in Chapter 4, some researchers have suggested that the higher rates of mental disorder in Britain found in people of African-Caribbean origin may be the result of differential diagnostic processes.

One of the most influential sociological works in this societal reaction tradition is that of Scheff (1966). He argued that when people's behaviour departs significantly from the expectations of others, and where other explanations of their behaviour fail, they are likely to become labelled as 'mentally ill'. Such labelling is influenced by factors such as the amount, visibility and intrusiveness of the symptoms. Family and friends will tend to accommodate, and even deny, very strange behaviour for long periods of time before they resort to defining their partners or relatives as mentally ill.

A key role is played by stereotypes of madness that are learned in early childhood and reinforced by the mass media and in ordinary social activities. In the crisis surrounding labelling someone mentally ill, these stereotypes of madness clarify and 'make sense' of the strange and unpredictable behaviour. Research by Philo *et al.* (1996) found that media images were more likely than not to demean and stigmatise mental illness, with two-thirds of all such items linking mental illness and violence. However, Link and Phelan (2001) have suggested that mental illness labels might also have a de-stigmatising effect. If mental illness labels lead to effective and supportive professional treatment, then patients *can* feel less stigmatised with the realisation that their problems are not of their own making and that treatment may help them. However, outside the clinic or consulting room in everyday life, they still experience both 'felt' and 'enacted' stigma (Chapter 2).

While societal reaction theory tells us little about the origins of the behaviour that results in someone being defined as suffering from a mental illness, it can help health care professionals focus on the consequences of these diagnoses. For example, in the process of 'making sense' of mental illness in everyday life, a person's past behaviour may be selectively reconstructed, and signs of individuality and previously acceptable idiosyncrasy become reinterpreted as signs of incipient madness. Professional health workers, including psychiatric nurses, are also prone to reinterpret a person's behaviour in terms of their label of mental illness (Rosenhan 1973). Many of those who become labelled as mentally ill also know the common stereotypes surrounding their condition and may come to accept their applicability to themselves and incorporate them into their self-conceptions and behaviour. Once they have been defined as mentally ill patients are 'rewarded' for playing their role 'properly' – that is, doing what doctors and nurses want them to do. Treatment regimes may lead to loss of independence and individuality, especially in hospital settings, and non-compliance may lead to 'punishments' in the form of further curtailments of activity and autonomy.

Self-harming behaviour

One of the major dangers of mental disorder and mental breakdown is the increased risk of deliberate self-harm. In this section we look at two of the most prevalent forms of self-harm in contemporary societies: suicidal behaviour and eating disorders.

Suicide

In England and Wales over the past few years just under 6000 deaths a year have been recorded as suicides, a rate of just over 11 per 100,000 population (Figure 8.1). Suicide is the second most common cause of death in people under 25 and, according to the statistics, males are three and a half times more likely to kill themselves than females. However, it would be wrong to view suicide and self-harm as a predominantly male problem. Females are more than twice as likely to attempt suicide as males and certain forms of chronic self-harm, such as eating disorders and self-mutilation, are much more common in women. So it would be more accurate to say that self-destructive impulses tend to express themselves differently in males and females.

While the official statistics provide a useful guide to patterns of suicidal behaviour, they significantly underestimate the number of suicides. Many 'suicidal' deaths are simply not recorded as such in the official statistics (Chapter 1) and it is generally accepted that suicide rates underestimate the true rate of suicide by about 50%. Further, in Britain an estimated 150,000 people each year commit serious acts of deliberate self-harm that would have led to death without medical and nursing intervention.

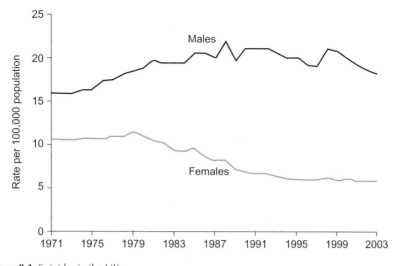

Figure 8.1 Suicides in the UK.
Source: Office for National Statistics. National Statistics website: www.statistics.gov.uk.
Crown copyright material is reproduced with the permission of the Controller of HMSO.

Suicidal behaviour

Research into the ways that people in modern societies go about harming themselves has contradicted some of the 'common sense' assumptions typically made about suicide. A common error, often made by doctors and nurses, is to assume that a clear distinction can be made between 'genuine' suicidal acts (aimed at death) and 'false' suicidal acts (cries for help). Detailed reconstruction of the circumstances of suicidal acts has proved this assumption to be false. The majority of acts of deliberate self-harm, including many that end in death, are desperate gambles with life and death where the result is decided by factors outside the individual's control. In his pioneering research, Stengel (1973) showed that most suicidal acts are not simply aimed at death and dying, but also at life, survival and contact with others. In most cases suicidal individuals give warnings of their intentions and try to communicate their unhappiness and growing despair to others. For example, most suicidal acts take place in a setting (usually the home) where others are present, and use a method (usually poisoning) where rescue is possible.

The observation that most suicidal acts are undertaken with ambivalent intent, and are often preceded by attempts to communicate unhappiness and despair, has implications for prevention and for nursing suicidal and potentially suicidal patients. Indications of possible suicidal intent may include:

- direct warnings of suicidal inclination;
- a preoccupation with death and dying;
- expressions of worthlessness and of being a burden;
- dramatic mood swings;

- significant change in behaviour;
- giving away treasured possessions;
- calls to say goodbye to people.

Understanding of these 'suicidal clues', coupled with known risk factors, such as depression, unemployment, little social support (Chapter 2) and a history of a self-harming behaviour, can help the nurse to make a reasonable assessment of suicidal risk (Skegg 2005).

Intervention and care

Suicide is a particular risk among those suffering from depressive disorders, especially those who are coming out of their depressive state. Yet, despite the association between mental disorders and suicide, the majority of those who deliberately harm themselves do not have a clinically defined mental illness. Most are suffering from an emotional breakdown, often triggered by some personal crisis, and have come to see suicide as the only solution. The observation that suicidal behaviour is not necessarily a symptom of psychiatric illness has implications for intervention and support. The therapy offered by doctors, psychiatrists and nurses can be invaluable in helping to manage psychiatric conditions. However, the tendency of many people to 'medicalise' unhappiness and take their emotional problems to doctors can be counterproductive (Chapter 2). Not only are drugs unlikely to be effective in the long term, as unhappiness and emotional problems are not diseases, but there is the possibility of iatrogenic consequences, such as dependency and overdosing. While medication can be helpful for people in emotional crises, a greater proportion of suicidal and potentially suicidal patients and clients need to be listened to rather than medicated. In such cases, psychological approaches may have more to offer than biological ones.

Partly as a result of their mistaken beliefs about the intent of people who overdose, nurses and doctors tend to be impatient with such patients. They are often treated harshly in casualty departments, ignored on the wards, and made to feel they are wasting staff time. Such reactions, although understandable, are likely to reinforce the low self-esteem of suicidal patients and make a re-attempt more likely.

Suicidal behaviour can raise a number of legal and ethical dilemmas for nurses. Attempting to commit suicide has not been illegal in Britain since The Suicide Act of 1961, but it is still a criminal offence under the Act to assist someone to commit suicide. Most ethical issues concerning suicide revolve around the contradictions that can arise from a person's autonomous right to determine their own life and the obligation on the part health professionals to protect a person believed to be incapable of making a rational decision for themselves. The observation of patients believed to be at risk of harming themselves and others typically falls on nurses. Not only does this involve practical problems of surveillance and restraint, but it can also be seen as a violation of patients' rights and a contradiction of the consumerist ethos of the modern health service (see Chapter 10). However, even though some may feel it is ethically wrong to restrain a potentially suicidal patient, legally a nurse who does not take reasonable care to protect a patient known to be a suicidal risk can be sued in the civil courts for negligence.

Eating disorders

An eating disorder is a condition where there is a serious disruption of eating habits leading to clinical harm. Eating disorders have one of the highest mortality rates of all psychiatric illnesses (Becker 2004). Here we look at two of the most common eating disorders: anorexia and bulimia nervosa.

Anorexia

Anorexia literally means a nervous loss of appetite but this is rather misleading because many sufferers have a voracious appetite which they are struggling to control. Anorexia is hard to define precisely because so many people in contemporary societies are preoccupied with food, diet and losing weight, but in 1987 the American Psychiatric Association (APA) identified the following criteria:

- a body weight at least 15% below that expected;
- a morbid fear of becoming overweight;
- a disturbed perception of body weight, where a person 'feels fat', even though she is obviously underweight;
- in women, an absence of at least three consecutive periods.

The majority of those diagnosed with anorexia are young, between 12 and 22 years, and over 90% are female. There are no official statistics on anorexia but survey research in Britain and the USA has suggested that between 0.5 and 1% of young females have suffered from anorexia at some time in their lives (Hoek and van Hoeken 2003). While the majority of those diagnosed either recover or live with the condition, about 15% of sufferers are hospitalised and about 10% of these eventually die from starvation or organ failure.

Bulimia

Bulimia is an eating disorder characterised by periods of binge eating (often in secret) followed by induced vomiting, excessive use of laxatives or diuretics to lose weight. Bulimics tend to be older than anorectics, the majority being in their twenties or early thirties. While bulimia is less likely than anorexia to be life threatening in itself, it is more likely to be associated with other forms of self-harming behaviour, such as alcoholism, drug abuse or self-mutilation. It has been suggested that between 1 and 2% of women aged 20–40 have suffered from bulimia and, like anorexia, over 90% of bulimics are women.

The precise causes of eating disorders are not clear but most researchers suggest they may be due to a combination of biological, socio-cultural and psychological factors.

Biological explanations

A great deal of biological research has focused on an area of the brain called the hypothalamus, which seems to play a part in regulating 'basic' human actions such as eating, sexual function, aggression and mood. Different parts of the hypothalamus produce hunger (lateral hypothalamus) and depress hunger (ventromedial hypothalamus) and these work alongside each other to produce a 'weight thermostat'. Some research has suggested, but not yet convincingly demonstrated, that a malfunction of the hypothalamus upsetting the 'weight thermostat' may be an underlying cause of anorexia, bulimia and obesity.

Biochemical research has also shown that eating disorders, like depression, are associated with low levels of the neurotransmitter serotonin, and many sufferers have been treated successfully with serotonin uptake drugs. However, it is possible that low levels of serotonin are a consequence rather than a cause of eating disorders. Another problem with biological theories is that they have difficulty in explaining both the apparent increase in anorexia and bulimia over the past two decades and the fact that they seem to occur almost exclusively in modern industrial societies. Sociologists suggest that some of the answers to these questions are to be found in the cultural norms of contemporary societies.

Socio-cultural theory

It is in affluent industrial societies where food is plentiful and cheap that there is most 'social pressure' to be thin (Littlewood 2004). While the health promotion industry warns of the dangers of being overweight, the diet, fashion and entertainment industries positively extol the virtues of thinness, bombarding the public with images of glamorously starving supermodels, singers and film stars. Being thin, especially for girls and women, has become associated with being attractive, successful and healthy, while being overweight has become the secular equivalent of sin. Socio-cultural theory suggests, and survey research has confirmed, that the result of this culture of thinness is that more and more women are dissatisfied with their body shape and that dieting has become a way of life for millions of them. For some, dieting can become an obsession that leads to anorexia.

Socio-cultural theory seems to explain why the majority of those afflicted by eating disorders are girls and women. Further support comes from a number of cross-cultural studies linking eating disorders to industrialisation. For example, the onset of eating disorders in Japan correlated with increasing industrialisation and exposure to idealised 'Western' body images (Pike and Borovoy 2004), while immigrants to industrialised countries from cultures where anorexia is rare are just as likely to develop the disorder as the indigenous population. However, socio-cultural theory does not explain why only some women suffer from eating disorders while the majority living in the same culture do not. Many researchers have suggested that some answers to this question are found closer to home in the family experiences of sufferers.

Family theories

Family theories argue that eating disorders are a product of various forms of problematic or dysfunctional family relationships (Lock 2004). For example, a great deal of research has shown that a disproportionate number of girls and women who develop eating disorders have either suffered traumas in childhood such as neglect, or physical or sexual abuse, or grown up in very 'controlling families', where parents make decisions for them and place constant pressure on them to be the best at everything. The consequence of such dysfunctional family relationships is that children are more likely to reach adolescence with a confused sense of personal identity (Chapter 2) leading to troubled states of mind, such as a low sense of self-esteem, feeling out of control or having a fear of growing up and reaching sexual maturity. In this context, a number of contemporary researchers, following pioneering research by Bruch (1978), have argued that for sufferers, eating disorders provide a 'solution' to these anxieties (Table 8.2).

Treatments

The first stage in the treatment and care of anorectics and bulimics is to try to restore normal patterns of eating and, in the case of some anorectics, to bring them back to a safe body weight. In extreme cases they can be hospitalised and, if deemed necessary, force fed. However, it is more common for sufferers to be treated in specialised residential institutions where there is a strict regime of rewards and punishments for eating or not eating. These regimes are generally successful, but they are only short-term solutions. Longer-term treatments today usually involve a combination of cognitive-behavioural therapy, family therapy and pharmacotherapy.

A particular difficulty with anorectics is that they often have strongly held but irrational perceptions of themselves. For example, many anorectics believe they are fat when they are really very thin, or believe they are academic failures even though they have achieved A grades in their exams. Cognitive-behavioural therapies have been found to be successful in challenging these beliefs and helping clients begin to change some of their thought processes and behaviour. Another important aspect of therapy for anorectics and bulimics involves focusing on what patients themselves feel they *gain* from controlling food intake or binging and purging, and trying to find less lethal ways of achieving these goals. In an analysis of different treatment programmes

Table 8.2 The anorectic solution.

Expressed emotion	Eating 'solution'
I am no good	Self-punishment
I have no control over my life	Controlling food intake gives me a sense of control of my body and my life
I don't want to grow up	Not eating keeps you small and periods stop

Kong (2005) suggested that nurses have a crucial role to play and maintaining empathetic involvement with the patients throughout their period of care and in helping to establish alliances between patients and carers.

Like suicide, the treatment and care of people with eating disorders can raise important ethical conflicts between respecting the autonomy of the patient (the right to control what they eat) and acting in the patient's best interests (forcing them to adopt 'normal' patterns of eating). In the short term, best interests usually prevail, especially if the patient is young, but people cannot be detained and made to eat indefinitely and health care professionals have to accept that sufferers must eventually be allowed to return to the outside world, even though a proportion of them will die.

Care of the mentally disordered

In modern societies the care of people with mental disorders continues to be organised primarily around psychiatric diagnoses and interventions. This is most evident in the hospitalisation of those with mental disorders but, even in the community, psychiatric and medical definitions constrain and influence the behaviour of other health care workers, social workers, lay carers and, as we have seen, the mentally disordered themselves and their families. Although, in practice, many people with severe mental disorders regularly move between hospital and community settings, the following sections consider these separately.

Hospital care

Once defined as mentally ill a person may be treated by their GP or as an out-patient at a psychiatric unit attached to a general hospital. Most psychiatric hospital care is now delivered in acute psychiatric units of general hospitals, often in a series of short admissions and discharges. When a person is severely disturbed and considered to be a risk to themselves or others, they may be compulsorily admitted to a hospital and they can be treated without their consent. While the vast majority of mental health admissions are technically voluntary, recent research in Britain has shown that one-third of voluntary patients felt coerced and two-thirds were not sure whether they were allowed to leave hospital (Bindman *et al.* 2005). Greater age, less insight and non-white ethnicity were associated with *perceived* coercion.

Sociological studies of mental hospitals have been particularly concerned with the ways in which admission procedures and the organisation of the hospital can undermine patients' sense of autonomy and identity. For example, in a highly influential study, Goffman (1991) argued that admission to a mental hospital may result in what he called a 'mortification' of the patient's self-concept. The restrictions on movement, the need to fit into the ongoing routines of hospital, having to ask permission for, or help with, things previously taken for granted can erode the patient's self-esteem and sense of autonomy. In some cases this results in a state of child-like dependency that could then be interpreted by nurses as *further* evidence of mental illness and psychological deterioration. A particular danger for chronically ill psychiatric patients is that they might become so used to long-term hospital care that they become 'institutionalised' and unable to function in the community. Indeed, the confusion and apathy often found amongst patients in mental hospitals and residential homes may be the result of long-term institutional care and excessive medication, rather than of mental disorder.

Growing realisation that the structure and organisation of mental hospitals were essentially pathogenic led to a number of reforms in the UK from the 1950s, with more mental hospitals developing 'open door' policies, workshops and half-way houses. One of the most radical reforms was the development of 'therapeutic communities' in the 1960s and 1970s, where hospital routines were made more flexible and egalitarian, and attempts were made to break down some of the hierarchical divisions between staff and patients. The 'group' became a therapeutic tool, decisions were made collectively and patients were encouraged to create their own treatments, often by redefining everyday events as part of therapeutic work. As mental hospitals continued to contract and close, the pressure on existing beds increased. Many of these reforms had to be abandoned and mental hospitals began to lose their therapeutic functions and reverted to the warehouses for storing the mentally disordered that they had been in the first half of the twentieth century.

De-institutionalisation and the rise of 'mental health problems'

Between 1950 and 1990, the number of residents in mental hospitals in England and Wales fell from almost 150,000 to under 50,000. During the 1990s and into the twenty-first century the numbers continued to fall, but much more slowly and there was an increase in numbers in 2003/04 (Table 8.3).

There are many reasons for the declining number of residents in mental hospitals in the second part of the twentieth century. First, the development of psychoactive drugs in the 1950s, particularly chlorpromazine, helped control the symptoms of many psychotic conditions, enabling more patients to function outside hospital. Secondly, the cumulative weight of evidence about the negative aspects of long-term institutional care contributed to the movement towards community care. Thirdly, governments confronted by the

Table 8.3 Number of patients under the care of mental health specialists in NHS hospitals.

Year	Number of patients
2001/02	31,006
2002/03	28,605
2003/04	31,230
2004/05	26,097

Source: NHS Information Centre, Crown copyright 2006.

escalating costs of health care, came to favour care in the community as a cheaper option.

It is also important to appreciate the consequences of de-institutionalisation as well as its causes. The asylum (literally meaning 'without cure') represented a clear physical *and* symbolic division between the 'sane' and the 'insane' and its decline has helped to blur this boundary. On the one hand, some conditions previously seen as mental disorders have been 'normalised' (see below); for example, people once seen as 'imbeciles' or suffering from 'mental retardation' are now seen as having 'learning difficulties'. On the other hand, an increasing number of deviant behaviours once seen as odd, immoral or criminal have now been re-classified as symptoms of mental disorder. Between 1975 and 1995 the American Psychiatric Association 'discovered' almost 200 new mental disorders.

Kutchins and Kirk (1997) argue that this process was brought about by psychiatrists looking for a new focus of enquiry with the decline of the asylums. They give a number of examples of what they consider to be non-diseases, such as 'frotteurism' (touching others on public transport) and 'fugue' (travelling abroad under an assumed identity) and 'generalised anxiety disorder' (simply being worried). One of the latest of these new diseases is oniomania, or compulsive buying, a disorder apparently now affecting between 2 and 8% of the adult population in the USA. A major consequence of this development is that millions more people have access to the 'sick role' (Chapter 2) and are therefore not held responsible for their actions.

In short, the decline of the concept of the asylum and the idea of insanity and the rise of the language of mental health problems has brought about a change in the way mental health and mental disorder are conceptualised in contemporary societies. Mental disorder (insanity) and mental health (sanity) are now seen as two poles of a continuum, with the majority of people located somewhere in between (Keys 2002). In contemporary societies few people are really mad, but comparatively few are in good mental health.

Community care

There are many definitions of community care but, in general terms, it means non-institutional care. The idea behind community care is, wherever possible, to give people with mental (and physical) disorders greater autonomy and self-determination, by enabling them to live in the community and, as far as possible, to make choices about their own lives. However, community care does not just refer to a set of policies; it also describes the organisation and delivery of non-institutional care in the real world. It is therefore important to distinguish between community care in *principle* and community care in *practice*.

The principles of community care

The first and most basic principle of community care is to ensure there is suitable accommodation for those with mental disorders living in the community.

This involves support for people who live with their own families, and developing facilities for those who do not, ranging from highly staffed 'hostel wards' and group homes, through shared accommodation with some professional support, to single person flats with minimal support.

A second key principle is to 'normalise' mental disorders as far as possible. This was originally developed with reference to people with 'mental handicap', now called learning disabilities, and later extended to other aspects of mental health where medical intervention, particularly biologically based approaches, had little or no tangible benefit. Normalisation strategies aim to enhance cognitive and social skills and promote ordinary life in three main ways, by providing:

- positive role models;
- a range of practical instruction and skill enhancement activities; and
- by attempting to integrate people with mental disorders into the community.

This involves developing more sources of support within the community, such as day care centres, and modifying social and physical environments in order to preserve or enhance functioning in spite of continuing disabilities. However, despite the laudable aims behind normalisation, ex-patients who are insufficiently independent should not be left to make choices and decisions of which they are incapable. It is, therefore, very important that community nurses make a careful assessment of what can, and cannot be, realistically achieved by a client.

A third key principle of community care is 'de-medicalising', as well as de-institutionalising, the management of care for the mentally disordered. This involves some transfer of responsibility from the NHS to local authorities. Professional intervention, from being the exclusive concern of health care professionals, has now become a multidisciplinary responsibility. The Care Programme Approach (CPA) was introduced in 1990 as a framework for the integrated care of people with mental disorders. Its key elements are:

- the systematic assessment of individuals' health *and* social care needs;
- the formulation of a care plan to address those needs;
- the appointment of a key worker to monitor the delivery of care;
- regular review and, if necessary, amendment of the care plan.

The CPA is based upon collaborative working between health and social services and other relevant local agencies to offer 'front-line' care, casework with long-term chronic cases and 'crisis management', including psychiatric referrals in acute cases. It also stresses the importance of trying to involve service users and their carers in decision making.

The practice of community care

Accommodation

Although there is a legal requirement that people with mental health conditions who are homeless have a 'priority need', available accommodation has not kept up with need. It had been estimated that people with mental disorders are between 30 and 50 times more likely to be homeless than the general population, and that between 30 and 50% of homeless single people have mental health problems (Warnes *et al*. 2003).

Many people with mental disorders are cared for by their families. While some families cope willingly and effectively, others experience great difficulties. Manifestations of mental disorder such as confused speech, muteness or unpredictability may be disruptive, upsetting and difficult to cope with. Families may also be more indirectly affected through the stigma (Chapter 2) they acquire, or feel they acquire, because of their relationship with the ex-patient, and may try to hide the fact of the ex-patient's hospitalisation, and distance themselves from them in various ways.

Normalisation

The success of 'normalisation' strategies and the community care of the mentally disordered, people with learning disabilities and others whose behaviour is unacceptable or difficult to relate to, depends upon their genuine integration into everyday social life. Their mere presence in a community does not equate to *integration* into that community. The evidence is not encouraging. People with mental disorders, and especially ex-mental patients, may be confronted by negative attitudes, discrimination and social exclusion in the community (Corrigan 2005). Such attitudes contribute to the difficulty of setting up 'halfway houses' and other community based treatment schemes for people with mental disorders. The idea that such conditions are essentially incurable persists, and so even people who have recovered from a mental disorder may be avoided and find it difficult to resume their previous work and family roles. It is thus not surprising that a common strategy followed by many former patients is that of 'passing' for normal by hiding the fact of their illness from others. Thus, community care requires more than government action and good health care, it also requires fundamental changes in social attitudes. It is very important that those working with people who have, or have had, mental disorders do not unintentionally 'conspire' with these negative views by unintentionally stigmatising them.

Integration of care

While an integrated approach to community care makes sense in principle, it has been difficult to achieve in practice. A number of critical studies have argued that the CPA is not only failing to provide effective and integrated care but that it was never adequate for the purposes for which it was introduced. Simpson *et al*. (2003) suggest that the main reasons for its failings included a top heavy authoritarian management structure alienating front-line clinical staff, the dedicated pursuit of unrealistic performance targets, inter-agency conflict and poor communication.

Underlying many of the problems associated with the inadequate care of people with mental disorders has been lack of adequate resources. In 2000 the government attempted to address this by designating mental health as a priority in its NHS plan (Chapter 11). Investment in mental health rose from £3.3 billion in 2001/02 to £4.5 billion in 2004/05. However, a great deal of this investment has been absorbed by increased demand (Chapter 10), long-term debts and increasing staff costs, and therefore it has had relatively little impact on improving the delivery of front-line services (Rogers and Pilgrim 2005).

Although institutional care and community care are often seen as alternatives, with the latter increasingly replacing the former, it is also important to appreciate how they are linked in practice. As a result of the diminishing number of hospital beds, a large number of acutely mentally disordered people are either not admitted to hospital or are discharged very quickly after admission. This means that an increasing number of community mental health workers have to spend more of their time managing emergency cases at the expense of their primary and long-term casework. The irony of this is that community mental health teams, specifically set up as an *alternative* to institutional care, have become a major route back into hospitals.

Re-institutionalisation

The movement from institutional to community care should not be exaggerated. First, while the numbers of psychiatric inpatients in Britain have declined sharply since 1955, NHS hospitals remain a major place of treatment, and the estimates of the number of residents in mental hospitals actually rose from 29,900 in 2000 to 31,550 in 2001. Secondly, rates of admission to mental hospitals have risen and patient throughput has more than doubled in the past 10 years, with many hospitals stretched to breaking point and exceeding their 100% occupancy rates. It is now common for patients to be discharged very quickly, only to return to hospital after a period in the community, in a 'revolving door' pattern of care: 15% of discharged patients are re-hospitalised within 3 months and 70% of all admissions are re-admissions. Thirdly, a consequence of the depopulation of long-stay mental hospitals has been a growth in the institutional care of mentally disordered people in prisons and in the private sector (Simpson 2000). In short, not only are many people with mental disorders still being treated in hospitals, but many others have simply exchanged one form of institutional care for another.

With mental hospitals now so overcrowded, criticisms of inadequate care in the community and increasing public fears about the dangers posed by some mentally disordered people, it is impossible to escape the conclusion that while the old asylum system institutionalised too many people, the brave new world of community care has too few hospital beds. It seems that this is a lesson government and health policy makers are starting to learn. The number of forensic beds in the UK is increasing, there are more privately funded secure units and the number of compulsory admissions to psychiatric care has risen. Reviewing the evidence, Priebe and Turner (2003) concluded that 'a new era in mental health care has started – reinstitutionalisation'.

Care or control?

Underlying the work of mental health professionals are two core assumptions: first, there *is* a specific category of diseases called mental disorders and, secondly, those suffering from a mental disorder can, in certain circumstances, be detained and treated without their consent. These two assumptions were challenged in the 1970s and 1980s by a movement that was labelled as 'anti-psychiatry' and some of the issues it raised continue to be relevant for mental health work in contemporary society.

The concept of mental disorder

One of the most influential and radical of the anti-psychiatrists is Szasz (1987) who claimed that there were no such things as mental disorders. He argued that if a person had a recognisable lesion, as in dementia for example, then they have a disease and not a 'mental disease'. However, in mental disorders where there are no identifiable lesions, such as depression, anxiety or various personality disorders, Szasz argued that these are not diseases in any scientific sense because their diagnoses are based on the subjective judgements of psychiatrists about their patients' *behaviour* rather than on any objective evidence of *bodily* symptoms.

Szasz' critique is logical and valid in some areas, but in others it has been overtaken by new research evidence in neuroscience. First, magnetic resonance imaging (MRI) scans are demonstrating beyond reasonable doubt that an increasing number of mental disorders, such as certain types of schizophrenia, are associated with recognisable lesions in the brain. Thus, diagnosis that a patient has schizophrenia can now be based on more than subjective judgements about their behaviour. Secondly, the plausibility of Szasz' critique is based on making a fundamental distinction between mind and body: bodies can be diseased but minds cannot. This view is now increasingly challenged by accumulating evidence that states of mind affect bodily processes and vice versa (Chapter 2). Thus, rather than ruling out the legitimacy of disease of the mind, most researchers today adopt a much more 'interactionist' view of the relationship between mind and body.

Ethics and psychiatric intervention

The second strand of the anti-psychiatry critique concerned the ethics of imposing psychiatric treatment on people. Szasz argued that although the idea of 'mental disorders' had little conceptual validity, it persisted in modern societies because it fulfilled important social functions. First, by defining behaviour that departs from social expectations as 'disease' and offering to cure it, the psychiatric professions are helping to reinforce accepted ways of thinking and behaving, and are sanctioning intolerance of deviation. Secondly, by labelling individuals whose behaviour departs radically from social norms as 'sick' and persuading or compelling them to have 'treatment', psychiatry and psychiatric nursing are acting on behalf of 'societies' rather than 'mentally disordered' patients. From this point of view, psychiatry is much more about the social control of deviant behaviour than about the care of 'sick' individuals.

This critique is still relevant to mental health work in contemporary societies (Chapter 10; Rogers and Pilgrim 2005). The basis of medical and nursing ethics is that health care professionals act as agents of their patients or clients. The fact that many people have not chosen to be treated in mental hospitals, but are there because others, such as family members, managers of residential institutions or the courts, want them there, seems to strike at the heart of this principle. Practices such as the hospital treatment of alcoholics and those with eating disorders, the compulsory admission of mental patients, and the widespread administration of major tranquillisers given without informed consent, raise important ethical issues about the rights of patients and responsibilities of mental health workers.

Anti-psychiatry argued that there should be no ethical or legal distinctions between the care of so-called mental patients and any other patients, and that it is unethical to impose treatment on *any* patient who refuses it. For example, while every effort should be made to help the anorectic patient who is starving herself to death, there is no ethical justification for effectively imprisoning her in a hospital and feeding her against her will. To do so is to impose what Szasz called the 'tyranny of psychiatry' over a defenceless patient.

However, for most commentators, the ethics of such a case are not so clear-cut. The management of a patient who refuses to eat involves a *conflict* between the ethical obligation to respect a patient's autonomy and to act in the patient's best interests. From this basis, taking away a patient's autonomy in the short run (not to eat) may be justified ethically by trying to safeguard their best interests in the longer term (not dying and possibly recovering). If it is judged that a patient's capacity to make a rational autonomous decision is compromised by age, weakness or a distorted body image for example, then it is more likely that health professionals' view of the patient's longer-term best interests will prevail. But this does not mean that mental health workers and the courts can simply ignore patients' wishes whenever they feel they know better. The power to control patients is strictly limited. For example, detaining and forcibly treating a seriously ill anorectic patient would only be ethical and legal providing:

- the patient is judged to be incapable of making a fully autonomous decision;
- the measure is only short term;
- there is no viable alternative.

The value of the anti-psychiatry movement is that it raised neglected questions about the status of mental disorder and the indiscriminate ways that mental health legislation was being used. Indeed, it played a part in helping to change both ethical guidelines and mental health legislation towards greater patient autonomy. However, its weakness was that it made a blanket criticism of psychiatry and all mental health legislation, which it saw as a universally repressive form of social control. Today, the key debate is not about whether psychiatry is a form of social control – something accepted by most mental health professionals – but rather about *how* that social control operates and whether it works in the best interests of patients and wider society in particular cases. It is also important to appreciate that criticisms of psychiatric control have to be balanced against alternatives, such as leaving very disturbed people to fend for themselves, face imprisonment and possibly harm themselves or others.

Summary

Mental disorder covers a wide range of conditions from recognised diseases to behavioural problems that are being treated as if they are diseases. Explanations of mental disorder and models of treatment are mainly based upon biological and psychological theories. Sociological research has drawn attention to the role of wider social influences on the origins and recognition of mental disorder and on the organisation of care. Suicide and eating disorders are recognised complications of mental disorders and it is now generally believed that both are influenced by a combination of biological and social factors. The management and care of self-harming behaviour raises important ethical issues as there may be a conflict between the patient's autonomy and best interests. From the middle of the twentieth century, there was widespread criticism of the institutional care of the mentally disordered, many of whom were seen as needing social care rather than medical treatment. The numbers of people in mental hospitals declined dramatically throughout the second part of the twentieth century and more people were cared for in the community. However, not only has community care failed to live up to the expectations vested in it, but many of those with mental disorders have simply exchanged one form of institutional care for another. More profoundly, the concept of mental disorder is itself contested and some critics have suggested that psychiatric care is more about controlling people than caring for them. However, such critiques have to be balanced against the lack of viable alternatives for the care of people with mental disorders.

References

Beck, A. (1991) Cognitive therapy: a 30 year retrospective. *American Psychologist*, 46, 382–9.

Becker, A. (2004) New global perspectives on eating disorders. *Culture, Medicine and Psychiatry*, 28(4), 433–7.

Bindman, J., Reid, Y., Szmukler, G., Tilley, J., Thornicroft, G. and Leese, M. (2005) Perceived coercion at admission to psychiatric hospital and engagement with follow-up – a cohort study. *Social Psychiatry and Psychiatric Epidemiology*, 40(2), 160–6.

Brown, G. and Harris, T. eds (1989) *Life Events and Illness*. Unwin and Hyman, London.

Bruch, H. (1978) *The Golden Cage: The Enigma of Anorexia*. Open Books, London.

Corrigan, P. ed. (2005) *On the Stigma of Mental Illness*. American Psychiatric Association, Washington DC.

Evans, J., Middleton, N. and Gunnell, D. (2004) Social fragmentation, severe mental illness and suicide. *Social Psychiatry and Psychiatric Epidemiology*, 39(3), 165–70.

Goffman, E. (1991) *Asylums: Essays on the Social Situation of Mental Patients and Other Inmates*. Penguin, London.

Hoek, H. and van Hoeken, D. (2003) Review of the prevalence and incidence of eating disorders. *International Journal of Eating Disorders*, 34(4), 383–96.

Hooley, J., Woodberry, K. and Ferriter, C. (2005) Family factors in schizophrenia and bipolar disorder, in J. Hudson and R. Rapee (eds) *Psychopathology and The Family*. Elsevier, New York, 205–23.

Keys, C. (2002) The mental health continuum: from languishing to flourishing. *Journal of Health and Social Behaviour*, 43(2), 207–22.

Kong, S. (2005) Day treatment programme for patients with eating disorders: randomised control trial. *Journal of Advanced Nursing*, 51(1), 5–14.

Kutchins, H. and Kirk, A. (1997) *Making Us Crazy*. Free Press, New York.

Laing, R. and Esterson, A. (1964) *Sanity, Madness and the Family*. Penguin, London.

Link, B. and Phelan, B. (2001) On stigma and its consequences. *Annual Review of Sociology*, 27, 363–85.

Littlewood, R. (2004) Globalisation, culture, body image and eating disorders. *Culture, Medicine and Psychiatry*, 28(4), 597–602.

Lock, J. (2004) Family approaches for anorexia and bulimia nervosa, in J. Thompson (ed.) *Handbook of Eating Disorders and Obesity*. Wiley, New Jersey, 218–31.

Philo, G., Secker J. and Platt S. (1996) Media images of mental distress, in T. Heller, J. Renolds, R. Gomm, R. Muston and S. Pattison (eds) *Mental Health Matters*. Open University, Buckingham.

Pike, K. and Borovoy, A. (2004) The rise of eating disorders in Japan: issues of culture and limitations of the model of 'westernisation'. *Culture, Medicine and Psychiatry*, 28(4), 493–531.

Priebe, S. and Turner, T. (2003) Reinstitutionalisation in mental health care. *British Medical Journal*, 326, 175–6.

Rogers, A. and Pilgrim, D. (2005) *A Sociology of Mental Health and Illness*, 3rd edition. Open University Press, Buckingham.

Rosenhan, D. (1973) On being sane in insane places. *Science*, 179, 250–8.

Scheff, T.J. (1966) *Being Mentally Ill: A Sociological Theory*. Aldine, Chicago.

Simpson, A. (2000) Private care's win, win. *Mental Health Nursing*, 20, 6–9.

Simpson, A., Miller, C. and Bowers, L. (2003) The history of the care programme approach in England. Where did it go wrong? *Journal of Mental Health*, 12(5), 489–504.

Skapinakis, P., Lewis, G., Araya, R., Jones, K. and Williams, G. (2005) Mental health inequalities in Wales: multi-level investigation of the effect of area deprivation. *British Journal of Psychiatry*, 186(5), 417–22.

Skegg, K. (2005) Self harm. *Lancet*, 366, 1471–83.

Stengel, E. (1973) *Suicide and Attempted Suicide*. Penguin, Harmondsworth.

Szasz, T. (1987) *Insanity: The Idea and its Consequences*. Wiley: New York.

Warnes, A., Carne, M., Whitehead, N. and Fu, R. (2003) *Homelessness Factfile*. Crisis, London.

Further reading

Busfield, J. ed. (2001) *Rethinking the Sociology of Mental Health*. Blackwell, Oxford.
A collection of original articles by leading sociologists on conceptual and diagnostic issues, mental health policy and professional practice.

Pilgrim, D. and Rogers, A. (2005) *A Sociology of Mental Health and Illness*, 3rd edition. Open University, Buckingham.
A general review of the key areas of sociological research, including theories and perspectives, social divisions, mental health work and psychiatry and legal control.

Video/DVD

Eating disorders from Halovine [www.halovine.com]

Websites

The Mental Health Foundation: www.mentalhealth.org.uk
www.mind.org.uk
www.samaritans.org.uk – *provides a lot of data on suicide and self-harm*
www.nationaleatingdisorders.org

Chapter 9

Death and dying

Death has both real and symbolic significance in our society, raising questions about the meaning of life, the definition of death, moral and ethical questions about euthanasia, end of life care and disclosing that a patient is dying. All these occur in the context of an ageing, multi-cultural, society where different groups have different beliefs, values and priorities in relation to death. Nurses are the main group of staff involved in the care of people who are dying in all settings of care and thus are intimately involved in and affected by these questions and dilemmas.

This chapter begins by considering one of the main determinants of the experience of dying: where dying and death occur. It also considers influential models of dying and bereavement, communication about and awareness of dying, and end of life issues. While miscarriage, stillbirth and the deaths of infants and children are of concern, in this chapter we concentrate upon adults, especially at older ages, as this is when most deaths occur. The chapter will:

- summarise the historical context of death in Britain;
- identify and discuss patterns of dying in different settings;
- discuss changing patterns of communication about, and awareness of, dying;
- discuss current models of bereavement;
- discuss euthanasia and end of life care.

Death in contemporary Britain

Over the course of the twentieth century dramatic changes occurred in the patterns of death and dying in Britain. In 1901 life expectancy at birth was 49 for women and 45 for men, which has now increased to over 80 for both sexes, mainly because of the decrease in infant mortality from 19–13% in 1901 to less than 1%. Life expectancy of adults increased more slowly, but by the century's end over 80% of the population could expect to reach the age of 65. In the twenty-first century survival beyond 65 continues to increase, with a substantial minority of the population over the age of 80 (Chapter 6). Over 80% of deaths in contemporary Britain occur in those aged 65 or older. Acute infectious diseases have been superseded by long-term chronic conditions as the major causes of death. Whereas formerly people would experience a number of deaths among those with whom they were closely associated, in the present era children rarely experience the death of a close friend or family member, and even for adolescents and adults such deaths are uncommon. Deaths from drug and alcohol abuse among young people are increasing rapidly and suicide is now the major cause of death among those aged below 35.

Most deaths result from chronic and degenerative diseases affecting primarily middle-aged and older adults. At the start of the twenty-first century, diseases of the circulatory system account for about 30% of all deaths, cancer is the cause of about 25%, and diseases of the respiratory system account for about 22% of all deaths. Most of the attention to death and dying of adults in contemporary Britain has focused upon cancer. Cancer patients receive the bulk of hospice and specialist palliative care services, but there has been an increasing recognition that those (generally older) people dying from heart disease, strokes and respiratory diseases are equally in need of specialist palliative care (Skilbeck and Payne, 2005). In 2005 the British government explicitly acknowledged that access to such specialist services should be based upon need rather than diagnostic category and must be extended to other disease categories.

Individualisation and medicalisation

Another major change during the twentieth century was the institutionalisation and 'medicalisation' of death. With the shift of the normal place of death from the home to a hospital or other institution, the management and control of death and dying increasingly shifted from lay management and religious authority to the medical profession. Death came to be defined as a medical event that must be validated by doctors, and dying came to be thought of primarily in terms of the management and treatment of disease. In 2003 only 18% of deaths occurred at home and 80% occurred in hospitals, hospices or nursing or residential homes (Table 9.1). Men are significantly more likely to

Table 9.1 Place of death, England and Wales, 2003.

Place of death	Male (%)	Female (%)	All (%)
NHS hospital	60	56	58
Nursing homes	7	13	10
Residential homes	4	10	7
Hospice	4.5	4	4
All institutional*	76	83	80
At home	21	15	18
Other	3	1.5	2
Number of deaths	253,852	284,402	538,254

* Includes non-NHS psychiatric hospitals.
Due to rounding, percentages do not sum to 100.
Source: Calculated from table 17, Mortality Statistics, General: Review of the Registrar General on Death in England and Wales 2003, Office of National Statistics: www.statistics.gov.uk

die in their own home than women, who are much more likely to die in a nursing or residential home. This is explained partly by the greater longevity of women.

Relatively few people in our society die as a result of sudden and unexpected deaths. The majority of unexpected deaths of young people are caused by accidents, only a minority of which reach a hospital. Among older people, heart attacks and strokes are the main causes of sudden, unexpected death. Again, most victims die prior to entry to the hospital, and those that do reach hospital may be treated in intensive or coronary care units.

A number of scholars have suggested that dying and mourning became highly individualised in modern societies as a consequence of the reduced immediacy of death and the decline of religion, meaning there were few of the collective family and community rituals that in previous eras made sense of death and supported the bereaved (see Seale 1998). Thus, when they are faced with coping with their own death or that of someone close to them people had to come to terms with this unfamiliar event without the help of clear collective rules, and with little support from the wider community. An important source of 'meaning making' in contemporary society may be the plethora of media stories and autobiographical accounts (usually about cancer) that provide 'templates' for how to manage a 'good dying' and 'appropriate mourning'. In contemporary Britain dying from cancer is particularly feared, and seems to act as a metaphor for more general and widespread anxieties about dying and death and provides a model for the 'good death' (Seale 1998).

Illich (1990) claimed that the increasing 'medicalisation' of life undermined people's ability to manage their own health and to cope with the pain and suffering that are an inevitable part of the human condition (Chapter 2). It also meant that death is seen less as an inevitable part of life and much more as a failure of treatment, signalling the end of 'natural death'. Brown and Webster (2004) identified three consequences of the medicalisation and clinical definition of death in late modern society. First, the process of dying is prolonged by the use of life-extending technologies [most dramatically in intensive care units (ITUs)]. Secondly, the loss of control over death experienced by dying people (especially by elderly people and in institutional settings). Thirdly, and more contentiously, is the medical administration of death, 'whereby the dying and the dead need to be accounted for in terms of the economic costs their end of life clinical care will incur'.

Although death is no longer a 'taboo' subject in contemporary Britain, it remains largely hidden from public view (Seale 1998). The solution for many people is to place the onus for dealing with death and dying upon doctors and nurses, although doctors and nurses may themselves have difficulty coping with the wider questions about the meaning of death. An important element of nursing work with dying people and their families involves dealing with such questions. Timmermans (2005) argues that medical authorities 'now broker the existentially frightening and ambiguous aspects of death and dying', making a death culturally acceptable and explaining its inevitability. 'Death brokering' involves establishing 'the acceptable line between curing or letting go' and achieving a 'good' rather than a 'bad' death.

The main places of care

This section focuses on the places where dying occurs, and the role of nurses in the care of the dying. The places where dying occurs are not necessarily the same as the place where people actually die: while less than a third of deaths occur in the places where people live, the majority of care takes place in these domestic and care homes. Seymour *et al.* (2005) provide an excellent review of the places of end of life care for older people. There may be a lot of interchange between home, hospital and hospice, with the involvement of a wide range of hospital, community and specialist palliative care services over the course of an advanced condition. The co-ordination of these various lay, statutory, voluntary and commercial sources of help (Figure 9.1) to provide 'joined up' or 'seamless' care for those who are dying has been recognised by government in its National Service Frameworks, as central to effective end of life care.

Dying in a hospital

NHS hospitals are the major sites of death in our society. Most of these deaths are of adults beyond middle life. The shift towards community care (Chapters 8, 10) has meant that NHS hospitals have mainly become places of acute, intensive, short stay treatment with long-term care being managed in the community (including residential and nursing homes). Hospital specialist staff (including nurses) working with patients with chronic advanced conditions are likely to be involved in the management of their care in the community. In 2003 circulatory diseases accounted for two-fifths of all hospital deaths, cancers for one-fifth, and respiratory diseases for just under a fifth. A significant number of deaths in hospitals occur over a relatively short period of time and death is a rare occurrence in many hospital settings. However, people in their last year of life take up nearly a quarter of hospital beds.

Our understanding of dying in hospitals is largely based upon studies of cancer settings, where dying took place over a long period of time and death was anticipated by the staff, and sometimes by patients (but see Field 1989, Seymour 2001). Many of the insights from the early studies of cancer deaths are still valid. For example, the *time* over which death occurs and its *predictability* are still major factors affecting how staff experience terminal illness and treat dying patients (Glaser and Strauss 1965). In general, hospital staff have most difficulty in dealing with quick and unexpected deaths and are most comfortable with deaths that are predictable and which can be prepared for. Another important factor is the *age* of the patient. In our society people find it is easier to accept the death of old people than of young people. In particular, nurses find it psychologically difficult to nurse infants and young children who are terminally ill, and people of their own age with whom they may identify, such as those with cancer or AIDS. Finally, as discussed below, communication and disclosure of information are central to the care of dying patients.

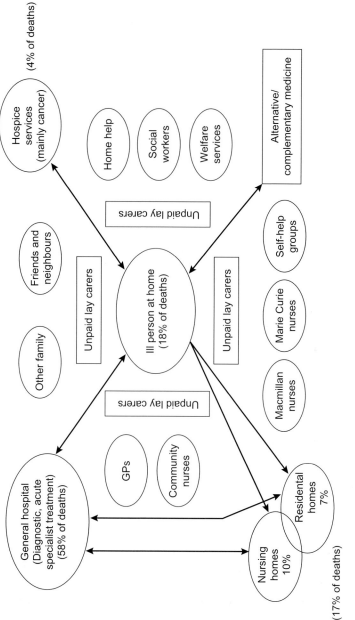

Figure 9.1 Sources of help for people who are dying.

Source: Field, D. and James, N. (1993) Where and how people die, in D. Clark (ed.) *The Future for Palliative Care*. Open University Press, Milton Keynes. Reproduced by permission of the Open University Press.

A number of developments, especially in more effective and reliable pain and symptom control, more widespread understanding of the benefits of palliative care and the introduction of specialist palliative care teams have improved the care of dying hospital patients, although this still seems to vary widely, both within and between hospitals. The number of staff involved in such care has increased, and the co-ordination of the various elements of the treatment of terminal conditions has become more complex. This means that the interdisciplinary co-ordination of care is important. Nurses, who are at the centre of care delivery, may thus be confronted with delicate and difficult tasks of negotiating potentially conflicting treatments and 'do not resuscitate orders' with doctors and others. Because of their continuous and close contact with the dying patient, nurses may become aware of the need for a shift to palliative care before doctors. It seems that it is still often difficult for the latter to move from therapeutic, and possibly aggressive, management of disease towards a pattern of care where other needs of patients and their quality of life are seen as primary.

The continuing development of clinical technology and knowledge has led to sophisticated interventions into matters of living and dying, and demands on trained nurses continue to increase (Chapter 12). However, Timmermans (2005) and Seymour (2001) suggest that this allows hospital staff to orchestrate an apparently 'natural' and inevitable 'good' death. For nurses, hospital deaths may raise questions of skill mix and responsibility, and cause difficulties in delivering patient-centred terminal care in accordance with the knowledge and expertise which nursing has developed. Changes in working patterns also affect the emotional involvement that develops between nurses and patients, perhaps making these more transitory and less intense. Yet, given the nature of nursing work, emotional involvement with some dying patients, especially long-term patients in specialist units, is likely to develop, with a sense of loss when the patient dies. However, while nursing a dying person may be stressful, Vachon's (1995) comprehensive review of the evidence suggests that the main source of such stresses is the work environment; for example, unclear boundaries and responsibilities and pressures on nurses to achieve managerial targets for discharging patients (Chapter 12).

In their study of nursing dying people in hospital, Hopkinson *et al.* (2003) described a number of commonalities and tensions. One source of tension is between the ideals that nurses had for providing good care and a 'good death' and the actual things that they saw and did in that care. For example, rapid or unexpected deterioration could be distressing. Another source of tension were things that were outside the nurses' knowledge or experience that they had to grapple with, such as responding to the question 'Am I going to die?'. Some of these could be addressed by asking advice from other, more senior, nurses. A final source of tension was the sense of 'aloneness' resulting from the unique experiences that nurses had with dying patients and their relatives. The 'personal reality differed for each of the nurses and, like the personal ideal changed across time with new experiences of caring for dying people' (Hopkinson *et al.* 2003: 529). Hopkinson *et al.* identified three factors that could prevent or resolve the tensions of nursing dying patients: supportive relationships with other staff; making assumptions about what course of action they should follow; and controlling their emotions. These allowed the nurses to be personally comfortable and to accept and be satisfied with their care and the subsequent death of a patient.

Care in the home

Although less than one-fifth of deaths occur in the domestic home, about 90% of the care of these people will take place in their own homes with the help and unpaid work of their close family and friends ('lay' carers, Chapter 10). Gomes and Higginson (2006) found that frequent home care visits from health care staff, living with a relative and being able to count on support from the extended family were strongly associated with cancer patients dying at home. Men are much more likely to die at home than women, especially older women (Storey *et al*. 2003). People who die at home will normally do so as the result of a long-term illness, often marked by persistent and distressing symptoms. It is thus highly likely that at some time they will have been admitted to a hospital or (in cases of cancer) a hospice for treatment of their condition.

While home deaths are seen as desirable, it must be recognised that carers and patients have different needs and attitudes. For the dying person the main advantages are that the familiar environment can provide psychological comfort, reassurance and support. They are also more likely to be able to retain greater autonomy and control of what happens to them than in an institution, at least during the time they retain mobility and mental clarity. For their lay carers, caring can be rewarding, maintaining and perhaps reinforcing family ties. It has been suggested that lay carers will cope better with their bereavement if they can take an active part in care, and this is easier at home than in a formal institution.

The *possibility* of a 'home death' depends primarily on the human resources available to help both patients and carers, and input from community nurses often plays a crucial role (Storey *et al*. 2003, Gomes and Higginson 2006). However, the physical and social costs for those caring on their own or with little outside help may be substantial, making their care work tiring and even a burden. Although many carers wish to look after their relative at home, a range of factors may make this difficult or impossible. The two main problems for home care are the adequate control of symptoms (where community nurses play a major role) and the constant attendance and extra domestic work that such care entails. Failure in either or both of these will lead to institutional care. Another factor is that some carers (and patients) feel that a home death would make it difficult for them to continue living in their home following the death.

Changes in population and social structure mean that there are now more people without family or relatives to provide unpaid home care (Chapter 10). Older women are particularly likely to be affected by this. The physical help and social support given by general practitioners and community nurses and their access to other resources of help is thus vital. Having an outsider to talk to and to ask advice from can be a source of social support and may help lay carers keep a sense of perspective. A community nurse may also be very important in negotiating inpatient care when it is necessary and in helping lay carers to come to terms with the fact they can no longer manage on their own.

In their systematic review of the factors influencing home deaths of terminally ill cancer patients Gomes and Higginson (2006) identified a number of illness-related, individual and environmental factors that influenced the likelihood of dying at home or in a hospital (Figure 9.2). Environmental factors were the most influential. Low functional status, an expressed preference for a home death, the presence of home care (with frequent visits), living with relatives and being able to count on support from the extended family were all strongly associated with death at home. They suggest that 'patients with non-solid tumours may be less likely to die at home because they have multiple options for treatment, even in the advanced stage of their disease. Their transition and referral to palliative care is often blurry and missed'. This is similar to patients with chronic cardio-pulmonary conditions (Exley *et al.* 2005) and it seems likely that these factors would also influence where terminally ill patients with long-term chronic conditions die.

External support is more available for cancer patients and their carers than for those dying from chronic non-malignant conditions. This partly reflects the higher priority given to people with cancer and partly the difficulty of recognising when dying is imminent for people where the continuing benefits of therapeutic admissions to hospital may persist until the admission during which the patient dies (Exley *et al.* 2005, Skilbeck and Payne 2005).

Hospice care

Hospice care in the UK originally focused around inpatient centres of excellence providing a 'good' pain free and aware death made possible by attending to the physical, psychological, social and spiritual needs of dying people ('holistic care') in a homely environment. Since the mid-1960s, when there were only a few, mainly inpatient units, hospice and specialist palliative care services have expanded dramatically and now take a variety of forms (Table 9.2). Hospices have now become integral to national plans and policies for the delivery of palliative care services and have strongly influenced the care of dying people in other settings. For 2003/04, the Hospice Information Service estimated 58,000 hospice admissions and 155,000 patients seen by community services. Hospice services are mainly offered to cancer patients (95%) but people with other conditions, such as motor neuron disease, may also be referred to them. Older people and those from minority ethnic groups (Firth 2001) are underrepresented among users of hospice and specialist palliative care services.

Referral to a hospice or specialist palliative care service is an important signal that an illness is regarded as 'terminal', conveying the message that death, if not imminent, is not too far away. This may lead to discussions with the person who is dying about their concerns and wishes. Talking about the

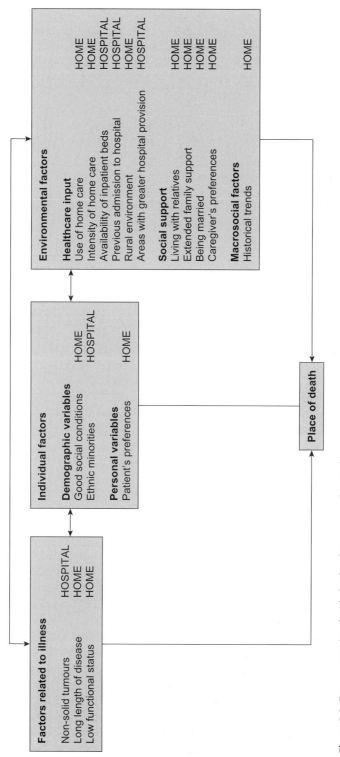

Figure 9.2 Factors associated with death at home or in a hospital.

Source: Gomes, B. and Higginson, I. (2006) Factors influencing death at home in terminally ill patients with cancer: systematic review. *British Medical Journal*, 332, 516–21, Figure 4, Reproduced with permission from the BMJ Publishing Group.

Table 9.2 Hospice and palliative care services in the UK and Ireland, 2006.

Voluntary inpatient units (2515 beds)*	158
NHS inpatient units (665 beds)	63
Children's hospices (242)	34
Day care hospices/centres	257
Home care services	356
'Hospice-at-Home'	114
Hospital nurses	47
Hospital support teams	305

*Includes three services (50 beds) exclusively for HIV/AIDS.
Source: Hospice Information Service: www.hospiceinformation.info/factsand figures.asp

person's death and dying is expected to be one of the strengths of hospice staff and is central to addressing psychological, social and spiritual aspects of dying. The hospice approach of holistic care aims to encourage the expression of all forms of pain so that they may be attended to. Thus, the nurse's role in supporting the patient is based on an understanding of the patient's emotions and not simply a narrow focus upon their physical pain. This inevitably leads to some emotional involvement with patients and those close to them, although this is more likely to be seen as rewarding than as a source of distress. Important components of coping with the inevitable deaths of patients are staff support and 'permission to grieve' (which may be denied to nurses in other settings). The supportive environment of the hospices and their focus on agreed goals of care should mean that there are fewer major difficulties of workplace stress than elsewhere (Vachon 1995).

The nature of referral as an inpatient to hospices has changed significantly, with many patients admitted for short-term symptom management. Continuing symptom appraisal and management may occur as part of hospice day care visits. An important result of this changing pattern is that the length of time that inpatients stay in hospices has reduced significantly, but that re-admissions are more common. Another significant change is that the proportion of inpatients with difficult to manage and distressing symptoms has increased. One such group are patients with bodies that are disfigured, with seeping fluids or unpleasant smells: what Lawton (2000) describes as 'unbounded bodies'. She describes how such patients move from being socially valued individuals to increasingly isolated objects of self-disgust as their bodily disintegration leads to their social and physical separation from others and their withdrawal from social interaction. Nursing such 'dirty' dying patients is a challenge to the hospice philosophy of enabling patients to live until they die with all their needs attended to, and challenges the ability to achieve the desired 'good' and dignified death.

Dying in an institutional care home

Changes in the NHS since the 1990s have meant that nursing homes have largely replaced long-stay hospital wards for longer-term symptom management and nursing care. Greater numbers of dying people are now admitted to nursing homes from NHS hospitals than previously, and inpatient hospices are also referring patients for admission to nursing homes. In 2003 17% of all deaths (11% of all men, 23% of all women) died in nursing and residential homes (Table 9.1). These were mainly people over the age of 65. The new elderly resident often sees entry into the care home as the final move of their life. As Froggatt (2004) notes, such a move may involve a number of losses, including companionship from family and friends.

In their discussion Field and Froggatt (2003) point out that most people living in institutional homes are there either because they have no one to care for them at home or because such carers can no longer do so. They note that the challenge for care homes is to provide supportive care for both their 'fit' and 'frail' residents and end of life care for those approaching death. Perhaps the most fundamental challenge is the pattern of morbidity and the nature of dying found in care homes. Compared to those living in their own or a relative's home, care home residents are more likely to:

- be suffering from chronic and long-term conditions;
- have significantly greater restrictions of their activities;
- have higher levels of mental confusion;
- have higher levels of incontinence, impaired sight and hearing.

The majority of residents die from chronic conditions other than cancer and are likely to have long-term multiple clinical conditions which may make it unclear whether or not they are actually dying (Froggatt 2004). Katz and Peace (2003) found that 42% of the deaths in their study were the result of 'general deterioration' (51% in nursing homes) and that only 9% were from an already recognized terminal illness. Thus, it may be difficult for residents to become involved in decisions about how their end of life care should be managed.

Care homes typically have very limited resources and only nursing homes have trained nursing staff and health care assistants. The low level of trained staff means that it may be difficult to manage the needs of residents living with ongoing chronic conditions, and adds to the difficulties caused by the disease profile of residents for recognising and meeting their needs for end of life care. General practitioners and community nurses may play a vital role in the care of residents, and the contributions – or lack of them – from external sources significantly influence the care of dying residents. For example, general practitioners are the primary resource for pain control and referral to palliative care services. However, if nursing home staff are trained for end of life care but general practitioners are not, conflicts can occur, for example over pain management.

Admission from care homes to hospitals is less likely to occur than from domestic homes. When hospitals (and hospices) transfer patients with advanced diseases to nursing homes this may occur so close to death that it is inappropriate. Few care homes use hospice and specialist palliative care services, although there are a number of initiatives to improve specialist input (Froggatt 2004). Although local hospices are potential sources for the management of difficult symptoms and for terminal care, access to them may be difficult for care home residents, particularly those with conditions other than cancer.

In many homes acknowledgement of death and dying is not overt. In part this may reflect negative societal attitudes towards older people (Chapter 6). Where death is accepted and integrated with living (e.g. in homes run by religious organisations), staff, residents and relatives may be able to talk openly about forthcoming events, including the possibility of dying. In such homes the bereavement needs of other residents are also more likely to be appreciated and attended to.

Communication and disclosure

Talking with dying people and their carers about a patient's terminal illness is a difficult, although often rewarding (Field 1989), part of nursing work. The seminal work of Glaser and Strauss (1965) identified four types of 'awareness contexts' that have profound consequences for the experiences of dying patients. These are:

- *closed awareness*, where staff kept patients in ignorance of their impending death, usually with the co-operation and agreement of their relatives;
- *suspicion awareness*, where patients suspected that they were dying and tried to get staff and relatives to confirm this suspicion;
- *mutual pretence*, where all parties knew that the patient was dying but did not acknowledge this, pretending that 'everything was normal'; and
- *open awareness*, where all parties knew about and acknowledged that the patient was dying.

They found that 'closed awareness' contexts were preferred by staff for a number of reasons, including their uncertainty about when death might occur and to 'protect' patients from adverse psychological reactions to disclosure, such as depression and anxiety. Closed awareness also allowed hospital staff and relatives to avoid the emotionally difficult task of talking about the terminal diagnosis and its meaning for the patient. However, closed awareness was hard to sustain and it tended to 'break down' and become transformed into 'suspicion' or 'mutual pretence'. Their work, and that of other researchers, suggested a number of negative consequences of the closed awareness context for patients:

- the physical and social withdrawal of staff and relatives from the patient;
- isolation and loneliness;
- increased uncertainty and anxiety;
- a sense of betrayal resulting from the restricted information and communication about their condition and its progression.

Open awareness contexts are thought to prevent or resolve these negative consequences, to enable more informed and more effective management of pain and other symptoms and to facilitate patient acceptance of, and preparation for, their death. However, this is a distinctly 'anglophone' perspective. In other cultures (e.g. Italy and Japan) closed awareness is seen as protecting the

---

Box 9.1 Types of open awareness

- **Suspended open awareness** Here, although the information has been given, the tacit understanding is that the patient's impending death will not be discussed or publicly acknowledged. This may be a temporary, initial, reaction or it may persist. Suspended open awareness may re-appear in situations where unexpected decline or improvement occur.
- **Uncertain open awareness** This results from the tendency of doctors to control the information given to patients by withholding, softening or otherwise modifying the 'clinical truth' about prognosis. A key element is the attempt by doctors and nurses to use uncertainty about outcome to maintain a 'margin for hope'.
- **Active open awareness** All parties understand and accept that recovery from the impending death is not possible and try to come to terms with this (Glaser and Strauss's original concept).

---

dying person from distress and many groups within culturally diverse societies such as Britain and the USA also take this view.

In practice, 'open awareness' appears to be ambiguous and conditional, with patients at one moment recognising, acknowledging and preparing for their death and at a subsequent time apparently denying that they are dying. Timmermans (1994) argued that reactions vary within and between patients and distinguished three types of open awareness (Box 9.1). Copp and Field (2002) suggested that within the overall context of open awareness patients may use 'denial' and 'acceptance' of dying as strategies to avoid threats and to preserve existing relationships.

Despite the evidence that in contemporary Britain both health workers and the general public prefer the management of dying in an open awareness context, this is often difficult to achieve, especially in long-term non-malignant conditions where uncertainty about the likely time of death may persist and where timing the move from an essentially 'curative/restorative' focus of treatment to 'palliative care' may be difficult to determine. Many nurses and doctors find the task of actually transmitting this information very difficult and stressful, and few have received adequate training in appropriate communication skills. Even when nurses believe that talking openly about death is the right thing to do, if they are uncomfortable about doing it they are likely to avoid or limit their contact with dying patients. This is especially likely to occur where death is uncommon, where there is little team support to nurses, and where there is no clearly formulated policy regarding disclosure.

In their day-to-day encounters with dying patients, research has found that health workers moderate and back away from automatic disclosure of a terminal prognosis (Field and Copp 1999). Reasons given for withholding or modifying the information given to terminally ill patients are:

- the patient's level of comprehension;
- the stage of the illness;

- the mental competence of patients;
- the severity of illness;
- to maintain hope;
- moral scruples.

Field and Copp (1999) suggested that a pragmatic and responsive pattern of communication and disclosure that recognises the rights of patients to full information and open awareness, while acknowledging that not all patients will want this, seems appropriate. This may be particularly important with patients from some cultural and religious backgrounds. However, one danger of adopting this approach is that nurses and doctors might not provide opportunities for patients to discuss their dying, thus preventing them from voicing their wishes and needs, which may remain unrecognised or misunderstood and unmet. Nurses must balance the advantages of openness and the respect for the emotional, cultural and informational needs of patients who do not wish to receive full disclosure, in such a way as to facilitate responsive, informed patient choice.

Bereavement

Both dying and bereavement have personal and social aspects: not only are personal attachments lost, but so are social relationships, connections and activities. For example, both the dying person and their partner will lose their relationship to each other and the shared social activities in which they participated as a couple. Attachment to others is a source of emotional and psychological strength and support, and a source of social cohesion (Chapter 2), but it is also a source of pain, loss and distress when attachments are under threat or severed. Further, as noted above, the experiences of dying and grieving, both before and after the death, are greatly affected by social and physical circumstances, such as where dying and death takes place, the types of communication between those involved, and the social support available.

The care received by the deceased person during their terminal illness has an important influence upon the bereaved person's experience of bereavement. In hospitals the main focus of nursing work and concern with dying people is with specific individuals, with little sustained provision (or capacity) to care for the grief and mourning of relatives and friends. These are more likely to be the province of general practitioners and community nurses, although the research evidence suggests that most bereaved people have no sustained bereavement-related contact with professional carers.

Psychological approaches

In contemporary Britain the education of nurses about bereavement has drawn primarily from psychodynamic, individual-centred understandings of grief and loss, although it is recognised that social dimensions such as age, gender, community affiliation and social attachment shape and influence individual responses to bereavement (Payne *et al.* 1999). 'Psycho-dynamic' models typically portray bereavement as a process during which the grieving individual passes through a number of phases or stages over a period of time (Payne *et al.* 1999: 70–83). 'Normal' reactions to bereavement have been described as occurring in approximately sequential but overlapping phases lasting about 2 years, although there are differences between people in terms of both the duration and form of each phase.

Typically the initial shock, disbelief and 'numbness' following the death may last from a few hours to a week. This is often followed by a chaotic period characterised by anger, distress, restlessness and 'searching' for the lost person. Denial may also occur. In this period of acute grief, the bereaved person may vacillate between seeking reminders of the dead person to assuage their sense of loss and avoiding them in order to escape from their grief. Familiar places, activities and sounds may all vividly recall the dead person, and many people report talking with, hearing or seeing the dead person. This is seen as a crucial stage where the reality of the death becomes confirmed and accepted. The bereaved person may experience a number of physical symptoms, such as weight loss and sleep disturbance.

This period is followed by a time marked by disorganisation and sometimes despair as the person comes to grips with their various losses and changes of activities, begins to learn new skills and develops new patterns of living. Finally, it is proposed, a stable pattern of life may be achieved when the person has resolved the problem of retaining their connection with the dead person while 'letting them go' and continuing with their own life. Individuals may become 'stuck' or move 'backwards' and 'forwards' between stages, and emotions may fluctuate over time. This generic model suggests that the 'work' of grief involves a process of 'letting go' of the dead person in order to return to normal social and psychological functioning.

The dual-process model (Stroebe and Schut 1999) draws upon theories of stress and coping to move beyond the view of bereavement as a generally unilinear progression of the individual through time. In particular, it criticises the pyscho-dynamic emphasis on intra-psychic processing (thinking and feeling) and its neglect of interpersonal relationships. Bereavement involves not only the loss of the dead person but also the subsequent changes that happen to the bereaved person. They stress that there is an oscillation between a 'loss orientation' (focusing on the deceased and the death, confronting and dwelling upon their loss) and a 'restoration orientation' (the practical tasks of adjusting to a new pattern of life). Both of these aspects must be dealt with, and healthy adaptation is a dynamic process involving both expressing and controlling emotions and dealing with concurrent life changes. Both 'loss' and 'restoration' related behaviours are important in coming to terms with bereavement and will vary according to gender, social and cultural background and personal circumstances. By moving the focus of explanation away from loss, the dual-process model directs attention to the variety of emotional and practical 'coping tasks' involved in adjustment to bereavement. However, despite the acknowledged role played by social factors, the focus remains firmly upon the individual.

Social approaches

During the 1990s sociological analysis of how grief is shaped by the social contexts and relationships of the bereaved strengthened our understanding of the centrality of the social dimensions of bereavement. The work by Riches and Dawson (2000) on parental and sibling responses to the death of a child shows how parents draw upon social networks and cultural ideas to make sense of and adapt to their grief. It also integrates existing evidence with their own research to show how the different socially patterned responses of men ('stoic' control of emotions, focus upon practical tasks) and women (expressing emotion) to their loss may create strains between partners.

Talking to other people about the deceased is an important way of establishing the meaning of relationships (Walter 1999). In his analysis of the variety of ways that bereaved people reshape their relationships with those who have died Walter challenged the assumption that grief is 'resolved' by 'moving on' from and 'letting go of' one's connection with the person who has died. On the contrary, many people want to 'hold on' to and remember those who have died and continue to include them in their lives in a variety of ways. To do so does not mean that they have somehow 'failed' to resolve their grief, or are grieving 'pathologically'.

Secular and religious ceremonies associated with the disposal of the dead body perform both psychological and social functions by confirming and reinforcing the fact of death. They also serve to validate the social worth of the deceased, to confirm the relationship of the mourners to them and to each other, and may mobilise social support for the bereaved. These are important functions because grieving may become complicated when the fact of death is uncertain or denied, e.g. when there is no body, and social isolation and lack of support are associated with difficulties with grieving. Elaborate rituals extending over a period of time can be found in some communities. These may serve to limit and guide mourning and to shape social support by providing a structure in which there is a gradual tapering off of the connection of the bereaved with the dead person. Secular ceremonies have become increasingly common in contemporary Britain.

Despite the significant developments in understanding grief and bereavement outlined above, most health workers and counsellors appear to work with implicit 'stage/phase' models that see bereavement as something to be 'worked through' to guide their understanding of bereavement and their work with bereaved people who need their help. It is important that nurses are aware of these new developments and that they become integrated into their practice, they are to assess the extent of the impact of the loss of bereavement, the nature of people's responses to it and recognise when it is appropriate to offer additional bereavement support services (Box 9.2).

End of life issues

An important consequence of the increasing ability of medical intervention to influence and control the process of dying is that death has become more

---

Box 9.2 Social aspects of bereavement

- Experiencing loss is a normal part of everyone's life and most people are resilient and have sufficient resources, in terms of their personal experiences of coping, existential and spiritual understandings, and a social network of family and friends to draw upon.
- Bereaved people will draw upon their cultural, social and spiritual understandings to provide meaning for their loss and to determine their behaviour and expression of their grief. These may be different from those of the nurse.
- Bereaved people display their grief in different ways in different environments, and these displays are largely socially prescribed. A failure to appear distressed when meeting a nurse does not mean that they can not or will not display their distress elsewhere, nor does it imply that they do not feel distressed.
- Grief hurts both physically and psychologically, and because of the loss of the dead person, bereaved people sometimes may no longer have their normal sources of social support. Socially isolated people may be in need of additional support.
- Bereaved people experience changes in their social roles, e.g. a wife becomes a widow, a parent may become childless, which changes how they are perceived by others and eventually how they perceive themselves. Adjusting to these new and changed social roles may be difficult and take time to accomplish.
- Providing an opportunity for a bereaved person to talk about the dead person and the process of their dying and death may be helpful, especially when they have concerns about the adequacy of the care provided to the deceased.
- Talking through experiences with bereaved people may help them to construct a narrative (a story) about the dead person and their final illness that will help them both to make sense of the death and to integrate their connection with the person who has died into their future life.

Source: Field, D. and Payne, S. (2004) Social aspects of bereavement. *Cancer Nursing Practice*, 2, 21–5.

---

ambiguous and harder to establish. Medical technologies have increasingly allowed death to be delayed, reversed or suspended, and for organs from the recently deceased to be used to save or improve the lives of others. The ever-increasing capacity of contemporary medicine to extend life, regardless of the quality of that life, highlights a number of moral dilemmas and practical concerns that have been debated in professional and legal settings and in the mass media. At the turn of the century such dilemmas were thrown into sharp focus in the UK by a series of medical scandals, such as the mass killing of elderly patients by the GP Harold Shipman and the retention of organs of dead children by NHS hospitals without parental consent. Three dichotomies encapsulate these dilemmas:

- the sanctity of life versus the quality of that life;
- patient rights versus professional responsibilities;
- 'active' intervention versus 'passive' inaction.

Given the demographic composition of our society, the changing economic and social climate, increasing cultural diversity, advances in medical technology and a continuing emphasis on individual rights (Chapter 10), end of life issues will become harder to ignore and more difficult to resolve.

Euthanasia

Euthanasia can be defined as the act of intentionally bringing about a person's death in order to relieve intractable suffering. It is usually administered by a doctor and differs from *physician assisted suicide*, where the person who dies causes their own death with the help of a doctor (e.g. providing lethal drugs). A distinction is often made between 'passive' and 'active' euthanasia. *Passive euthanasia* is where patients are allowed to die, and may involve withholding treatment or removing life support equipment. *Active euthanasia* is where something is done to a person to bring about their death. Whereas passive euthanasia is legal in certain circumstances in Britain, active euthanasia is illegal. However, the so-called 'double effect', whereby a physician can prescribe treatment that may hasten death, is legal, provided that the primary intention is to relieve distress.

Another important distinction, related to consent, is between voluntary and involuntary euthanasia. *Voluntary* euthanasia is where the person themselves requests death. With *involuntary* euthanasia the person is usually incapable of either doing this or giving consent. In contemporary Britain it appears there is growing support for voluntary active euthanasia (i.e. at the patient's request) in clearly defined circumstances (e.g. intractable pain). However, fear of the involuntary euthanasia of older and/or mentally incapacitated people 'for their own good' by doctors and nurses remains.

The main grounds advanced for legalising voluntary euthanasia are to relieve uncontrolled suffering and to respect the rights and autonomy of individuals to make their own choice about when to die. The main grounds for opposing euthanasia are presumptions about the sanctity of life and fears that the legalisation of euthanasia will lead to a 'slippery slope' whereby vulnerable people, such as the mentally infirm and the elderly, will be coerced into agreeing to their lives being ended. Opponents of active euthanasia view it as a failure to provide good care, whereas its proponents see it as allowing the assertion of personal control and individual choice. Personal beliefs about the sanctity of life are also important in shaping attitudes towards the acceptability of euthanasia.

The debate about euthanasia in Britain has been influenced by the powerful lobby against it from the palliative care movement and by practice elsewhere, particularly in The Netherlands. The palliative care lobby argues that providing good palliative care, especially pain relief, will obviate the wish for euthanasia. However, Seale (1998) challenges this assertion, arguing that unacceptable levels of dependency are more significant. His research found that dying people receiving hospice care were twice as likely to want euthanasia than those who were not. It seems likely that hospice practices and philosophies that facilitate open awareness, the expression of fears and encourage patients to exercise choice may partly explain this finding.

After a long period when it had been practised under clear guidelines and protocols, voluntary active euthanasia was legalised for adults and children over 12 in The Netherlands in 2001, provided that:

- the request is voluntary and well considered;
- the patient is suffering from intolerable chronic pain;
- the patient has a clear and correct understanding of their situation and prognosis;
- a second doctor's opinion has been obtained;
- appropriate medical procedures are used to cause the death.

Onwuteaka-Philipsen *et al.* (2005) found that between 1995 and 2001 there had been a 'gradual stabilisation of end of life practices' in The Netherlands. They suggested that 'end of life decision making' has become a recognised part of the care of many patients who are facing death, with two-fifths of all deaths preceded by 'a medical decision that probably or certainly hastened death'. Along with active voluntary euthanasia, these included the use of possible life-shortening alleviation of symptoms and decisions not to treat (Table 9.3). Physician-assisted suicide and ending a patient's life without their explicit request ('involuntary euthanasia') comprised less than 1% of the cases. The deliberate administration of deaths was rare, and usually by explicit request from the patient. They found that the proportion of voluntary euthanasia deaths and patient demand for physician-assisted death had not increased from 1995 to 2001. Euthanasia was mainly restricted to patients who did not have cancer, were younger than 80, and were cared for by a family physician. Physicians seemed to have become more reluctant to participate in assisted deaths.

Other surveys have used the Onwuteaka-Philipsen (translated) questionnaire, including one of UK medical practitioners (Seale 2006). Table 9.3 compares

Table 9.3 End of life decisions for non-sudden deaths in The Netherlands and the UK.

	The Netherlands (2001/02)	UK (2004)
Doctor-assisted dying:	5.12%	0.54%
Voluntary euthanasia	3.89%	0.17%
Physician-assisted suicide	0.31%	0.0%
Ending life without explicit request from patient	0.90%	0.36%
Alleviation of symptoms with possible life-shortening effect	30.1%	36.3%
Non-treatment decisions	30.1%	33.4%
All end-of-life decisions	*65.4%*	*70.2%*
No end-of life decisions	*34.6%*	*29.8%*

Source: Seale, C. (2006) National survey of end of life decisions made by UK medical practitioners. *Palliative Medicine*, 20, 1–8.

results from The Netherlands and the UK. In terms of decisions to take action, Table 9.3 shows an extremely low level of the three types of doctor-assisted dying in the UK. None of the UK doctors in Seale's survey reported engaging in physician-assisted suicide, and the majority of the 51 doctors who commented (82%) supported the legal ban on medical involvement in euthanasia and physician-assisted suicide. Over one-third of the deaths (35%) were the result of the 'double effect', where the alleviation of symptoms had hastened death.

Table 9.3 also shows that in both countries around one-third of all deaths where end-of-life treatment is considered resulted in decisions to withhold and/or withdraw treatment (non-treatment). This contrasts strongly with Italy where the equivalent proportion was just over 5%. According to Seale (2006: 6) the low level of doctor-assisted deaths and the high proportion of non-treatment decisions in the UK 'suggests a culture of medical decision making informed by a palliative care philosophy'.

Advanced directives

Voluntary euthanasia requires that patients are able to express their wishes, usually when death is in prospect. Advance directives (or 'living wills') allow individuals to assert their preference to refuse life-saving treatment in specific circumstances *before* death is an imminent possibility. These originated in the US, where they have legal status. They have become increasingly common in contemporary Britain, reflecting the wider societal emphasis upon individual autonomy and the right to choose (Chapter 10) and concerns about being kept alive by life support technology in a 'vegetative' state. Mass media reportage of high-profile cases where the medical continuance of life has been challenged on the grounds of 'poor quality of life', and the availability of proforma 'living wills' from organisations such as the Voluntary Euthanasia Society, have also contributed to their increased use.

Although there is some confusion about the legal status of advance directives in Britain, in the 1990s a series of legal judgements led the BMA in 1999 to recognise that the oral or written advance refusal of life-saving treatments (e.g. cardiopulmonary resuscitation, CPR) is fundamentally the same as a patient's legal right to refuse other treatments. However, it argued that advance refusal of basic life-sustaining care (e.g. oral hydration and nutrition) should not be seen as binding.

Do not resuscitate orders

There has also been concern about decisions made by health professionals not to resuscitate patients (DNR) for whom such action is deemed futile or detrimental to their quality of life (the ethical principle of malfeasance). Media reports of such decisions have suggested that they reflected ageism, and discriminate against older patients. They also seem to present an over-optimistic view of the success of CPR. Davey's (2001) study of an acute surgical unit found that communication between staff and with patients about DNR was poor and that patients' views were rarely sought (thus denying their autonomy). The ward nurses felt that there were, in fact, too few rather than too many DNRs, and that these were often too late to protect their patients from futile and harmful CPR attempts. There was no direct evidence of ageism, although age was certainly a factor in arriving at a DNR decision. The major long-term US study of seriously ill hospitalised patients (SUPPORT 1995) found that although 80% of hospital patients who died had a DNR order, almost half of these were written in the 2 days before they died, suggesting that these also may have been 'too late'.

Summary

NHS hospitals remain the main places of death in British society, but most of the care of people who are dying takes place in their own home. Institutional care homes for the elderly have become more important as places where people live and die, and the role of hospice and palliative care services is expected to expand further. Good end of life care in the twenty-first century will require better co-ordination between services to work across these settings. Nurses have an important role to play in this co-ordination as they are usually centrally involved in caring for people who are dying. Interpretations of how dying and bereavement are experienced have been framed in terms of the 'working through' of emotions in order to reach acceptance and adaptation to the death. However, more recent models have questioned the validity of this framework for bereavement, recognising the continuing bonds that may be retained with the dead.

As we move into the twenty-first century the wider societal pressures for greater patient involvement in the decisions about their end of life care will persist. The 'privileged' position of those dying from cancer is likely to be challenged and palliative care services extended to those with non-malignant chronic conditions and other excluded groups, such as members of ethnic minorities. The need to respect the autonomy of patients from diverse cultural backgrounds is likely to become increasingly important, with more patients demanding consultation about resuscitation orders and the choice of euthanasia, while a sizeable minority may wish to remain minimally involved in such decisions. Finally, the tension between the medical control of dying and the rights of dying people to exercise some control over decisions made about their treatment and death is likely to persist, but it seems unlikely that doctors and nurses will lose their central role in its management.

References

Brown, N. and Webster, A. (2004) *New Medical Technologies and Society. Reordering Life*, Chapter 6 Technologies of death and dying. Polity Press, Cambridge.

Copp, G. and Field, D. (2002) Open awareness and dying – the use of denial and acceptance as coping strategies by hospice patients. *Nursing Times Research*, 7, 118–27.

Davey, B. (2001) Do-not-resuscitate decisions: too many, too few, too late? *Mortality*, 6, 247–64.

Exley, C., Field, D., Jones, L. and Stokes, T. (2005) Palliative care in the community for cancer and end-stage cardio-respiratory disease: The views of patients, lay-carers and health professionals. *Palliative Medicine*, 19, 1–8.

Field, D. (1989) *Nursing the Dying*. Tavistock/Routledge, London.

Field, D. and Copp, G. (1999) Communication and awareness about dying in the 1990s. *Palliative Medicine*, 13, 459–68.

Field, D. and Froggatt, K. (2003) Issues for palliative care in nursing and residential homes, in J.T. Katz and S.M. Peace (eds) *End of Life in Care Homes: A Palliative Care Approach*. Oxford University Press, Oxford.

Firth, S. (2001) *Wider Horizons. Care of the Dying in a Multicultural Society*. National Council for Hospice and Specialist Palliative Care Services, London.

Froggatt, K. (2004) *Palliative Care in Care Homes for Older People*. The National Council for Palliative Care, London.

Glaser, B.G. and Strauss, A.L. (1965) *Awareness of Dying*. Aldine, Chicago.

Gomes, B. and Higginson, I. (2006) Factors influencing death at home in terminally ill patients with cancer: systematic review. *British Medical Journal*, 332, 516–21.

Hopkinson, J.B., Hallett, C.E. and Luker, K.A. (2003) Caring for dying people in hospital. *Journal of Advanced Nursing*, 44, 525–33.

Illich, I. (1990) *Limits to Medicine: Medical Nemesis: The Expropriation of Health*. London, Penguin.

Katz, J.T. and Peace, S.M. eds (2003) *End of Life in Care Homes: A Palliative Care Approach*. Oxford University Press, Oxford.

Lawton, J. (2000) *The Dying Process. Patients' Experiences of Palliative Care*. Routledge, London.

Onwuteaka-Philipsen, D.J., van der Heide, A., Koper, D., *et al.* (2005) Euthanasia and other end-of-life decisions in the Netherlands in 1990, 1999, and 2001. *Lancet*, 272 (9381), 395–9.

Payne, S., Horn, S. and Relf, M. (1999) *Loss and Bereavement*. Open University Press, Buckingham.

Riches, G. and Dawson, P. (2000) *An Intimate Loneliness. Supporting Bereaved Parents and Children*. Open University Press, Buckingham.

Seale, C. (1998) *Constructing Death. The Sociology of Dying and Bereavement*. Cambridge, Cambridge University Press.

Seale, C. (2006) National survey of end of life decisions made by UK medical practitioners. *Palliative Medicine*, 20, 1–8.

Seymour, J. (2001) *Critical Moments – Death and Dying in Intensive Care*. Open University Press, Buckingham.

Seymour, J., Witherspoon, R., Gott, M., *et al.* (2005) *End-of-life Care. Promoting Comfort, Choice and Well-being for Older People*. Policy Press, Bristol.

Skilbeck, J. and Payne, S. (2005) End of life care: a discursive analysis of specialist palliative care nursing. *Journal of Advanced Nursing*, 51, 325–34.

Stroebe, M.S. and Schut, H. (1999) The Dual Process Model of coping with bereavement: rationale and description. *Death Studies*, 23, 197–224.

Storey, L., Pemberton, C., Howard, A. and O'Donnell, L. (2003) Place of death: Hobson's Choice or patient choice? *Cancer Nursing Practice*, 2(4), 33–8.

SUPPORT, Principal Investigators (1995) A controlled study to improve care for seri- ously ill hospitalised patients: the study to understand prognoses and preferences for outcomes and risks of treatment (SUPPORT). *Journal of the American Medical Association*, 174, 1591–8.

Timmermans, S. (1994) Dying of awareness: the theory of awareness contests revis- ited. *Sociology of Health and Illness*, 16, 322–9.

Timmermans, S. (2005) Death brokering: constructing culturally appropriate deaths. *Sociology of Health and Illness*, 27, 993–1013.

Vachon, M.C.S. (1995) Staff stress in hospice/palliative care: a review. *Palliative Medicine*, 9, 91–122.

Walter, T. (1999) *On Bereavement. The Culture of Grief*. Open University Press, Buckingham.

Further reading

Clark, D. and Seymour, J. (1999) *Reflections on Palliative Care*. Open University Press, Buckingham.
  Still the best review of policy issues from a sociological perspective.

Seymour, J., Witherspoon, R., Gott, M., *et al.* (2005) *End-of-life Care. Promoting Comfort, Choice and Well-being for Older People*. Policy Press, Bristol.
  Provides an excellent general overview and review of the main issues for end of life care for older people.

Part IV

Health care

Chapter 10

Health care in contemporary Britain

The organisation and delivery of health care, like patterns of health and disease, do not exist in a vacuum but are shaped by the societies in which they operate. The characteristics and problems of health care in contemporary Britain take place within organisational contexts that are themselves shaped by wider social processes. This chapter will:

- outline some key social changes in contemporary British society;
- identify some of the increasing pressures on the delivery of health care;
- discuss recent changes in the organisation of health care;
- examine recent changes in the culture of health care.

Social and cultural changes in contemporary societies

Individualism and identity

We observed in Chapter 1 that a key sociological problem involves exploring relationships between individuals and societies and how these relationships change over time. One of the major social changes of the past few decades, especially in affluent societies like Britain, is increasing 'individualisation'. Organisations that previously provided authoritative social control over people's lives, such as the police, Christian churches, schools and the professions, are losing some of their authority, and many of the social institutions that once shaped people's behaviour and their sense of identity, such as family, community, social class and gender, have become less influential.

The dominance of received truth – traditional, religious and scientific – has also been challenged by easier public access to information and competing opinions, including access to competing ideas and explanations about health and illness, with the development of the electronic 'world wide web'. Both scientific and religious knowledge may be challenged and found wanting. The rapid expansion of the availability of the internet, mobile phones and other forms of 'instant communication' at a distance has, among other things, transformed the nature of time and space which now extend well beyond the immediate local setting. The 'disembedding' of individuals from their localities is a key feature of contemporary societies, contributing to the greater choice and freedom of action for individuals and forcing them to become more self-aware in deciding their choice of behaviour (Giddens 1991).

Sociologists are not agreed about whether these developments are part of a major social transition from a 'modern' to a new type of 'post' or 'late modern' society. However, they are generally agreed that contemporary societies are characterised by weakening social conventions coupled with greater individual material resources, leading to more individuals having much greater choice over how they live their lives. Many of the lifestyles characteristic of previous eras are absent in contemporary societies, individuals' identities are less dependent upon their social backgrounds and social attributes, and they feel freer to construct their identities through the lifestyle choices they make. For example, an increasing number of people no longer feel they have to get married, have children or stay in relationships that are not working for them. Similarly, increasing numbers of people no longer feel that age, gender or ethnicity constrain them to act or dress in particular ways or take up specific household or occupational roles. In terms of health behaviour and health care, this type of analysis may help to make sense of the growing emphasis upon individuals as consumers of health services and the commodification of such services through the introduction of market principles (see below). It also partially explains the increased emphasis upon individuals taking responsibility for their own health and illness choices, and increasing expectations of health care.

Changing family patterns

Although there are many different types of family structure, by the mid-twentieth century in Britain (like most Western societies) the dominant family type was the nuclear family; that is a married couple with a small number of dependent children. The nuclear family was not only the statistical norm, it was also the moral norm and was seen by the prevailing ideology of the day as a 'good thing'. Men were supposed to be the 'providers', women the 'nurturers' and an array of emotional and educational indicators suggested that children who had 'stable' two-parent home backgrounds did rather better academically and emotionally than those who did not.

One of the consequences of the greater individualism described above has been an increasing fragmentation and diversity in family life (Beck-Gernsheim 2002). In contemporary Britain, marriage declined as a valued social institution, with people marrying later or not marrying at all. Cohabitation has become much more common, especially among younger people, and divorce is also rising. At the turn of the century Britain had the highest divorce rate in Europe, five times higher than it was in the 1960s, with 40% of marriages ending in divorce. People are also having fewer children, and in 2001 the birth rate of 1.64 children per woman was the lowest recorded since records began in 1934.

These developments have also changed the relationship between families and households. In the middle of the twentieth century most households were family based. Today, with increasing relationship breakdown, many more people have ties with family members living in other households and an increasing number of households are not based on traditional family ties. At the start of the twenty-first century a quarter of couples had no children and it is predicted that 25% of the current generation of women of childbearing age will not have any children. There has also been an increase in friendship-based households, and more people are choosing to live alone. In the 1960s 4% of households were comprised of single people, but by 2004 this had risen to 12% (Office of National Statistics 2006).

These changes in marriage, divorce and parenthood are bringing about a much greater diversity in families and households. Two of the major changes have been the growth of one-parent households and the increasing number of step or reconstituted families. Nearly a quarter of children under 16 live in one-parent households, typically headed by a woman. Historically these have been associated with teenage illegitimacy and poverty and are most commonly found in inner city areas. However, since the 1990s an increasing number of older, economically secure, single women have chosen to become single mothers.

Step-families were rare in the middle of the twentieth century and were largely brought about by the death of one of the marriage partners, but at the start of the twenty-first century step-families comprised just over a fifth of British households and 10% of children were living in them. There may be ambiguities and tensions about social relationships within step-families arising from emotional commitments to members of previous family units. Continuing relationships, for example with grandparents, can be a source of tension, and relationships with wider kin, for example old and new aunts and uncles, may be ambiguous. These issues may blur the responsibilities for the provision of lay health care and social support between step-family members.

State welfare

As British society has become individualistic, the state welfareism that characterised it in the third quarter of the twentieth century has begun to decline. The philosophy behind the 'modern' welfare state, outlined in the Beveridge Report of 1942 and established following the Second World War, was that access to basic human 'rights', such as work, housing, education, health care and financial support in sickness and old age should be guaranteed by the state and not left to the inconsistencies of the market. However, by the 1970s these principles were being increasingly questioned in principle and diluted in practice, as successive governments struggled to finance the escalating costs of state welfare in the face of economic recession (Glennester 2000).

The principle of trying to maintain full employment was abandoned in 1976, an increasing number of benefits became subject to means testing and a great deal of state housing stock was sold off and not replaced. Those who can afford it are now expected to contribute more financially towards their own health care, pension plans and their children's education (especially higher education). In the past two decades both Conservative and New Labour governments have encouraged a 'marketisation' of welfare; first, by encouraging more private investment and secondly by attempting to make those services that remain in state control, particularly education and health, more responsive to market forces (see below and Chapter 11).

Pressures on the NHS

The National Health Service (NHS), which began treating patients in July 1948, was the 'jewel in the crown' of the new British post Second World War welfare state. Its main aims were to provide:

- universal access to health care;
- free health care at the point of access to all British citizens;
- equality of health care regardless of social background or place of residence;
- professional autonomy and clinical freedom for doctors.

In 1949 the NHS consumed under 4% of Britain's gross national product (GNP) or national wealth. Throughout its life it has expanded and consolidated its key role in British society. Despite fluctuations in the national economic fortune, since the 1960s around 6% of Britain's GNP has been spent on health services, which is still less than that of most other comparable countries. This proportion is planned to rise to 9.4% by 2007/08, to bring Britain into line with other European Union countries. Although there has been a growth in private health care organisations, over 80% of Britain's health care is currently provided by the state.

The founders of the NHS naively believed that its costs would stabilise once a pool of sickness had been 'mopped up'. However, its costs have continued to increase above the rate of inflation and it is now accepted that the demand for health care is potentially limitless. Between 1977/78 and 2000/01 NHS spending doubled in real terms to £50 billion, rising to £63 billion in 2003/04, and a projected £84 billion in 2006/07 (Table 10.1).

However, despite continuingly increasing government investment, the NHS is rarely out of the news and most of it is bad news: health professionals

Table 10.1 Government Expenditure on the NHS.

Year	NHS cash spending (£ million)
1999–2000	48,362
2000–2001	53,039
2001–2002	59,880
2002–2003	66,314
2003–2004	74,928

Source: Office of National Statistics.

complaining about lack of resources compromising care, lengthening waiting lists, health care trusts facing bankruptcy, cancelled treatments and individuals being denied potentially life-saving treatment. The paradox of the British public paying more each year for an apparently deteriorating health service cannot simply be explained by deficiencies *within* the NHS. They are largely the result of increasing pressures *outside* the service. Here we discuss four of these pressures: the UK's ageing population, developments in medical technology, changes in the health care workforce and changing public expectations of health care.

An ageing population

The increasing numbers of older people in Britain is a continuing pressure on the NHS. As we saw in Chapter 6, life expectancy has increased significantly and older people now constitute a higher proportion of the population than ever before. In 2001 over 7% of the population were 75 or older, compared to 4.5% in 1971, and the number of over 85s continues to increase, projected to reach 2 million in 2020.

NHS expenditure per head is highest at birth and in old age (Figure 10.1). On average, people aged 75–84 cost the health service more than four times the national average, with those over 85 nearly seven times more expensive. This is not because older people are abusing the health service, but simply because they are more vulnerable to long-term illness and disability. Acute infectious diseases have been superseded by long-term chronic conditions as the major sources of illness and death in our society, and the burden of disease comes primarily from cancers and from long-term chronic conditions and their disabling effects (Chapter 7). These are conditions that primarily affect middle-aged and, especially, older adults. Over half of people over the age of 60 living in domestic homes (as distinct from residential homes) have a limiting long-standing illness.

The rising burden of disease, coupled with diminishing resources for lay care brought about by changes in family life and patterns of employment, have important implications for the health service. There are also significant costs to local authorities providing or paying for statutory social services for old people, and to the families and 'lay carers' of sick and disabled people. A common estimate is that the NHS requires an annual increase of 1% in its real income to keep pace with the additional costs resulting from the increasing number of old people in the population.

Medical technology

Within the medical sphere the continuing and seemingly ever-quickening pace of development of medical, surgical and pharmacological technology has made new (and more expensive) forms of treatment possible, and led to more powerful and sophisticated interventions into matters of life and death.

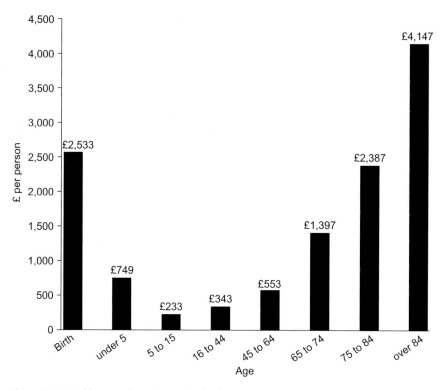

Figure 10.1 Health expenditure by age, England 2002–2003.
Source: Figure 2.15 in Yuen, P. (2005) *Compendium of Health Statistics 2005–2006*. Radcliffe Publishing, Oxford. Reproduced with permission from the Office of Health Economics.

The development and marketing of new drugs increases costs in both hospitals and community general practice. Even technological developments that reduce the costs of treatment in the short run, for example by preventing heart disease or allowing day care treatment instead of hospitalisation, tend to increase costs in the long run as simpler and cheaper treatments become more widely available and more patients are treated. Developments in medical practice have therefore tended to increase health care costs. The influential Wanless Report of 2002 (Wanless 2002) estimated that medical technology added between 2 and 3% a year to the growth in health spending. The establishment of the National Institute for Clinical Effectiveness in 2000 to scrutinise the effectiveness of clinical treatments was driven partly by the recognition that costly new treatments should be monitored for their 'cost-effectiveness' before being approved for general use.

At the same time that medical intervention has become more powerful, it has also become more complicated and dependent upon a growing range of specialists, thus making it more difficult to co-ordinate the various elements of treatment. The development of such techniques has been partly responsible both for the concentration of secondary medical practice in large general hospitals since the mid-1960s and the ever-increasing costs of hospital medicine. Advances in medical specialisation and high-technology medicine have also led to the development of a greater range of nurse and other paramedical specialists. This has altered the boundaries of nursing work, increased the demands on nursing staff and led to a greater range of skill mix in nursing care (Chapter 12). It has also resulted in hospitals becoming primarily concerned with acute care, with long-term care moving to other settings, such as nursing homes, which may be outside the NHS.

Changes in the health care workforce

Throughout its life the main cost for the NHS has been its workforce, accounting for nearly 70% of its budget. With over a million workers, it is the largest employer in Britain. The costs of skilled staff in the NHS have historically risen faster than the general rate of inflation. Health care is labour intensive and government plans for improving the service have acknowledged that one of the main constraints upon delivering an improved service is the difficulty of recruiting staff at all levels. For example, one of the major difficulties in providing effective health care has been the lack of specialist nurses. While significant expansion of the workforce is required if the government plans are to be achieved, the difficulties in achieving such an expansion have included increasing competition in the labour market, especially for more highly qualified workers, and the relatively long time-frame required to educate and train skilled staff (Chapter 11).

The expectations that staff hold about their pay and working conditions have altered significantly over the life of the NHS, with the long hours expected of, for example, nurses, junior doctors and general practitioners no longer being acceptable. This is partly due to changing societal attitudes to the balance between work and leisure and family life. The increasing numbers of women occupying specialist positions also means that a greater proportion of health workers are taking career breaks in order to bring up their children. In combination, these two factors mean that greater numbers of health workers are required to staff the service.

Changing public expectations of health care

The expectations that patients and the general public hold about the health service is another source of increasing health costs. Peoples' ideas of what constitutes 'health' and illness change over time (Chapter 2), and for the majority of Britain's population good health has come to be seen as a right, rather than as a matter of social status or chance. Health expectations have risen with the general increase in standards of living and quality of life since the 1960s, leading to more health seeking behaviour, such as preventive screening, and higher expectations of the outcomes of care. Whereas current older generations appear to have lower expectations of health and functioning, those born since the advent of the NHS expect better levels of health and demand more from the health services. The introduction and success of the NHS has been a major factor leading to such raised expectations. Yet, despite the well publicised and real benefits to individual patients of procedures such as renal dialysis, hip replacement and cataract surgery, there is debate about the contributions that changes in medical technology have made to the improved health and increased longevity of the British population since the establishment of the NHS (Chapter 2).

The pressures on health care we have discussed in this section have contributed to both the ever-increasing costs of health care and to continuing concerns about the delivery of health care by the NHS (Figure 10.2). Since the 1990s increasing concerns about the costs, effectiveness and equity in the provision of NHS care have led to changes in the mixed economy of health care in Britain, particularly an increasing role for the private sector (Chapter 11).

The organisation of health care

As we have seen in the previous section, many of the difficulties of delivering comprehensive and universal health care in contemporary Britain are located not in the NHS itself but in the wider societal context within which it operates. The net effects of continuously increasing expectations of health care and the ever-increasing costs of providing such care means that the NHS requires more money each year simply to keep pace with the additional pressures being placed on it. Partly as a response to these pressures there have been some significant changes in the past two decades in the way that health care is organised and delivered (Chapter 11). In this section we look at the mixed economy of health care, hospital care and care in the community.

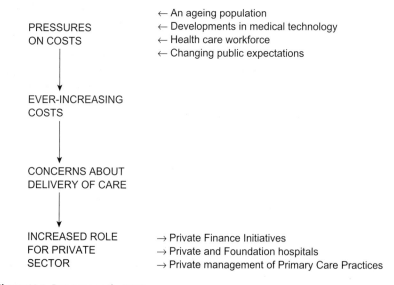

Figure 10.2 Pressures on the NHS.

The mixed economy of health care

The original philosophy behind the NHS was that health care should be provided by the state free at the point of use and that access to care was determined by need, not by ability to pay. However, although the NHS was the major source of health care, it was not the only source of such care. During the latter part of the twentieth century the role of lay care in the community (see below) and of voluntary organisations came to be increasingly recognised, and an expanding role for commercial enterprise was encouraged.

In Britain and in many other Western societies there has been a shift towards a greater 'market orientation' in the provision of health care. Markets are institutions in which people freely exchange commodities (goods and services) for money. Those on the political right believe that free market organisations are generally more efficient and give consumers more choice than centrally planned, state run organisations. However, these arguments do not necessarily apply to health care (Tudor Hart 2006). First, a market system of health care, as in the USA, often fails to allocate adequate health care to those who are most in need of it – the poor and the elderly. Secondly, private health care systems which are in competition with each other tend to be less efficient and have higher administrative costs than state funded systems such as the NHS. Thirdly, the consumers of health care do not have the expertise to make informed choices about their treatment and so inevitably rely heavily on the advice of health professionals. Finally, under a market system people may be persuaded to undergo treatments that they do not need, for example it has been estimated that one-third of operations performed in the USA are unnecessary (Blank and Burau 2004, chapter 3).

There has been increasing commercial involvement in health care in contemporary Britain since 1980. The Conservative governments of 1979–1992 introduced a 'market orientation' into the provision of health care by introducing compulsory competitive tendering for ancillary services such as catering, cleaning and laundry. In 1979 private contractors undertook only 2% of NHS ancillary services. By 1985 the figure had risen to 40%, falling back to less than 25% following concerns about the quality of work and standards of hygiene, concerns that persist into the twenty-first century. Subsequent governments introduced and expanded Public Finance Initiatives, under which companies contracted to provide facilities and services to NHS purchasers (Chapter 11). In 2002 the New Labour government reaffirmed its intention to use the private sector to work in conjunction with NHS services to expand capacity, increase access and promote diversity in the provision and choice of health services (Department of Health, 2002).

Although there has been a substantial expansion of private sector health care, it accounted for only 18% of total spending on health care in 2005, significantly below that in other contemporary affluent societies (Yuen 2005). Private sector involvement is much higher in areas such as non-acute surgery, long-term care of the elderly and reproductive medicine, and many nurses are finding employment in nursing homes and other private sector institutions in preference to employment within the NHS. Around three-quarters of all

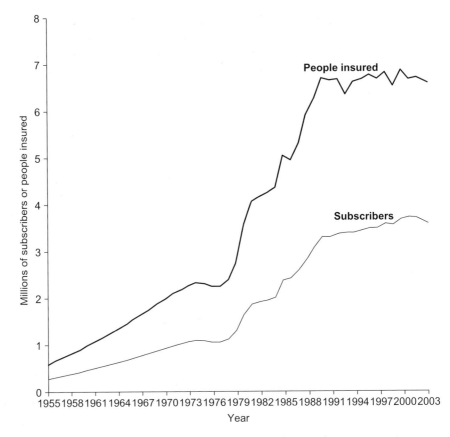

Figure 10.3 Private medical insurance subscribers and people insured, UK 1955–2003.
Source: Figure 2.19 in Yuen, P. (2005) *Compendium of Health Statistics 2005–2006*. Radcliffe Publishing, Oxford. Reproduced with permission from the Office of Health Economics.

those using private health care outside the NHS pay for it with health insurance, usually purchased by their employers. The Wanless Report (Wanless 2002) estimated that private health insurance amounted to 1.2% of GNP. In 1971 2.1 million people had private health insurance, this increased rapidly during the 1980s, reaching almost 7 million by 2003 (Figure 10.3). The growth of private health insurance for individuals is explained partly by government initiatives to encourage private health insurance and partly by people's perceptions about failings of the NHS, such as long waiting lists. There appears to be a trend for more people to make 'one off' payments for individual treatment episodes (e.g. cataract surgery) in order to avoid long waiting times.

Hospital care

Hospital care has been at the centre of the NHS since its inception, with over 60% of the NHS budget being spent on the hospital sector from the mid-1960s, peaking at 68% in 1972/73. The second half of the twentieth century saw 'a decline in the numbers of hospitals and hospital care yet increased rates of hospitalisation' (Armstrong 1998). A number of continuing concerns have led to a fundamental reappraisal of the current role of the hospital:

- the high costs of hospital care;
- iatrogenic complications such as cross-infection;
- negative physiological, psychological and social effects of long-term stays;
- ever-improving surgical techniques requiring shorter periods of hospitalisation.

At the start of the twenty-first century hospitals remain at the centre of the NHS, although their organisation and pattern of work has changed. Economies of size and the increasing complexity of hospital care have led to decreasing numbers of hospital beds, the closure of smaller hospitals and the centralisation of services into larger hospitals with a greater range of specialist staff and equipment. Improved techniques, greater use of day care and outpatient clinics and the extension of hospital services into the community have reduced the time patients spend as inpatients (although there is concern that some inpatients are now discharged too soon). Thus, hospitals have been largely transformed into centres dealing mainly with acute care, with the rapid turnover of more patients through fewer beds. The three-tier pattern of care proposed in 1995 for cancer services has become the template for the treatment of other conditions. Centres of excellence with 'leading edge' technologies based in large specialist hospitals offer highly specialised interventions and the treatment of rare conditions; general hospitals with recognised specialist units manage common conditions; and the care of chronically ill patients in the community is increasingly managed through hospital departments rather than by GPs and community nurses.

As in any organisation, hospital activities are underpinned by a number of beliefs about what is important and how work should be done, and these change over time. While the bio-medical model remains dominant in shaping hospital work, there have been attempts, especially by nursing and other paramedical staff, to supplement it with approaches that pay more attention to social and psychological aspects of patient care. Effective information and communication are central to patient management, patient well-being and clinical recovery, and improvements in this area are seen by government as central to increasing patient choice (Department of Health 2005a). Within hospitals, nurses are particularly well located to contribute to effective communication with patients, as they have most continuous contact with and knowledge of them, and they play a central role in co-ordinating the range of tasks and activities involved in clinical and care work (Chapter 12).

The hospital has been seen as a place of safety where patients can recover in bed from their illness or their treatments. While this is still the case to some extent, there is now increasing awareness of the dangers of hospitals. Stories of medical errors, bureaucratic incompetence, violence and patients left for long periods without care are now common currency in the media. While media stories usually focus on the health care professionals involved, many of these problems are caused institutionally, rather than individually, by the growing pressures on limited hospital beds. Another area of concern is that hospitals are seen as places where patients may be at danger of infection or damage from their clinical care. An increasing number of hospital-acquired infections are becoming resistant to antibiotics and this is most dramatically illustrated by the rise of the MRSA (methicillin-resistant *Staphylococcus aureus*) superbug (Department of Health 2005b). The pressures on beds and the iatrogenic dangers of hospital care, coupled with the adverse consequences of bed rest itself, has reduced the average time a patient spends in hospital and has led to those requiring long-term care being looked after in the community rather than the hospital.

Care in the community

Although the hospital remains the focus for acute interventions and the treatment of complex conditions, there has been a progressive shift in the care of certain categories of people requiring long-term care to community settings. The movement to 'de-institutionalise' the care of people with learning difficulties in the 1960s spread to the care of the mentally ill, culminating in the closure of many long-term wards and institutions in the 1980s (Chapter 8). While these changes seem to have been largely based upon the view that care in the community was more appropriate for such people, governmental stress upon community care also seems to have been motivated by the view that it would be cheaper care. It was at least partly due to the high costs of hospital care for long-term conditions that care of people with physical disabilities and of the elderly in the community (e.g. in nursing homes) also became priorities. More recently, the development of day surgery and 'hospital at home' initiatives has shifted some of the care of the acutely ill into the community. The care of non-threatening acute and chronic conditions has always taken place primarily in the community, managed by general practitioners, community nurses or simply through self-care at home.

The 'mixed economy' of health care lies at the heart of health care provision in the community, although the boundaries and responsibilities between statutory, voluntary and commercial providers of care are not always clear. One of the main difficulties is in articulating the contributions of various care providers. Within the health service the differing interests of hospital-based staff, primary care teams and institutional homes (most of which are commercially run) makes joint planning difficult. Both health and social services workers may be involved in the provision of care, and there may be difficulties co-ordinating between them, especially for categories of patients such as those with long-term disabilities, where it is not clear which service is responsible for funding care (Chapter 6). Such ambiguity has long been recognised as a serious detriment to effective and responsive care in the community, and in January 2006 the government published plans for a more integrated care system, aimed at helping more people live in the community (Department of Health 2006a). Voluntary groups contribute to community care and can make significant contributions to improving the lives of patients and their lay carers, yet liaison between lay and professional carers may be problematic.

Lay care

While paid workers provide key elements of care *in* the community, the major source of care *by* the community is unpaid care from families, relatives and friends. As noted earlier, this resource of 'lay' or 'informal' care has been affected by the increasing fragmentation and diversity of family life described earlier. Although there is no evidence that contemporary families are abandoning their familial responsibilities of care, the reduction in family size and the fragmentation and complexity of modern family structures, and the increased number of women working, means that there are proportionately fewer people available to provide such care. Further, members of step-families, cohabiting couples or divorcees may feel less obliged to care for sick or aged relatives and ex-kin.

According to the 2001 census there were about 6 million lay carers in the UK, most them are adults, although there are also over 100,000 children providing care, 8% of whom were spending at least 50 hours a week on caring. Most carers spend over 20 hours a week on caring, and one-fifth (1.3 million) spend at least 50 hours a week (Bajekal *et al.* 2006). Both sexes take part in lay care, although women are more likely to be the sole or main carer, to spend more than 20 hours a week in caring and to receive less outside help. While community nurses and social services staff may provide invaluable support to carers, there are many, especially in older couples where the deterioration of one partner may not be noticed, who do not receive sufficient external support.

Becoming a lay carer is usually a result of family relationships, and most carers (93%) look after a relative (Maher and Green 2002). Older, chronically sick, terminally ill, physically handicapped and mentally ill people are particularly likely to receive lay care in their family on a long-term basis. Some of these suffer from long-term conditions and may be severely disabled, bedridden, incontinent or confused. Constant attention to therapeutic regimes and monitoring of symptoms may be required. Such caring may be hard work – literally a 'labour of love'. Carers often experience a heavy round of daily tasks, a reduction of their social lives, and increased social isolation. They are frequently cut off from other carers and from the formal health care system. Financial costs for them may include missed job opportunities.

Lay carers typically have responsibility for most, or even all, aspects of their patients' welfare, although they are rarely qualified or trained for their caring work. Lay care may be both open-ended and demanding and many carers are 'on call' at all hours of the day and night. Over a third of lay carers have no help with their caring work from others. The costs of care – financial, physical and emotional – to these lone carers, who are usually women, may be considerable. Half of all carers have a long-standing illness themselves, and over a third (35%), rising to nearly a half (47%) among elderly carers, have limiting long-standing illnesses (Maher and Green 2002). During the

1990s the important role of unpaid lay carers in looking after chronically and terminally ill people in their own homes was increasingly recognised, with parliamentary legislation in 1995 establishing the provision of services to meet the needs of carers. However, there are few pressure groups to represent their interests, or opportunities for them to meet others in like situations, and the extent to which they are supported by professional workers varies, despite recognition that they are entitled to such support.

The changing culture of health care

The changes in the organisation of health care that we looked at in the previous sections have been accompanied by changes in the beliefs, ideas and practices of health care. In this section we look at three recent changes in the culture of health care: the challenge to medical dominance, the influence of individualism in health care and the rise of consumerism.

Challenges to medical dominance

For the past two centuries health care in Western industrial societies has been dominated by medical science and the power of the medical profession. When doctors negotiated with the architects of the NHS they were in a powerful position to extract a number of important concessions from the government, including the right to treat private patients. The final agreement between the government and the medical profession:

- guaranteed the professional autonomy and clinical freedom of doctors;
- gave doctors a major voice in the allocation of health care resources;
- confirmed the power of doctors over other health workers, including nurses.

During the past three decades there have been increasing challenges to this medical dominance. At the basis of these challenges has been a growing realisation that the returns of clinical medicine have not always matched the significantly increased levels of investment. A number of research studies have suggested not only that medicine has done rather less to improve human health than was generally believed, but that it has also created iatrogenic disease (Chapter 2). Public confidence in medicine has also been eroded by a number of high-profile scandals about medical mismanagement, failures, abuses of power and an unevenness of care between different regions and hospitals. The challenges to medical dominance arising out of these concerns have come from the public and consumer groups, other health professionals and governments.

Lay public

Patients are no longer the passive recipients of health care that they once were, and today, the old adage 'doctor knows best' is no longer universally accepted. Not only do medical errors now receive much more publicity than they once did, but magazines, newspapers, TV programmes and, above all, the internet, have made information about health, illness and treatment options available to an increasingly wide section of the general public. For example, in 2000 there were over 70,000 websites disseminating health information (Cline and Haynes 2001). The consequence of this is a process that sociologists call lay skilling, where increasing numbers of people (rightly or wrongly) feel they are better informed to question, challenge and increasingly complain about medical decision making (Henwood *et al.* 2004).

Other health workers

Another challenge to medical dominance has come from other health professionals, including nurses. The medical profession has maintained its dominance over these groups through two main strategies. Some groups, such as nurses, have been subordinate to medical control. Their roles have been largely delegated to them by doctors and they have had little scope for autonomy, independence or self-regulation. Other professional groups, such as dentists and pharmacists, have had their activities limited to a specified range of activities, with the medical profession playing a key role in their registration procedures. However, as they sought greater autonomy in their education and work, nursing and other professions allied to medicine have successfully challenged the medical claim to exclusive expertise and have asserted their own areas of specialised skill and competency. Nursing has been aided in this respect by government initiatives to relieve the pressure of work on medical staff by reallocating clinical activities, such as prescribing routine diagnostic procedures, and providing other sources of help and information to patients, such as the NHS Direct telephone advice service.

   The growing popularity of alternative therapies is another challenge to medical pre-eminence. Initially, the medical profession simply dismissed most alternative medicines as 'quackery' and warned the public of the dangers of being treated by 'unqualified' practitioners. However, in spite of these warnings, alternative medicine grew in popularity and by the turn of the century it was estimated that between a fifth and a quarter of the British population had used some form of alternative medical treatment (Saks 2006). The widespread use of alternative medicine has meant that it has had to be taken more seriously, and this was formally acknowledged in Britain in 2000 by the House of Lords Select Committee on Science and Technology that looked at complementary and alternative therapies (CAM). This identified three main groupings (Box 10.1), recognized the great diversity of standards within this disparate set of therapeutic practices and recommended measures such as licensing of herbal products (now occurring) and a single regulatory body for each discipline.

   The challenge to medical dominance posed by CAM has to be put into context. First, although a substantial minority seek help directly from non-orthodox practitioners, most users continue to use conventional medicine and receive concurrent treatment for their condition within the NHS. Secondly, some 'alternative' practices have been incorporated into medical practice For example, osteopathy and acupuncture are now available to some NHS patients, and other therapies are widely used in nursing homes and hospices. It is likely

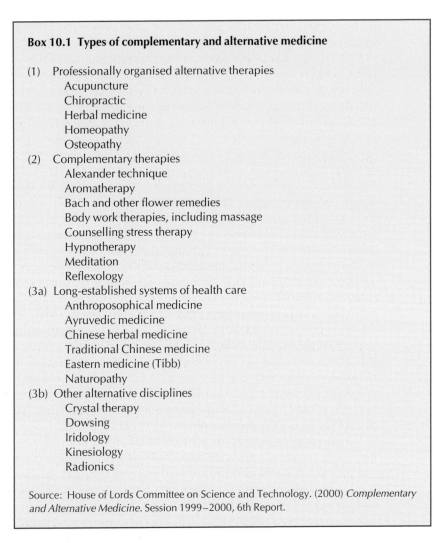

Box 10.1 Types of complementary and alternative medicine

(1)   Professionally organised alternative therapies
          Acupuncture
          Chiropractic
          Herbal medicine
          Homeopathy
          Osteopathy
(2)   Complementary therapies
          Alexander technique
          Aromatherapy
          Bach and other flower remedies
          Body work therapies, including massage
          Counselling stress therapy
          Hypnotherapy
          Meditation
          Reflexology
(3a) Long-established systems of health care
          Anthroposophical medicine
          Ayruvedic medicine
          Chinese herbal medicine
          Traditional Chinese medicine
          Eastern medicine (Tibb)
          Naturopathy
(3b) Other alternative disciplines
          Crystal therapy
          Dowsing
          Iridology
          Kinesiology
          Radionics

Source: House of Lords Committee on Science and Technology. (2000) *Complementary and Alternative Medicine*. Session 1999–2000, 6th Report.

that some CAM therapies will become an increasingly important source of health care in twenty-first century Britain, and the more they become incorporated into mainstream health care and become 'complementary' rather than 'alternative', the less threat they pose to medical dominance (Mizrachi *et al.* 2005). Thus, in his evaluation of the challenge posed by alternative and complementary therapies to modern medicine Saks (2006: 87) concluded that 'this consumer-led challenge (to medicine) has not as yet fundamentally subverted the material foundations of professional dominance of British medicine, even if it has generated a greater degree of questioning of its approach'.

Government control

The greatest challenge to medical power has come from government reforms of the NHS. The ever-increasing demand for health care outlined in the second section of this chapter has led successive governments to try to control costs and attempt to make clinicians more accountable for the resources they use.

In the early 1990s the Conservative government initiated a programme of reforms of the health service designed to transfer much of the decision making over resources from doctors to managers (see Chapter 11). The subsequent New Labour government adopted a different strategy. While devolving decision making from the centre to Primary Care Teams and hospitals, and appearing to give health professionals more discretion to make clinical judgements, these decisions had to operate within the new systems of accountability and regulation set out by the government (Department of Health 2000, 2002). Doctors and other health professionals have become much more accountable to government for the resources they use, and their clinical activities are more closely monitored than ever before. The establishment of the National Institute for Clinical Excellence, the Commission for Health Improvement and National Service Frameworks exemplify the attempt to shift power from the medical profession to government agencies through the greater regulation of their activities. In 2006 the Chief Medical Officer recommended a more rigorous system of regulation of medical practice, including reform of the General Medical Council, a clear standard to define a good doctor and new measures to identify poorly performing doctors. Although medical power has certainly been challenged and to some extent eroded on a number of fronts, the British health care system is still dominated by medical science and the bio-medical approach to treatment. Doctors, especially specialists, continue to enjoy considerable power and status, and maintain their authority over other health workers. Medicine may be challenged but it is likely to retain its dominant position for the foreseeable future.

The consequences of these recent changes for nursing are less clear and may be a little more paradoxical (Chapter 12). On the one hand, as we observed above, there are new opportunities for nurses to expand their role by doing things that were once the exclusive preserve of doctors, such as making independent clinical judgements and prescribing medicines. However, nursing professional autonomy has also become eroded in some areas. Like doctors, nurses' judgements are now subject to increasing challenge and complaint from patients and, like doctors, their work is now monitored to a much greater degree by government regulation. However, perhaps most worrying for the nursing profession (and patients!) is the current policy of transferring tasks previously done by trained nurses to unskilled health care assistants. This is called 'skill mix' but, for some, 'de-skilling' would be a more accurate description. A possible consequence of this development is that nursing may well become increasingly fragmented, with relatively few nurse specialists at the top and a much larger number of relatively unskilled 'nurses' at the bottom.

Individual rights and responsibilities in health care

The more individualistic nature of contemporary societies and the decline of state welfareism that we described in the first section of this chapter are reflected in the culture of health care by the increasing importance now given to patients' rights and individual responsibilities for health.

Rights

The 1990s saw a growing concern within Britain for the rights of individuals to good standards of service and to clear information about goods and services. Within health care, the concept of the rights of patients to minimum standards of service and informed choice was most clearly signalled by the introduction of the now defunct 'Patient's Charter' in 1991. In 2002 the commitment to patient rights was reaffirmed as a central aspect of the restructuring of the NHS (Department of Health 2002). At the local level, providers of health services, such as NHS Hospital and Primary Care Trusts, have been required to produce their own written standards and, like schools, are now evaluated in terms of a number of performance indicators, the results of which are open to the general public. There has also been increasing openness with patients about diagnosis and prognosis. For example, many (but by no means all) patients have access to their own medical records, although whether this improves clinical management of their conditions has yet to be established.

It would, however, be wrong simply to conclude that patients today have more rights than they did in the relatively recent past. They have rights to more choice, information and complaints, but they no longer *necessarily* have a right to health care itself. Increasingly, health care is being rationed (Chapter 11) and some patients are being denied access to health care on grounds of the age, their inappropriate health behaviour (e.g. smoking, excessive alcohol intake), the nature of their condition or whether their health authority is willing to finance the treatment they need.

Responsibilities

While people have demanded, and have been given, more rights in health care, they have also been held more responsible for their own health. Many of the major diseases of contemporary British society are increasingly being attributed to lifestyle and behaviour, and maintaining health and preventing illness have become more explicitly defined by government and health professionals as the active responsibility of individuals (Chapter 2). As many areas of everyday life, such as diet, alcohol consumption and exercise, have become subject to medical intervention, the clients of medicine and nursing are no longer simply people who are ill, but potentially all of us, as witnessed by the health education and health promotion campaigns which exhort us to 'look after ourselves' to eat and drink 'sensibly' and to lead healthier lives. These developments are changing the work context and focus of many nurses and other health professionals, especially those working in the community, who are becoming increasingly involved with monitoring and regulating lifestyles and behaviour.

Consumerism

Another significant change in contemporary societies has been the rise of the ethic of consumerism (Bauman 2002). This view holds that as patterns of consumption in contemporary affluent societies are increasingly determined by choice, want, and preference rather than need, consumers have more power and authority at the expense of producers. Underpinning this view is the belief that the market always 'knows' best, and that 'success' depends on pleasing the consumer. These consumer values are now having a significant influence on the delivery of heath care. A number of policy changes are transforming the public service culture of the health service into something much closer to a commercial enterprise as attempts are made to remould professional–patient relationships in the image of provider–customer relationships in the free market.

The rise of consumerism

The increasing similarity between seller–consumer and professional–patient relationships can be seen in a number of ways. First, those selling goods and services in the free market have to find out what customers want through market research, and now the NHS has to do the same. In 1998, just a year after it came to office, the Labour government ordered the first national survey of the NHS and 150,000 people from every part of the country were asked for their views about the service. Doctors and nurses are now expected to research their patients' lives and expectations in order to provide the 'right' kind of service. Initiatives in medical and nurse education aimed at eliciting the 'patient's point of view' and modules aimed at developing better 'communication skills' in health care are good examples of this process.

Secondly, like any other customers, patients are now much freer to express any dissatisfaction with complaint and litigation. Patients have become more willing to challenge doctors' authority, with written complaints about NHS hospital and family services reaching 133,820 in 2004/05 (Department of Health 2006b). Thirdly, just as the market uses the supposed expertise of the informed consumer, so health care has developed the idea of the 'expert patient' who should be more active in the management of their own condition. For example, in Britain, Expert Patient Programmes are based on the idea that patients' expert knowledge of their own conditions is a valuable resource that has not been exploited enough in the care of chronically ill individuals. Nominated lay experts can empower other sufferers who would then operate in 'partnership' with doctors and nurses.

The consequences of consumerism

While governments and some patient organisations argue that greater consumerism in health care both empowers patients and leads to better practice from health care professionals, there are also reasons to be concerned about the effect of these developments on nursing and medicine and, ultimately, on patient care. First, according to some critics, the growth in health care education of subjects designed to elicit the consumer's view, such as social sciences, ethics and communication skills, has resulted in young nurses (and doctors) having inadequate technical skills in certain key areas (McNee *et al.* 2005). There is evidence that the growing culture of patient complaint and litigation is not only undermining the morale of health care professionals, it is also leading to more defensive health care practices where the primary consideration is not necessarily what is in the best interests of the patient, but what is the safest option for the person providing the treatment (Kessler *et al.* 2006).

Initiatives like Expert Patient Programmes may be based on expectation rather than independent evidence. Many patients are simply too sick, old or confused to participate expertly in their own health care and some research has suggested that many of those who can participate in principle have neither the inclination nor the knowledge to do so in practice (Prior 2003). Further, there are concerns that – like behavioural approaches to improving and maintaining health – expert patient programmes may be a disguised way of cutting or rationing health care services. After all, if increasing numbers of sufferers are really experts in their own health care why do we need so many health care professionals?

Summary

Demands upon the NHS are greater than ever before and the service is under increasing pressure from demographic change, developments in medical technology and practice, greater consumer expectations and the rising costs of the health care workforce. In response to these pressures governments have made a number of changes to the organisation of health care, the most important of which are encouraging the increase of private sector and voluntary health care, reducing the time people spend in hospitals and encouraging the growth of community and lay care. There have also been changes in the culture of health care: medical dominance has been challenged, attempts have been made to give people more rights over, and responsibility for, their own health care and, with increasing consumerism in health care, professional–patient relations are increasingly coming to resemble provider–customer relations in the free market. These changes in health reflect changes in wider society, particularly the growth of individualism and the decline of state welfareism.

References

Armstrong, D. (1998) Decline of the hospital: reconstructing institutional dangers. *Sociology of Health and Illness*, 20, 445–57.
Bajekal, M., Osborne, V., Yar, M. and Meltzer, H. (eds) (2006) *Focus on Health*. Office of National Statistics/Palgrave Macmillan, London. Available at www.statistics. org (accessed April 2006).

Bauman, Z. (2002) *Work, Consumerism and the New Poor*. Open University Press, Buckingham.

Beck-Gernsheim, E. (2002) *Reinventing the Family: In Search of New Life Styles*. Polity, Cambridge.

Blank, R. and Burau, V. (2004) *Comparative Health Policy*. Palgrave, Basingstoke.

Cline, R.J.W. and Haynes, K.M. (2001) Consumer health information seeking on the Internet: the state of the art. *Health Education Research*, 16, 671–92.

Department of Health (2000) *The NHS Plan: A Plan for Investment, A Plan for Reform*. The Stationery Office, London.

Department of Health (2002) *Delivering the NHS Plan*. The Stationery Office, London.

Department of Health (2005a) *Creating a Patient-led NHS: Delivering the NHS Improvement Plan*. The Stationery Office, London.

Department of Health (2005b) *MRSA Surveillance System*. The Stationery Office, London.

Department of Health (2006a) *The Health and Social Care System*. The Stationery Office, London.

Department of Health (2006b) Data on written complaints in the NHS 2004–05. Available at www.ic.nhs.uk/pubs/wcomplaints (accessed August 2006).

Giddens, A. (1991) *Modernity and Self Identity*. Polity, Cambridge.

Glennester, H. (2000) *British Social Policy Since 1945*, 2nd edition. Blackwell, Oxford.

Henwood, F., Wyatt, S., Hart, A. and Smith, J. (2004) 'Ignorance is bliss sometimes': constraints on the emergence of the 'informed patient' in the changing landscapes of health information, in C. Seale (ed.) *Health and the Media*. Blackwell, Oxford.

Kessler, D., Summerton, N. and Graham, J. (2006) Effects of the medical liability system in Australia, the UK and the USA. *Lancet*, 368, 240–6.

Maher, J. and Green, H. (2002) *Carers 2000. Results from the Carers' Module of the General Household Survey 2000*. The Stationery Office, London.

McNee, P., Clarke, D. and Davies, J. (2005) The teaching of clinical skills in the context of children's nursing. *Journal of Child Health Care*, 9(3), 208–21.

Mizrachi, N., Shuval, J. and Gross, S. (2005) Boundary at work; alternative medicine in biomedical settings. *Sociology of Health and Illness*, 27(1), 20–43.

Office of National Statistics (2006) *Social Trends 36*. Stationery Office, London.

Prior, L. (2003) Belief, knowledge and expertise: the emergence of the lay expert in medical sociology. *Sociology of Health and Illness*, 25, 41–57.

Saks, M. (2006) The alternatives to medicine, in D. Kelleher, J. Gabe and G. Williams (eds) *Challenging Medicine*, 2nd edition. Routledge, London.

Tudor Hart, J. (2006) *The Political Economy of Health Care: A Clinical Perspective*. Policy Press, Bristol.

Yuen, P. (2005) *Compendium of Health Statistics 2005–2006*, 17th edition. Office of Health Economics. Radcliffe Publishing, Abingdon.

Wanless, D. (2002) *Securing our Future Health: Taking a Long-Term View. Final Report*. HM Treasury, London.

Further reading

Kelleher, D., Gabe, J. and Williams, G. eds (2006) *Challenging Medicine*, 2nd edition. Routledge, Abingdon.
   A collection of original papers looking at challenges to medicine from a variety of sources.
Tudor Hart, J. (2006) *The Political Economy of Health Care: A Clinical Perspective.* Policy Press, Bristol.
   A critical evaluation of current changes in British health care.

Chapter 11

Health policy

Introduction

The previous chapters have shown that people's health and their ability to cope with illness are influenced by a range of social and cultural factors. This chapter considers another set of influences on health and illness, the impact of government health policy and of the health services that are available. As the provision of health care in contemporary Britain is the result of a long series of incremental changes and reforms, understanding health policy necessarily involves adopting an historical perspective. This chapter will:

- discuss the making of health policy;
- outline and discuss the major reforms of health policy in Britain;
- describe New Labour's health policy agenda;
- discuss key issues in contemporary health policy.

Health policy and the politics of health

Health is political – it matters both to states and populations. It is not something left entirely to individual initiative, voluntary action or private markets. Everywhere, health and health care are a major preoccupation of governments, and in all developed countries governments play a major role in regulating health care and access to it, providing finance and, in some cases, directly providing health services. In the UK, for example, around 8% of national income ('GDP') is spent on health care, nearly all of it by the government on the NHS. In many other countries, for example Canada, France, Germany and the USA, the figure is even higher. Data from the Organisation for Economic Co-operation and Development (OECD) show that, at £1547 per person spent on health care in 2003, the UK spends about 15% less than France, 21% less than Germany and about 11% less than the OECD average (Figure 11.1). However, among OECD countries the UK has seen one of the fastest rates of growth in health care expenditure as a proportion of GDP since 1990. The latest available data show that the proportion of GDP spent on health care per person is significantly above the OECD average (Yuen 2005).

In addition to financing health care to a greater or lesser extent, governments in most developed countries seek to regulate and modify individual

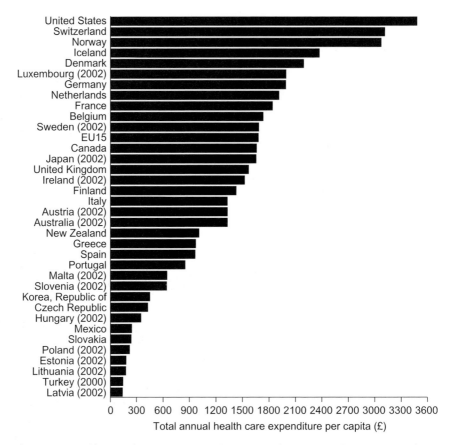

Figure 11.1 Health Expenditure per person in Organisation for Economic Co-operation and Development (OECD) and European Union (EU) countries, *c.* 2003.
Source: Figure 2.6 in Yuen, P. (2005) *Compendium of Health Statistics 2005–2006*. Radcliffe Publishing, Oxford. Reproduced with permission from the Office of Health Economics.

and group behaviour to promote health, for example by smoking bans, controlling access to alcohol, prohibiting the sale and use of 'hard' or addictive drugs, campaigns on sexual health, workplace health and safety laws, food safety standards, and environmental health laws and regulations. Therefore, health policy is something that nearly all governments engage in to varying extents and in different ways.

Health policy

The term 'health policy' is often used to refer to decisions and actions of governments in relation to health. In the UK this mainly takes the form of legislation (law-making), and decisions about funding and budgeting for health care provided by the NHS. It can also include proposals and statements of intent in the form of ministerial speeches, White Papers, advice and guidance from the Department of Health (DH), directives such as National Service Frameworks (NSFs) and decisions by such bodies as the National Institute for Health and Clinical Excellence (NICE). Health policy extends beyond the NHS and the delivery of health care and health services as it also embraces a wider health agenda that includes issues of public and preventive health.

It is important to make a distinction between 'health policy' and 'health care policy'. *Health care policy* is about individual care and treatment and the provision of services. *Health policy* is much broader, and arguably has more influence on health than health care policy as it involves a range of social as well as medical factors that impinge on the health of a population. However, health care policy is seen as more important for voters, public opinion and governments. As Klein (1989: 173) observed:

> *The NHS has . . . a political constituency: those whose income comes from working in it and those who, as patients, derive some direct benefits from its services. Prevention has no such constituency. Those who will benefit cannot be identified; moreover, the benefit itself is uncertain. For prevention is about the reduction of statistical risk, not about the delivery of certain benefits to specific individuals.*

While political parties and governments might believe that it would be better to spend public money on public and preventive health measures, the practicalities of winning elections demand that they spend money on improving health care and health services For example, by shortening waiting lists, increasing the numbers of doctors and nurses, and increasing the availability and uptake of new medical technology. Thus for policy makers, following the bio-medical model of health with its focus upon the cure and care of individuals may be a more immediately attractive option than following the socio-medical model that focuses on the health of the general public (Chapter 2).

It is also important to appreciate that health policy involves not only actions and deliberate decisions to do something, but also decisions to do nothing rather than something. For example, some issues may not come up for consideration, while the discussion of others may be postponed. Therefore, what is or what is not included on the agenda for discussion and decision is vital for an understanding of policy making (Ham and Hill 1984). For example, the Conservative government of the early 1980s decided not to act upon the advice of the Black Report (Townsend and Davidson 1982) to reduce socio-economic health inequalities, whereas the new Labour government in 1997 made the reduction of such inequalities a key component of its health policy.

Finally, it is important to distinguish between the formulation and planning of a policy, its implementation and its outcome. A policy does not really exist unless and until it is implemented, and there may be a 'gap' between its formulation and implementation. Further, policies do not always achieve their goals, for example, a policy goal of the NHS when it was founded in 1948 was to achieve equality of health for the UK population. However, the reality is that inequalities of various kinds still persist.

Making health policy

There have been major constitutional changes in the UK since 1998, resulting in political devolution to the four constituent countries, so that it is no longer possible to talk about a single UK health and NHS policy. There are now devolved governments with varying degrees of autonomy and responsibility in Scotland, Wales and Northern Ireland, and there are now, more clearly than before, four UK health systems, each with its own priorities and policies. English and Scottish policies for the NHS, for example, now seem to be quite different. In what follows the focus is on English developments.

In England, health policy is formally in the hands of the DH, headed by a Secretary of State, who is a politician. However, governments do not make health policy on their own. Much day to day health policy making is the outcome of a complex process of bargaining and negotiation, involving trade-offs and compromises, between the government and various interest, pressure and lobby groups that comprise the health policy 'community'.

The NHS itself and its constituent parts can have their own policies. Primary Care Trusts (PCTs), for example, can make their own policies about such issues as the treatments they will commission from hospital providers, or the resources they will devote to public health. Health policies are also influenced by a wide range of groups, agencies and organisations which influence health policy in various ways and to varying extents. These include Parliament, health care professions, local government, trade unions (including those in the health sector such as UNISON), voluntary organisations, such as MENCAP, MIND and Age Concern, patient groups and voluntary movements, such as the hospice movement. Other organisations include international agencies such as the World Health Organisation and the European Union (EU), international pharmaceutical companies, private health insurers and private health service providers. The totality of these groups and interests may be referred to as the health policy 'community'.

The DH may choose to consult groups and organisations, such as voluntary organisations and professional associations, before deciding on policy changes, either to seek their consent or acquiescence for proposed changes or because they may have expertise in relation to some issue. Organisations like the British Medical Association and the Royal College of Nursing are usually consulted by the DH as a matter of routine. Organisations may also actively try to represent their views to government, seeking meetings with ministers and civil servants, or submitting memoranda, or trying to enlist the support of the media or MPs to bring pressure to bear on ministers. In other cases, its membership of international or supranational organisations, such as the EU, impose obligations that the government must meet. An example is the European Working Time Directive which has limited the hours that junior doctors can work.

Health ministers are also accountable to Parliament, which has important scrutiny and oversight responsibilities. MPs can ask questions of ministers about the state of the NHS, or about issues affecting their constituents and the care they have received. In addition, there is a House of Commons Select

Committee which 'shadows' the DH, and has the power to summon and cross-examine witnesses, including ministers and civil servants. This committee reports on particular issues to which the DH is normally obliged to respond. Another source of policy influence are *ad hoc* expert committees of inquiry, set up by the government to look into particular issues, such as the Black Committee on health inequalities and the Wanless inquiries into NHS funding (Wanless 2002) and public health (Wanless 2004).

In recent years the British media have also become influential in affecting health policy: health and the state of the NHS are news. Ministers are acutely sensitive to the impact that media reporting on the NHS may have on government popularity, and this sensitivity has been increasing. For example, media campaigns about the lack of choice in health care, the 'postcode lottery' of access to care and the unavailability of potentially life-saving treatments have all influenced governments' health policy. Health service users and voters may also have some influence on policy, and that influence seems to have been increasing in recent years. However, the influence of the public is hard to distinguish from that of the media, since the former is shaped to some extent by the latter (Seale 2002).

Groups and interests in the health policy community are not necessarily equal in their power to influence policy. On the whole, policy has been dominated by provider rather than consumer or user interests. As we have seen in Chapter 10, the medical profession has been the most powerful interest group in relation to health policy because it has had the power to determine priorities. The priorities of the medical profession have been focused on acute care and a 'medical model' approach to sickness and ill-health. It has been suggested that the existence of this medical power has resulted in lower priorities being given to long-term illness and disability, public and preventive health, and the relative neglect of socially based inequalities in health.

Although dominant, the medical profession has been challenged in recent years by other groups, such as management, politicians and civil servants (Kelleher *et al.* 2006) (Chapter 10). The past 20 years in British health policy have seen a determined attempt on the part of policy makers to wrest control from the profession and to reshape agendas and priorities in new directions. As we shall see later in the chapter, policy makers have sought to change power relations within the NHS by emphasising and developing primary care and de-emphasising hospital care, and by taking a renewed interest in public and preventive health. Doctors and nurses have become subject to various forms of monitoring, audit, inspection and evaluation of their work. Some of these developments in auditing and inspection have been advanced by recent scandals, such as the exceptionally high child mortality rates at the Bristol Royal Infirmary and the case of the medical mass-murderer Harold Shipman. As a result, it has been suggested, the profession has been weakened and its capacity to block or thwart change has at least been challenged and may have been reduced. A further development challenging medical power has been the rise of the patient as a 'consumer', willing to challenge professional decisions (Chapter 10).

Thus, health policy is a process of change and conflict: a policy cycle in which certain health issues come to the top of the political agenda (for instance,

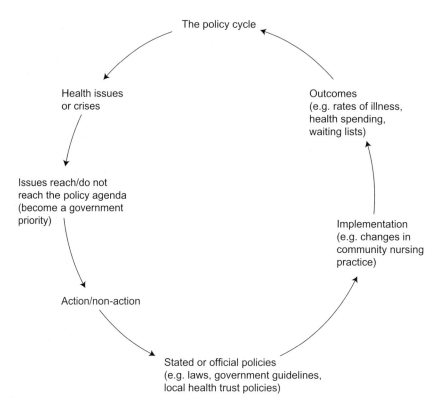

Figure 11.2 The policy cycle.

through media interest in 'health scares' or a health minister's interest in bringing about reform). These issues are either downplayed and side-tracked, or acted upon by government – with varying results in terms of implementation and outcomes (Figure 11.2).

While changes in health policy command the greatest attention, the maintenance and continuity of policy are equally important. There is a large element of inertia in public policy and introducing change can be difficult, especially in relation to an area like health where there are competing interests and conflicting demands on policy makers (Ham 2004: 153). Although there has been a large amount of what looks like radical change in the UK, and especially English, health system in recent years, some of this may be more apparent than real. As we will see, the similarities between New Labour policy after 1997 and Conservative policy before that are striking.

The NHS: origins and development

The National Health Service (NHS), the major provider of health care in the UK, was created in 1948, building upon the existing infrastructure of health service facilities and providers already in place – hospitals, GPs and a variety of local and community based services. By the standards of that time health care provision was of high quality, although it was not universally accessible and many hospitals were in severe financial circumstances. Government responsibility (at local and national levels) for individuals' health and welfare was more limited than today, and there was no centralised, co-ordinated set of health services. For instance, before the NHS, hospital services were provided by a patchwork of voluntary (charitable) foundations, municipal hospitals (run by local government) and private hospitals and clinics (Webster 1998).

The creation of the NHS involved changes in funding, entitlement and governance. The funding of health care was simplified, now coming from central government sources, and made up almost entirely of general tax revenues, with some contribution from National Insurance. The level of and increases in health care funding became entirely subject to central government discretion and its centrally imposed NHS budget. The private sector was greatly reduced, but retained a small and marginal role in both health care and health insurance. Entitlement to the use of health services became universal. Fees and charges were abolished and the service became 'free at the point of use', although prescription charges were soon introduced. Hospitals – both local authority and voluntary – were taken into national public ownership under the control of Boards of Governors or Regional Hospital Boards under the Ministry of Health.

The health care 'settlement' of 1948 involved a deal between the State and the medical profession, involving the entrenchment of professional power, the exclusion of popular, user or democratic representation, and the acceptance by politicians that they would take a back seat in the management of the service. Although many doctors were initially opposed to state medicine, they quickly realised that the NHS *consolidated*, rather than compromised, medical power and autonomy. Hospital specialists became salaried employees, with a generous system of merit awards to reward the most able and with the right to treat private patients in their now publicly owned hospitals. The division between general practice and specialised hospital medicine was retained and enhanced. The GP service, created with the introduction of National Health Insurance in 1911, was left largely unchanged, although access to GPs became universal. GPs retained their status as independent contractors to the state system, avoiding salaried service and what they saw as subjection to bureaucratic state control. Local authorities thereby lost many of their major health responsibilities, but retained responsibilities for community medical services and public health. The result was a divided 'tripartite' governance structure, in some respects a messy political compromise (Webster 1998).

After its creation the structure of the NHS remained relatively unchanged for over 30 years, as both major political parties and successive governments accepted the fundamental principles on which it was based (Chapter 10) and its tripartite structure and the dominant role of the medical professions within it. However, by the mid-1970s this political consensus was breaking down, and the election of a Conservative government in 1979 signalled the start of the first significant structural and managerial reforms of the NHS.

Conservative reforms

A Conservative government under Margaret Thatcher was elected in 1979, and the Conservatives were to remain in power for the next 18 years. This period was one of radical upheaval and challenges to the NHS. The Conservative health service reforms should be viewed in the context of their reform agenda for all of the public sector after 1987. Similar reforms were applied to education, housing and social care services. Much of this reform agenda was driven by a concern with efficiency and value for money (Bartlett and Harrison 1993).

While the Conservatives maintained the basic principles of a 'free' health service financed mainly by central government, they were determined to increase managerial control over health professionals and to make health care organisations more accountable for the resources they used. There was significant reform in the management of the NHS following the Griffiths Report in 1983 (Klein 2001, Ham 2004). This resulted in the introduction of 'general management', of the kind now familiar in the NHS. This managerial reform involved a new emphasis on performance, measured in terms of 'effectiveness' and 'efficiency', and on 'quality', as well as on innovation and change.

The most radical reform was the introduction of a competitive structure into the NHS, known as the internal market. This was based on the principle that money to pay for health services should 'follow the patient'. The NHS was divided into groups of 'purchasers' and 'providers' of health services. Health service providers, such as hospital trusts, were expected to compete against each other to provide their services to purchasing groups, such as health authorities and GP practices. Under these reforms some GPs became fundholders of their own budgets with the ability to 'purchase' hospital services for their patients.

The aim of the purchaser–provider split was to decentralise the system, to move services closer to the patient and also to enhance efficiency by increasing awareness of the cost of services. The more successful providers would attract more patients than the less efficient or cost-effective, and efficiency was thus rewarded with more money and resources. The new management culture and the internal market brought about significant changes to the work environment of health professionals, particularly by undermining their autonomy and increasing managerial control of their work. Under the Conservatives the private health sector also expanded in both its funding and in the provision of services. Private health insurance, private hospital care, private residential and long-term nursing care, and the contracting-out of a variety of ancillary, non-core hospital services, all developed in this period. Although the Conservatives did not rule out substantial privatisation of health care funding, they continued to defend the fundamental principle of free, state funded health care that had existed since 1948.

Other important changes included the introduction of the Patient's Charter, a basic list of entitlements for patients covering various aspects of service quality, such as waiting lists. This was part of a larger strategy for public sector services called the Citizen's Charter. The early 1990s also saw the beginnings of a general strategy for population health, involving an expansion of community care, a greater emphasis on health education and promotion, and financial incentives for GPs to carry out preventative work.

Evaluation of the impact and effectiveness of the Conservative reforms has been difficult, because the plans were modified in the process of implementation, and because the effects of the reforms are hard to disentangle from the effects of other policy changes occurring at the same time (Ham 2004: 44–7). Some improvements were noted, but criticism centred on the alleged creation of a 'two-tier' service, in part resulting from one of the most dynamic elements of the reforms, GP fundholding and commissioning. Fundholding practices demonstrated their ability to 'fast-track' patients to specialist secondary care. This showed that contracting and commissioning appeared to work in bringing about some improvements in patient care. One sympathetic observer of the reforms concluded that 'the change in behaviour and culture was nevertheless tangible . . . the separation of purchaser and provider responsibilities altered the organizational politics of the NHS leading to changes in the balance of power both within the medical profession and between doctors and managers' (Ham 2004: 46–7).

Many long-standing problems were left unaddressed by the Conservatives, notably the issues of NHS funding, health care 'rationing' or prioritising and health inequalities. In some cases these problems were made more serious through the effects of other public policies, such as the determination to limit tax and public expenditure increases. This was compounded by the rise in unemployment, the growth of poverty, increasing homelessness and the widening of income inequalities that was characteristic of the 1980s and early 1990s. To some extent New Labour has attempted to deal with these neglected issues. It has also adopted and adapted other aspects of the Conservative legacy of health care reform.

'New' Labour health policy

The New Labour government, elected in 1997, has carried forward the programme of reforms begun under the previous Conservative governments, but at the same time there have been genuine departures from Conservative policy. The main aims of the New Labour government's strategy has been to 'modernise' the NHS and to increase the volume and quality of care (Klein 2005: 52). Since 2000 the NHS has been in a constant state of change.

Resourcing the NHS

The early years of New Labour from 1997 to 1999 were years of relatively low growth in funding as a result of New Labour's election pledge to adhere to Conservative public spending targets. However, the NHS still received higher than average annual increases in funding (4.8% per year) in comparison with other services and compared with its historical average of 3%. In 2000, following a winter influenza epidemic that increased pressure on NHS hospital beds, the government announced that spending on the NHS would be doubled, with the aim of matching the European average by 2008. Some of this increased funding has been spent on increasing the number and pay of NHS staff. Since 1999, the NHS has employed an extra 56,700 more nurses, 5400 more consultants and 1900 more GPs (Klein 2005). Health care is a labour-intensive activity, and the bulk of health care budgets – almost 70% of the total – is spent on staff salaries. There have also been increased intakes in medical and nursing students. However, questions remain about how effective the increases in funding and NHS staff have been in securing improvements in the volume and quality of patient care. For example, it has been claimed that although 40% more was spent on the NHS between 1998 and 2003, this resulted in only a 5% increase in inpatient activity (Toynbee and Walker 2005).

Managing and regulating the system

New Labour originally rejected the Conservatives' internal market experiment, with its allegedly bad consequences for equity, co-ordination and planning (Department of Health 1997). However, it recognized that the purchaser–provider separation and the creation of primary care commissioning had brought some benefits. Although New Labour proposed the abolition of GP fundholding, in practice it has built on and extended the scheme. The concept of a 'primary care-led NHS', originally promoted by the Conservatives, was one that the government found acceptable, and it made all GPs 'fundholders'. All GP practices would henceforth become members of collective commissioning entities called Primary Care Groups (PCGs), later to become Trusts (PCTs), with devolved budgets which would be used to commission care from secondary providers. This was an implicit acknowledgement that the GP fundholding scheme had brought some benefits for those patients whose GPs were members of the scheme. The government aimed to give PCTs control of 75% of the NHS budget by 2004.

Other innovations included the introduction of NHS Direct, a 24-hour telephone and online consultation service, and the introduction of local walk-in centres, both staffed by nurses to provide basic advice and care. These were 'modernisation' measures aimed at increasing public access to health services. The government also introduced National Service Frameworks (NSFs) to set minimum appropriate standards of care and treatment for a range of conditions. As well as specifying standards of care and treatment, the underlying idea of the NSFs is to try to eliminate variations in treatment between areas and localities, and to ensure that the quality of treatment does not depend on where a patient lives. One effect of the introduction NSF standards has been to encroach on doctors' clinical freedom.

New Labour's health policy initiatives also included the creation of special agencies for evaluating and regulating health service performance, such as the National Institute for Health and Clinical Excellence (NICE) and the Healthcare Commission. NICE is concerned with evaluating medical technology (which includes all types of therapeutic interventions, drugs, procedures, surgical and other) in terms of their effectiveness and efficiency, permitting their use by the NHS or alternatively rejecting and prohibiting it. Like NSFs, NICE's directives also function to limit clinical freedom. Another important new organisation, the Healthcare Commission, has the task of inspecting and monitoring standards of care in NHS organisations.

Targets

Another major aspect of New Labour developments in the management of the NHS is the use of targets of all kinds. These represent an attempt to strengthen control from the centre (the DH in England). Targets also have their origins in the Conservative period of the early 1980s, with the development of Performance Indicators and the performance-related pay and fixed-term contracts of the Griffith management reforms, but go much further than these. An example of a target is that of reducing waiting times to 18 weeks from initial GP consultation to inpatient hospital operation, to be achieved for all conditions and specialisms by 2008 (Timmins 2005). Waiting lists are typically associated with elective, non-urgent, surgical procedures. Waiting lists and waiting times have been a key area for service improvements in the NHS since 1997, and the government has had some success in bringing these down. Money has been directed at these, possibly to the detriment of care and treatment in other areas.

Management has been strengthened ('micro-management' is the term favoured by those unsympathetic to this development). Such 'top-down' control is particularly associated with the enhanced power of the Treasury under New Labour over all aspects of domestic policy. However, in 2006 the government seemed to be moving away from the 'command and control', top-down managerial approach associated with the regime of targets and public service agreements, towards a looser, more arms-length regulation, relying on monitoring and inspection by agencies such as the Healthcare Commission to maintain and improve standards (Klein 2005: 52).

The NHS plan 2000

The NHS plan in 2000, which put forward a 10-year programme of development for the NHS, introduced some new emphases into health policy. The plan was a consensus-building exercise, involving wide consultation with the public, health professions, other NHS staff, patient groups, professional associations and researchers within the health care community. As well as reiterating the core principles of the NHS, the plan enunciated the basic aim of creating a health service 'designed around the patient'. The implication being that the NHS had failed to create a health service focused on individual patient needs. The government argued that this was due to, among other things, a long history of under-investment, the lack of nationally set and monitored standards, rigid demarcations between staff, the lack of measurable incentives and the disempowerment of patients.

The emphasis was on investment and reform. Elements of reform identified by NHS staff and public included:

- increased staffing;
- reduction in waiting times;
- more staff training;
- 'joined up' working with social care.

There were a large number of specific commitments, including cleaner hospitals, better hospital food, improved pay and working conditions, the development of intermediate care (Chapter 6) and links with social care, new consultant and GP contracts, the creation of 'modern matrons' in hospitals, more information and greater choice for patients and the commitment to cut waiting times for inpatient, outpatient and primary care. The management of the system was also changed, with national standards to be established by the DH with regulation and scrutiny by agencies such as the Commission for Health Improvement (now the Healthcare Commission) strengthened.

The government committed themselves more firmly than ever to the idea of a 'patient-led' NHS, to the expansion of patient choice and, in principle, to a greater devolution of decision-making responsibility to lower levels in the system. The creation of PCTs and 'foundation hospitals' (see below) exemplify this. However, underlying all these changes was the commitment to centralised regulation of the NHS, embodied in the NSFs, NICE and the Healthcare Commission.

In 2002 the DH announced the development of so-called 'foundation' hospitals (Department of Health 2002a). These looked suspiciously like the NHS hospital trusts promoted by the Conservatives in their 1990 legislation. 'Foundation' hospitals are supposed to enjoy a degree of independence and freedom from central control, although the degree of independence and autonomy was a matter of disagreement between the DH and the Treasury. This was, and remains, a controversial issue, with critics arguing they are a 'backdoor' to privatisation (Pollock 2004).

Choice of provider was a significant element in the 2000 reform package. This was highlighted by the Conservatives in their 1989 reform plans for the NHS (Department of Health 1989), but New Labour has gone much further in attempting to realise it. Choice of provider, whether primary care doctor, specialist, or hospital, is something that people in many European and other countries take for granted, but this has never figured prominently among the goals of the NHS. Patients are now to be allowed to choose their hospital provider from a list of four or five, and it is intended that from 2008 their choice will be unlimited. The choice agenda is to some extent a response to the Conservative Party challenge on this issue (Klein 2005: 58). 'Choice' is a controversial policy, rejected by traditionalist defenders of the NHS, who argue that 'choice' is incompatible with the basic goal of the NHS to provide equality of access to health care for all on the basis of need (Tudor Hart 2006). They suggest that not everybody can choose and that 'choice' is a policy that can only lead to a 'two-tier' service.

Another important innovation has been the introduction, in 2004, of a new system for paying health care providers (mainly hospitals) by results. This involved the construction of a reimbursement schedule of tariffs or fees for every medical procedure based on average costs for each procedure. Providers with below average costs can keep the surplus; those with above average costs will suffer a shortfall which will supposedly induce them to improve efficiency, but might have implications for the long-run financial viability of some providers (Klein 2005: 59–60). By this means, money is supposed to 'follow the patient'.

Private sector and public–private partnerships

The increasing involvement of the private sector in the NHS was discussed in Chapter 10. New Labour initially shunned collaboration with private sector health care providers but this began to be reversed in 2000 when the DH agreed a 'concordat' with the private sector, involving an agreement for the NHS to use independent sector facilities to treat NHS patients. The policy has developed further since then with the introduction of independent sector treatment centres (ISTCs), some supplied and staffed by commercial groups from overseas, to provide specialist treatment for routine elective conditions, such as hip replacements and cataract operations, where there are substantial NHS waiting lists. This is part of the government's supply-side strategy for increasing NHS capacity (Allsop and Baggott 2004). However, the introduction of such public–private partnerships has proved to be controversial.

Public–private partnerships take a variety of forms. They can involve collaboration between the NHS and private sector providers, either hospitals or ISTCs providing highly specialised procedures in bulk. A second wave of ISTCs is planned to provide an extra 1.7 million operations for the NHS by 2010. Another area of public–private collaboration is that of the Private Finance Initiative (PFI), which involves the use of private capital investment in the building and equipping of NHS infrastructure, such as hospitals. The PFI programme was launched by the Conservatives in 1992, but only bore fruit under Labour; no PFI deals were signed under the Conservatives (Tudor Hart 2006). By 2006 a large number of PFI deals had been signed with private sector consortia. The main advantage for government in these arrangements is a reduction in public-sector capital costs, which henceforth no longer appear in the government's capital budget. Other claimed advantages include better project management, faster and more efficient building and commissioning of new schemes to time and on budget, things rarely achieved in the days of public sector commissioning.

PFI schemes have been attacked by the government's critics, mainly on the left, who argue that ostensible, 'up-front' budgetary savings do not translate into overall lifetime savings on the projects. The growing numbers of hospitals and services financed by privately raised capital have to repay shareholders' investments and thus become increasingly subject to the laws of the market. Critics' fear is that they will inevitably focus on the more profitable treatments. The NHS is essentially renting the assets from the private consortia for a fixed period, until they eventually revert to public ownership, and it is argued that the costs in the long run will be higher (Pollock 2004).

Changing patterns of work in the NHS

The NHS is a major employer, and employment in it has expanded since 1997. In 2004 it employed approximately 1.3 million people, an average annual increase of over 39,000 staff since 1997. As well as doctors and nurses, it employs a myriad of different occupational groups in a variety of clinical and non-clinical support roles, and in a variety of settings, from teaching hospitals to community care (Figure 11.3). The twenty-first century has seen continual restructuring and reorganisation of the NHS, involving new ways of working and new incentives for its staff within a context of ever-changing and increasing demands. There has been a move towards integrated and managed care with the advent of PCGs and PCTs. Roles for health service workers such as nurses are in flux, with nurses and other professionals being encouraged to undertake a wider variety of roles (Chapter 12).

The emphasis in health care is shifting from the acute hospital to primary care and community settings, with the advent of NHS Direct, walk-in centres, the introduction of nurse prescribing and increases in numbers of primary care practice nurses. A DH document, *Liberating the Talents* (Department of Health 2002b), was concerned with promoting developed and expanded roles for nurses, midwives and health visitors working in primary care, for example by taking on work traditionally done by GPs and by providing more secondary

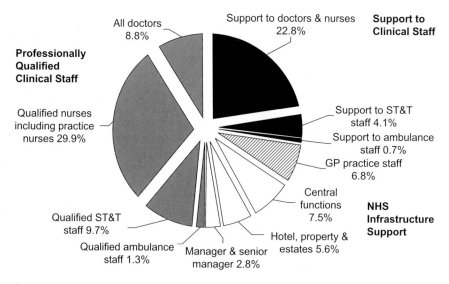

Figure 11.3 NHS staff 2004.
Source: Department of Health (2005) *Staff in the NHS 2004*. The Stationery Office, London. Crown copyright 2006.

care in community settings. Early research suggests that another consequence of this policy has been the devolution of some medical and nursing work in general practices to less qualified and cheaper personnel (Charles-Jones *et al.* 2003).

Patterns of acute hospital care are changing, with falls in lengths of hospital stay, higher bed occupancy rates and more intensive use of facilities. After a review of hospital bed provision in 2000 the DH accepted that care should be moved 'closer to home'. This required the expansion of intermediate care services to prevent acute hospital admissions. It has also suggested a reversal of its emphasis on centralising acute hospital services in larger facilities and maintaining local access – although the European Working Time Directive has made the staffing of small acute hospitals more difficult (Ham 2004: 90).

Staffing

The issue of staffing is of interest for a number of reasons. As has already been noted, NHS staff numbers, mostly 'front-line' staff, have increased in recent years. At the same time the European Working Time Directive has reduced the hours that can be worked by junior hospital doctors, thereby restricting the apparent expansion of medical labour supply. Another issue affecting staffing is immigration. Staff expansion in the NHS has been aided by the immigration of substantial numbers of overseas health workers to meet the shortfall in nursing (Chapter 12) and other staff. The NHS has always relied on people from overseas to fulfil its staffing requirements and actively recruited them in the 1960s and 1970s. However, this poses questions about fairness and human rights, because Britain appears to be meeting its shortfall in health care staffing requirements at the expense of the needs of developing countries, where most of the overseas recruits come from.

From the point of view of the work, pay and conditions of health service staff in the NHS, one of the most significant recent developments has been the launch of the *Agenda for Change* initiative in 2004. This is essentially a programme of job evaluation, linked to grading and pay, underpinned by a number of goals such as 'equal pay for work of equal value'. It can also be seen as another employer-sponsored attempt to promote flexibility and break down traditional demarcation lines in the system, and as a basis for modifying labour inputs into the caring process, substituting expensive labour (doctors) by less expensive (e.g. nurse practitioners) (Ham 2004: 60) (Chapter 12). Despite what looks like a focus on the interests of NHS employers, the programme seems to have been welcomed by health service unions like the RCN and UNISON, presumably because the associated pay increases have helped to make them acceptable.

Public and preventive health

New Labour has attempted to raise the profile of public and preventive health, with health improvement explicitly the first priority of the DH. The basis of the government's strategy was the consultation document *Our Healthier Nation*, published in 1997. This built on earlier Conservative initiatives, in particular the similarly-named *Health of the Nation* (1992). However, unlike the Conservative document, the New Labour document acknowledged the existence of health inequalities, placing emphasis on the socio-economic determinants of health. The document proposed four priority areas for improvements in health:

- heart disease and stroke;
- accidents;
- cancer;
- mental health.

Numerical targets were set for improvement by 2010 – a similar approach to the Conservative document. These targets were subsequently reiterated in 1999 with a new emphasis on improving health in later life with the aim of preventing 300,000 unnecessary and untimely deaths (Department of Health 1999). A Health Development Agency (subsequently incorporated into NICE) was created to realise these objectives.

One of the issues leading to the emphasis on public and preventative health was New Labour's concern about the persistence of socially based health inequalities and the need to reduce them. However, it is not entirely clear how far this is being realised in practice. Financial deficits and other priorities appear to have compromised public health efforts by diverting funds to acute care. In 2006 New Labour's public health policy seemed very similar to that of the preceding Conservative government, mainly emphasising individual responsibility for health: individuals should adopt healthy lifestyles, stop smoking, eat healthily and take exercise. This seems to reiterate the message of the influential Wanless Report of 2002, which considered various 'scenarios' for the long-term future of health spending, including what it called the 'fully engaged' future, in which the control of health care costs would require individuals to take more responsibility for their own health.

The final Wanless Report in 2004 explored the 'fully engaged scenario' further. It detailed policies for limiting the demand for health care by reducing the consumption of alcohol, smoking and salt in food. In response, the Department of Health (2004) attempted to strike a balance between individual and collective responsibility. Individual choice takes place in a social context, including education, housing, and employment, among many others, which public policy can influence. The DH said nothing about the distribution of income and its modification through taxes and benefits, although this has been argued to be one of the most important factors influencing health (Chapter 3). However, the government can claim that the tax and benefit systems have become more redistributive towards the less well-off since 1997, with the introduction and advance of so-called 'stealth taxes' and increases in social security benefits for the retired and families with children (Shaw *et al*. 2004).

The creation of Health Action Zones (HAZs), area-based strategies for health interventions in areas of high deprivation, demonstrates one government response to the health inequality issue. It also illustrates its interest in 'joined-up' strategies for social interventions generally, since HAZs require multi-agency partnerships and working. The HAZ strategy involves targeting geographically identifiable areas, populations or communities characterised by multiple deprivations and allocating resources accordingly. An example of this kind of area-based strategy focusing on inequality is the 'Sure Start' programme, which targets families in deprived areas with a mixture of health and social interventions designed to improve health. Substantial resources have been devoted to the HAZ programme and, although it has yet to prove its worth, the early indications are that it has raised the profile of health inequalities in local areas by raising the issues of hidden groups and has improved mainstream health services in some disadvantaged areas.

Rationing, priorities and health care

One of the original aims of the NHS was to provide equal access to its care for all citizens. A number of well-publicised cases of patients being denied access to essential treatment has brought this into question and raised the issue of rationing of health into the public consciousness. While the rationing of health services as an issue of public concern only came to the fore in the early 1990s, it has always existed. Rationing is universal and unavoidable. However, the words 'priorities' and 'prioritising' are sometimes preferred as more neutral terms to 'rationing' by some, for example by politicians.

Rationing in the NHS is nothing more than allocating or distributing health care in a context where ability to pay for treatment no longer operates, and where demand by professionals to drive up spending on health care is limited by fixed or 'global' budgets. In the NHS, which is governed according to the principles of need and equality, rather than the ability to pay, the allocation of health care resources takes place via the decision-making of professionals such as GPs and hospital consultants, by the managerial decisions of health authorities and PCTs about how their budgets should be spent on commissioning care for the populations being served, and by the decisions of Treasury and, in England, the DH officials and politicians who determine the level of funding.

The most visible manifestations of rationing are waiting lists for outpatient and inpatient non-urgent care and the time delays involved in consulting GPs. These are examples of 'rationing by delay', which has always existed in the NHS. Another type of rationing is by restricting access to particular treatments in the NHS. The availability of some procedures or interventions, such as in vitro fertilization (IVF), abortion and tattoo removal, has been restricted in particular areas, or been subject to varying criteria of eligibility. Recent media publicity about the denial and the restrictions of treatment to particular individuals has raised public concern about the prevalence of the so-called 'postcode' rationing. This is where the availability or quality of treatment varies from area to area, which is contrary to the NHS principle of providing equality of access to the best available treatment. High-profile media coverage of such inequalities in access to treatment (e.g. in the prescription of cancer drugs) have maintained public attention and concern. The impression created is that cost and affordability have become criteria for treatment rather than need, and that the fundamental NHS principles of universality, comprehensiveness, treatment on the basis of need and the absence of direct payment for treatment, are increasingly being called into question.

The scope of NHS services has become more restricted. Fundamental services such as eye care, dentistry, long-term nursing and rehabilitative care have increasingly been pushed outside the NHS in recent years, or become subject to charging and means tests. Some of this, as with dentistry, seems to have happened in an unintentional and piecemeal way, as dentists, increasingly unhappy with their NHS remuneration, withdrew from the service to practise privately. Other changes, such as the introduction of charges for eye tests, were the product of deliberate decisions.

Beyond 2006

At the time of writing, it is too early to gauge the overall effect of New Labour's health policy reforms. While New Labour has invested more heavily in the health service than any previous government, and can claim to be successful in a number of areas, such as increasing the material and human resources going into the NHS and improving the speed of treatment, concerns continue to be expressed about its 'modernisation' agenda. This is unsurprising because health and the provision of health care services have been a long-standing focus of concern in Britain, and changes to the NHS raise strong feelings and opinions. As was noted at the start of this chapter, health policy involves a process of change and conflict.

Two main concerns can be identified. First, poor management at the local level is compromising the modernisation agenda. In particular, it has led to financial deficits amongst hospitals and PCTs, accompanied by bed closures and job losses among their staff. Such NHS deficits affect local authorities' social care provision and in 2006 there were growing concerns about shortfalls in care budgets. It seems likely that funding and managing the NHS will continue to be practical and political issues. It has also been suggested that the continual process of change under New Labour since 2000 is undermining staff morale (Strachan-Bennett 2006) and reducing productivity.

Secondly, critics argue that New Labour's 'marketisation' of the NHS is undermining its original principles of providing comprehensive and equitable health care for all (Pollock 2004). A continuing concern is that the increasing involvement of the private sector in providing and managing health care is leading to a less equitable system of health care. For example, Tudor Hart (2006) argues that increasing marketisation of the NHS will lead to a system that is neither efficient nor equitable.

It is difficult to predict the consequences of New Labour's reforms on nursing, as some of its proposals are still at the discussion stage and, as we have seen above, there is often a gap between policy and implementation. However, three outcomes for nursing can be anticipated. First, nurses (and other health care professionals) can expect that their work will continue to be closely regulated and monitored. At the same time, the opportunities for some nurses to expand their roles and take on more responsibility are likely to grow (Chapter 12). Secondly, foundation hospitals are here to stay and, with the private sector now allowed to commission primary care, more nurses will be working in market-orientated organisational settings. Finally, the emphasis upon primary and preventative health care is likely to continue and, if the government's most recent plans for a major expansion of primary care are realised, large acute hospitals will no longer be the focus of the NHS. Thus an increasing number of nurses will work in primary care locations, such as GP surgeries, health centres and community hospitals.

Summary

Health is political, and in Britain, like most developed countries, the funding and regulation of health care is largely the responsibility of government. However, health polices are also shaped by a range of other interested parties, including health care organisations, professional bodies, and voluntary and commercial organisations. The NHS is the major provider of health care in the UK and its fundamental founding principles and structural organisation remained largely unchanged for over 30 years. Since 1990 there have been substantial changes in the organisation of the NHS, with the introduction of an internal market and the growth of private investment in health care. In many respects New Labour's health policies have continued these, while also introducing a programme of modernisation based on increasing management and regulation, greater inter-professional working, the expansion of primary and preventative health care, and the further expansion of commercial involvement in the NHS.

References

Allsop, J. and Baggott, R. (2004) The NHS in England: from modernisation to marketisation?, in N. Ellison (ed.) *Social Policy Review 16*. Policy Press, Bristol.

Bartlett, W. and Harrison, L. (1993) Quasi-markets and the National Health Service reforms, in J. Le Grand and W. Bartlett (eds) *Quasi-Markets and Social Policy*. Macmillan, Basingstoke.

Charles-Jones, H. Latimer, J. and May, C. (2003) Transforming general practice: The redistribution of medical work in primary care. *Sociology of Health and Illness*, 25, 71–92.

Department of Health (1989) *Working for Patients*. HMSO, London.

Department of Health (1997) *The New NHS*. HMSO, London.

Department of Health (1999) *Saving Lives*. HMSO, London.

Department of Health (2002a) *Delivering the NHS Plan*. HMSO, London.

Department of Health (2002b) *Liberating the Talents*. HMSO, London.

Department of Health (2004) *Choosing Health*. HMSO, London.

Ham, C. (2004) *Health Policy in Britain*, 5th edition. Palgrave, Basingstoke.

Ham, C. and Hill, M. (1984) *The Policy Process in the Modern Capitalist State*. Wheatsheaf, Brighton.

Kelleher, D., Gabe, J. and Williams, G (2006) *Challenging Medicine*, 2nd edition. Routledge, London.

Klein, R. (1989) *The Politics of the NHS*. Longman, London.

Klein, R. (2001) *The New Politics of the NHS*. Longman, Harlow.

Klein, R. (2005) Transforming the NHS: The Story in 2004, in M. Powell, L. Bauld and K. Clarke (eds) *Social Policy Review 17*. Policy Press, Bristol.

Pollock, A. (2004) *NHS plc: The Privatisation of our Health Care*. Verso, London.

Seale, C. (2002) *Media and Health*. Sage, London.

Shaw, M., Davey Smith, G. and Dorling, D. (2004) Health inequalities and New Labour: how the promises compare with real progress. *British Medical Journal*, 330, 1016–21.

Strachan-Bennett, S. (2006) Is nursing a job for life? *Nursing Times*, 12C(8), 16–19.

Timmins, N. (2005) Hewitt warns that failing hospitals will be closed. *Financial Times*, 14 May, 5.

Townsend, P. and Davidson, N. (1982) *Inequalities in Health*. Penguin, Harmondsworth.

Toynbee, P. and Walker, D. (2005) *Better or Worse? Has Labour Delivered?* Bloomsbury, London.

Tudor Hart, J. (2006) *The Political Economy of Health Care: A Clinical Perspective*. Policy Press, Bristol.

Wanless, D. (2002) *Securing our Future Health: Taking a Long-Term View. Final Report*. HM Treasury, London.

Wanless, D. (2004) *Securing Our Future Health: Taking a Long-Term View*. HM Treasury, London.

Webster, C. (1998) *The National Health Service: A Political History*. Oxford University Press, Oxford.

Yuen, P. (2005) *Compendium of Health Statistics 2005–2006*, 17th edition. Office of Health Economics. Radcliffe Publishing, Abingdon.

Further reading

Ham, C. (2004) *Health Policy in Britain*, 5th edition. Palgrave, Basingstoke.
A clear and comprehensive overview of the development of health policy in Britain by one of the acknowledged authorities in the field.

Chapter 12

Nurses and nursing

The UK health care system has been undergoing rapid and persistent reform and change over the past decade, as discussed in the previous two chapters, and the organisation and content of nursing work is undergoing major changes, presenting both opportunities and challenges for nurses. This chapter examines the implications for nursing of the development of flexible working practices, where the provision of care depends on staff skills rather than their job titles. It looks at changes in the health care division of labour and the ways these have affected the character and nature of nursing and its relationship with medicine and other health occupations. Following current conventions, the term nursing will be used to refer to nurses, midwives and health visitors unless otherwise specified. The chapter will:

- discuss nursing and the changing NHS;
- discuss changing roles in nursing;
- discuss the relationships between nurses and doctors and nurses and patients;
- examine nursing work in different contexts;
- discuss the effect on nurses of the new regulatory context.

Nursing and the changing NHS

The history of nursing is characterised by growing autonomy of practice as traditional hierarchies have slowly broken down both within the nursing profession and between nursing and medicine. The individual autonomy of nurses has grown alongside an increasingly complex and specialised division of labour both within nursing and between nursing and other health care occupations. However, even though individual nurses have greater autonomy in patient care than when nursing began, they also depend upon others more than ever before, and their work is regulated and constrained by government policies, managerial agendas and the increasing demands of patients. The relationship between these contradictory trends towards greater individual autonomy and responsibility and increasing regulation and control is central to understanding the work of nurses in the contemporary NHS.

At the centre of contemporary government health policy in the UK is radical change in the role of health care practitioners, involving both greater flexibility of practice and greater regulation and audit of their practice through targets (e.g. reduced waiting times) and protocols for the delivery of 'patient centred' health care (Chapters 2 and 10). These initiatives have created greater opportunities for nurses to expand their area of influence and to exercise greater control over their work, as have developments within nursing. The slow breakdown of traditional hierarchies between nursing and medicine (and those within the nursing profession) has led to increasing autonomy of practice for qualified nurses, within an increasingly complex and specialised division of labour both within nursing and between nursing and other health care occupations. This means that even though individual nurses now have greater autonomy in patient care than when nursing began, they also depend upon others more than ever before.

Government policies

Demand for health care has risen steadily since the inception of the NHS as a result of an ageing population, the development of medical technology and rising public expectations (Chapter 10), and the mismatch between supply and demand has become especially acute in recent years. For some time the NHS has experienced serious difficulties in providing the appropriate number of skilled staff to supply the service. This has been addressed primarily through significantly increased funding that has allowed the better remuneration of skilled NHS staff, but also through attempts to use NHS resources, such as staff and beds, more effectively. As discussed in Chapter 11, the most recent attempt to address this problem has been a proposed shift in care from acute to primary care and the expansion of community services (Department of Health 2006a). Nurses would play a central role in delivering this policy.

Since the 1990s the roles of nurses and other health professionals have been extended and expanded, professional boundaries have been blurred and inter-professional working encouraged (Colyer 2004). For example, *A Health Service of All the Talents* (Department of Health 2000) states that health care providers should no longer be thought of in terms of 'different professional tribes' and called for concerted action to develop more flexible working practices whereby the provision of care depends on the skills of staff rather than their job titles. Breaking the boundaries between professional groups – such as doctors and nurses – and developing flexible working have become new orthodoxies in health policy circles (Allen 2001) and is central to the 'modernisation' of the NHS.

This modernisation can be illustrated by developments in primary care where practice nurses (whose numbers have doubled since 1990), health visitors and district nurses working within general practice are engaged in a diversity of new roles in the interstices of traditional nursing and medical work. According to Peckham and Exworthy (2003: 16), 'role delegation and substitution between and within professional groups is changing the face of inter-professional relations in primary care'. Nurse practitioners are increasingly taking on roles that include diagnosis, telephone advice and home visits, as well as acute medical work. Charles-Jones *et al.* (2003) suggested that not only has health promotion and chronic disease management work been delegated to practice nurses but so has acute medical work 'which has "traditionally" been considered to be GP work'.

Nurse prescribing has become common throughout the NHS since 2002, with nearly 32,000 independent nursing and midwifery prescribers in 2005 (Nursing and Midwifery Council 2005), and is another example of the increased role of nurses in the NHS. From May 2006 such prescribers will be able to prescribe almost all licensed medicines. There were also almost another 6000 'extended' and 'supplementary' nurse prescribers. In their study of nurses taking a course to enable them to become nurse prescribers Bradley *et al.* (2005) found that the majority of these nurses were already prescribing 'by proxy', so the course simply formalised what they were already doing. However, they suggest that the development of nurse prescribing could lead to the professional development of nurses and improve both communication with and care of patients.

These and other changes in government policy are just one lever for change in nursing practice. In theory they open up the possibility for flexible working practices and new nursing roles that contribute to increased autonomy of practice. Change has also been stimulated by developments within nursing. Before considering these, we will look at the nursing workforce.

The nursing workforce

The size and composition of the nursing workforce in the NHS is a crucial factor in its ability to meet the demands of clinical governance, government targets such as reducing waiting times and the implementation of the National Service Frameworks.

In September 2004 1.3 million people were employed in the NHS, including 397,515 qualified nursing, midwifery and health visiting staff (315,440 whole-time equivalents (wte)) and 177,331 unqualified nursing staff, mainly nursing assistants/auxiliaries and healthcare assistants (126, 460 wte). The ratio of qualified to unqualified nurses (about 70 : 30) has remained constant since 1997. Taken together, these nurses comprised nearly 45% of the NHS workforce (Department of Health 2005). In addition, there were just over 3000 nurse learners, mostly on post-registration training courses, who were not included in the workforce statistics.

The size of the NHS nursing workforce has been increasing since 2002, mainly through recruiting overseas staff and retaining older staff and encouraging returners by better pay and improving the quality of working lives through family friendly and flexible working practices. In 2005 the Royal College of Nursing (RCN) reported that the NHS nursing workforce had increased by about a fifth since 1997 and the Nursing and Midwifery Council (NMC) (2005) reported increasing numbers of the total on their register for every year from 2002 to 2005.

Age, gender and ethnicity

It has been recognised that the NHS needs to tackle both indirect and direct discrimination by age, gender and ethnicity if it is to retain and develop an effective workforce. This is certainly true within nursing.

About 90% of nurses are women although the proportion of male nurses has increased since the 1990s. Since 2002 over 10% of registered practitioners have been men, compared to 8.5% in 1992 (Nursing and Midwifery Council 2005). This is expected to rise, as 15% of student nurses are men. Importantly, men are over-represented in senior nursing grades. This may reflect direct discrimination insofar as men are more likely to be selected for promotion on their basis of sex, and/or indirect discrimination, since women are more likely to work part-time and to take career breaks which are disadvantageous to promotion and further training (Whittock *et al.* 2002).

In 2005, nearly 18% of qualified nurses were from a minority ethnic group, mainly from Asian/Asian British and Black/Black British groups (Nursing and Midwifery Council 2005). This is above the national average. In 2002 over half of new entrants to the register (16,161) were from outside the UK, including 1091 from the European Union (EU). In 2004/05 this had reduced to 11,708, with 243 from the EU. Over the 5-year period 1998–2002, nurses from outside of the UK and EU rose rapidly, from 3621 to 15,064 in 2001, declining to 11,477 in 2005. In 2005 India replaced the Philippines as the main source of overseas nurses, with Australia and South Africa also providing significant recruitment. According to the Royal College of Nursing (2005), since 2001, about 45% of new entrants to the register have been from overseas. Despite the existence of equal opportunity policies, a national survey of NHS staff in 2005 found that 17% of black and minority ethnic staff said they had experienced discrimination because of their ethnic background.

The UK nursing workforce has become older. In 1996 over half of registered nurses were under the age of 40, whereas in 2005 nearly 60% of those on the register were over 40 and 16% were 55 or over, and therefore eligible for early retirement. Less than 5% were below 25, partly reflecting the exclusion of learners from these statistics. However, the lower proportion of younger nurses also reflects the greater range of other career possibilities for young women in contemporary Britain. This ageing of the nursing workforce is a major concern as older nurses are more likely to retire or reduce their hours of work (Royal College of Nursing 2005).

While this sub-section has focused upon the NHS, it is important to recognise that about 30% of registered (i.e. qualified) nurses work outside the NHS, mainly in independent care homes. Almost as many unqualified nurses (167,000) work outside the NHS as work within it (Royal College of Nursing 2005). While there is clearly interchange between the NHS and independent sectors, it is unclear how much cross-working there is and its effects. It is also important to note the increasing use of agency or 'bank' nurses in the NHS. While this may provide more flexibility for both nurses and NHS Trusts, it may lead to poorer quality of care (Hart 2004). It is also a source of financial strain for many Trusts and was a factor in the financial crises in a number of NHS hospital trusts in 2006.

Developments within nursing

The defining feature of a profession is generally considered to be its distinctive knowledge, based on credentials gained through advanced training. Distinctive knowledge is the basis for creating exclusive control over a particular area of work. Doctors, for example, have traditionally been able to establish control over substantial areas of health care work by successfully claiming that they alone possess the expertise to exercise the clinical judgement that is intrinsic to diagnosis and treatment. This is one reason why the medical profession has resisted governmental attempts to standardise care through the introduction of clinical guidelines into the NHS. Because nursing has struggled to establish a distinct knowledge base and area of expertise it has found it difficult to follow a knowledge-based 'professionalising' strategy (Hart 2004).

Nursing knowledge and nursing practice have always been difficult to define. In the mid-nineteenth century, Florence Nightingale commented, that 'the elements of nursing are all but unknown' and as recently as 1999 the UKCC stated that 'a definition of nursing would be too restrictive for the profession' (cited in Royal College of Nursing 2002). However, 3 years later the RCN produced the following 'carative' definition that emphasises both the ability of nurses to exercise clinical judgement and to be patient-centred in their work. Nursing is: 'the use of clinical judgement and the provision of care to enable people to promote, improve, maintain, or recover health or, when death is inevitable, to die peacefully' (Royal College of Nursing 2002: 1). The RCN stressed that nursing cannot be defined simply by the content of its work (e.g. by particular tasks). Rather, it is nursing's knowledge base that is central, especially exercising clinical judgement and clinical decision-making.

Central to nursing's professionalising strategy in the UK, and crucial to the its position and status, was the transformation of the education (rather than simply the 'training') of nurse entrants from what was essentially an 'apprenticeship' model whereby new entrants learned how to become nurses while working as part of the nursing workforce under the supervision of qualified nurses. The launch of Project 2000 in 1987 was an attempt to deal with this by moving nurse education out of the work environment into higher education. This was underpinned by a new philosophy which stressed nursing's unique contribution to patient care while drawing upon academic disciplines such as psychology and sociology to develop a distinctive body of knowledge and practice that separated nursing from other health occupations.

The main aim of this reorganisation of nurse education was to develop a knowledgeable workforce who were able to reflect critically upon their practice. Emphasis was placed upon patient-centred care, reflected in the 'nursing process' and 'primary nursing', which aimed to provide individually tailored care delivered by one nurse rather than a number of nurses each undertaking set tasks with every patient. However, this proved extremely difficult to implement and a modified 'team nursing' model using a mixture of trained and untrained nurses has often been adopted. However, Hart (2004) suggests that such models have been 'appropriated by management' because they continue to emphasise the role and responsibility of individual nurses.

Another equally important development within nursing was changes in the accountability and governance of nursing following the introduction of the UKCC *Scope of Professional Practice* in 1992. These have been described as a watershed development for nursing (Royal College of Nursing 2002). Changes in the accountability and governance of nursing in the early 1990s had profound consequences for the development of nursing in the UK. Prior to the introduction of 'Scope' nurses needed to have 'extended role' certificates signed by doctors before they undertook any work that was not included in their basic training. 'Scope' changed the professional agenda by disassociating the scope of practice with particular tasks, associating it instead with the knowledge and skills needed for safe and competent performance. There is no longer a list of tasks that a particular grade of nurse can or cannot perform, and in early 2003 the range of grades was replaced by a competency-based structure. Nursing jobs are now based upon the levels of knowledge and skill, responsibilities, and the physical, mental or emotional effort that they involve.

Developments in nursing have always interacted with government policies. This has been particularly evident since 1997 when 'New Labour' took office (a detailed examination is provided by Hart 2004). The implementation of the government's *Agenda for Change* programme in December 2004 exemplifies how opportunities for increased recognition, autonomy and role expansion for nurses are constrained by financial concerns and managerial constraints flowing from governmental policy. Although the establishment of a 'fairer' unified clinical scale within the NHS was initially welcomed as improving the status and income of nurses, it has not been universally welcomed. While it has meant that the work of nurses at the bottom of the scale was rewarded with much higher pay than previously, the results for qualified nurses were much more equivocal. Due to financial and managerial constraints many NHS Trusts restricted the number of re-gradings they allowed at the higher levels of the scale, meaning that nurses with similar skills and responsibilities were regraded at different levels on the scale, causing serious discontent. There are also concerns that *Agenda for Change* will undermine the role of qualified nurses by promoting the use of health care assistants to undertake some of their work (Hart 2004: 266–72).

Changing roles in nursing

'Scope' provided the opportunity for nurses to develop their practice in innovative ways and was the precursor to subsequent changes in nursing practice. There has been continuing debate about the distinction between 'extended' and 'expanded' nursing roles and their merits and implications for nursing practice. There are different occupational structures associated with extended and expanded roles and although, in reality, nursing work is likely to combine elements of both expanded and extended roles, as 'pure types' they are a useful way of thinking about the different directions in which new roles might develop and the tensions within them.

Extended roles

Extended roles refer to work that is delegated by doctors, i.e. nurses taking on what has traditionally been doctors' work. This is a form of labour substitution. Doctors shed tasks which, for various reasons, they prefer not to perform. This may be because they are seen as mundane or uninteresting, keeping them from what is considered to be more important and exciting work. In this context, nurses take on a more technical role. In the extreme scenario, nursing work can involve moving from patient to patient performing a series of discrete tasks such as taking blood or siting intravenous lines. In some contexts, this can be the best way of 'getting through the work' and making sure that patient needs are met. However, critics of the extended role approach stress that it leads to the fragmentation of care and abandons nursing's caring role. This point can also apply to more advanced forms of practice, such as clinical nurse specialists and nurse consultants, which take nursing closer to medicine.

Extended roles involve not only the delegation of doctors' work to nurses, but also the delegation of the work of trained to untrained nursing staff. Health care assistants (HCAs), who were introduced into the NHS in 1990, are expected to take on routine nursing work. Much of this involves basic patient care, such as help with eating and bathing, and helping trained staff with, or personally undertaking, procedures such as basic observations. Tensions at the HCA/trained nurse boundary concern the lack of value that is placed on 'caring work'. HCAs report feeling de-valued as professionals, something which is reflected in the lack of a career structure (Thornley 2001).

The extended role tends towards a hierarchical structure: HCAs are distinguished from trained nurses and basic grade nurses are marked out from those with higher training. A raft of senior or advanced roles – with a range of titles such as clinical nurse specialist, advanced nurse practitioner and nurse practitioner – have developed, with nurses in these roles working at a higher level of practice. Through these developments nursing retains, and may even be intensifying, its hierarchical structure. A hierarchical structure may benefit nursing by re-introducing the clear leadership structure at ward or unit level that was lost with the reforms of the early 1980s. For example, by the introduction of nurse consultants and 'modern matrons'. Conversely, it can be argued that this further divides the nursing profession along lines that mimic medicine and distance nurses from patients.

Expanded roles

Expanded roles refer to nurses retaining a distinctive nursing base of practice, but expanding this to encompass new skills and responsibilities. From the *expanded* role perspective, these developments are seen as nursing inappropriately mimicking medicine and adopting a bio-medical model of practice (Chapter 2). Proponents of the expanded role argue instead that new role developments should be embedded within a holistic model of care such as that embodied in primary nursing. Sloughing off nurses' caring role to HCAs is seen as undermining the ability of trained nurses to work effectively, because nursing work often involves the 'layering of conduct' (Latimer and Rafferty 1998) or 'strategic multi-tasking' (Allen 2001). Trained nurses often embed routine caring and 'housekeeping' work in their skilled work, for example bathing a patient as part of assessing skin care or tidying bed areas as they update patients' charts. Allen argues that from a caring perspective this is a pragmatic use of time that can 'make a vital contribution to the maintenance of a safe environment for patients'. From this perspective, caring work and clinical work are indivisible.

The expanded role stresses team work rather than a hierarchy of individuals in roles with different levels of skill and status, and emphasises partnerships with patients. The nurse's role is seen as a teacher or facilitator, enabling patients to marshal their own healing resources in the belief that 'involving patients as partners in care increased their knowledge and control of their health' (Salvage 2002: 13). In the current environment of the NHS, where care is organised by specialism and staff shortages inhibit innovatory practice, the delivery of holistic patient care through a participatory model is difficult to achieve in practice. However, many nurses justify the expansion of nursing roles in exactly these terms (Latimer and Rafferty 1998).

Gender

It has long been recognised that gender divisions are intrinsic to the health care division of labour (although in the twenty-first century, women are becoming equally common in UK medicine). Traditionally, nurses, who are predominantly female, have been the adjunct of doctors; the 'unacknowledged co-ordinators, the supporters, the moppers up of tears and fears' (Davies 2000: 348). In trying to shed this role and image, contemporary nursing has been split between adopting the conventional definitions of professionalism (as discussed above), which are embodied by medicine, and trying to develop its practice along other lines. Extended and expanded roles represent and draw upon these different approaches.

Extended roles are a route to nursing autonomy through inclusion within a masculinist bio-medical model of practice premised on personal autonomy and self-management, impartiality and emotional distance (Davies 2000). In coming close to the bio-medical model of practice, extended roles are seen by Davies and others as inappropriately adopting a masculinist approach to practice. Davies argues that instead of seeking inclusion in the 'masculine model', nursing should seek to transcend it by adopting a model of nursing that positively values feminine traits, recognises interdependence with others (colleagues and patients), has collective accountability for practice, an engaged and committed stance towards clients; and involves the investment of self in the clinical encounter. These are the values that underpin expanded roles and 'new nursing'.

Nurses, doctors and patients

Numerical increases in the NHS workforce since 2002 have been accompanied by changes in its clinical skill mix. Medical workforce capacity has been affected by the reduction in doctors' working hours and skill mix changes are seen by government as making an important contribution to the potential mismatch between the demand for doctors and their supply. In the most basic terms, the 'up-skilling' of nurses to take on clinical tasks that were once the province of doctors is a key solution to medical workforce problems. A more highly skilled, trained and flexible nursing workforce can also make a contribution to staffing problems within nursing.

Nurse–doctor relationships

In many ways nursing has been defined by its subordinate relationship to medicine. For most of the lifetime of the NHS doctors were usually able to make decisions about patient care free from external regulation by government and health care management. Patients were far less likely to question treatment decisions than they are now, and nurses were largely cast in a 'handmaiden' role. This relationship and the presumed infinite knowledge and expertise of doctors made it difficult for them to admit that they needed input and advice from nurses. Thus it was difficult for nurses to provide much input into clinical care, even though it was often needed, especially when junior doctors were unsure or made mistakes.

Over time, the relationship between nurses and doctors has developed into one of greater equality. Based on his research in a range of clinical areas in an urban general hospital between 1989 and 1993, Porter (1995) identified four kinds of nurse–doctor relations (Table 12.1). The first, *unmitigated subordination*, was where nurses adopted an unquestioned obedience to medical orders and had no direct input into medical decision making. He remarked that this has declined over time.

Table 12.1 Nurse–doctor relationships.

Type	Nurse's role	Doctor's role
Unmitigated subordination	Obey doctors' instructions	Take decisions Give orders
Informal covert decision making	Imply actions 'Steer' decisions	Take decisions 'Hear' suggestions
Informal overt decision making	Suggest actions Discuss decisions	Take decisions Discuss decisions
Formal covert decision making	Take decisions Negotiate joint decisions	Take decisions Negotiate joint decisions

Source: derived from Porter, S. (1995) *Nursing's Relationship with Medicine*. Avebury, Aldershot.

Informal covert decision making is where statements that nurses make about patient care are co-opted by doctors as their own. This can be seen as a step towards nurse autonomy as nurse–doctor relations began to lose their authoritarian characteristics.

Informal overt decision making is where nurses have an involvement in patient care, but this is not officially sanctioned. This type of interaction involves nurses suggesting, even requesting, that doctors (usually juniors) initiate or change an aspect of patient care. At the time of his research this was the predominant form of nurse–doctor relationships.

The final type, *formal overt decision making*, which nurses typically shied away from, involves taking formally sanctioned independent decisions about patient care. While this was uncommon at the time of Porter's research, nurse prescribing and other role changes mean it has become much more common in contemporary nursing practice.

While government policies have emphasised an increasingly autonomous role of nursing within the wider division of labour, there appears to be a large gap between policy and practice. Hart (2004) argues that the 'multitude' of new nursing roles has led to lack of clarity, the blurring of boundaries and responsibilities and increased stress for nurses. She claims that there has been no substantial change in the position of nurses who 'have been subjugated as a group, placed in a system where they are expected to subordinate their needs and take on a subservient role' (Hart 2004: 180).

Nurse–patient relationships

As with nurse–doctor relationships, we can identify a continuum in the relative control exercised by nurses and patients over their interactions. At one extreme, epitomised by intensive care settings, nurses are dominant and active while patients are passive and compliant. At the other extreme, found where nurses are employed to care for rich clients in their own home, the patient is dominant, the nurse is responsive to their requirements, and treatment decisions are jointly negotiated to comply with the patient's expectations. In between these extremes are situations where nurses guide alert and co-operative patients who may be able to 'steer' decisions about their care, for example in the treatment of infectious diseases or accidental injuries, and more equal relationships where nurse and patient discuss decisions about the management of relatively stable long-term conditions in the community. Finally there are cases where knowledgeable 'expert' patients actively guide nurses in the management of their condition (Chapter 7). Current nursing theory, with its stress upon patient-centred nursing, aims to move nurse–patient relationships to these more equal and co-operative patterns, emphasising (in line with government policy) the involvement and participation of patients in their care.

Nurse–patient relationships are influenced by a number of factors. The nature of the patient's *disease condition* is important. Where it develops slowly over a period of time patients are more likely to be able to discuss and participate in decision making as they may have already made some adjustments to it, or mentally rehearsed possible outcomes of seeking professional help for it. In particular, where a condition is chronic but stable, the patient may become more expert in both its technical management and in recognising signs of deterioration or danger than the nurse, and hence take the lead role in its management (Chapter 7). With a sudden onset, particularly if it is as a result of an accident, there is no such preparation time, and the patient may be more dependent upon nurses and doctors.

The *place* where nurses and patients meet is another important factor influencing the relative power and control exercised by each party. Patients are likely to have the most control and influence in their own home (where the nurse is in some sense a guest), and least power and control as inpatients in an NHS hospital. The nature of the condition and the places where nurses and patients meet seem the most powerful factors in producing the variations in the extent to which patients can become involved in decisions about their care. Nurses (and other health professionals) are most powerful, active and controlling in hospital situations where the patient is critically ill and literally dependent upon their actions. When the nursing care is provided in their own homes and is about a long-standing, well-managed physical condition, patients are most powerful, active and in control. However, even here Millard *et al.* (2006) found that the extent to which community nurses allowed patients to participate in discussions about the management of their conditions varied widely.

Nurse–patient relationships are also influenced by a number of other factors, such as the *personal characteristics* of the patient and the nurse, the relative *knowledge* each has about the condition and its treatment, and the *social status* and *cultural background* of patient and nurse. Although the personal characteristics of patients and practitioners are not supposed to intrude into or influence treatment, the evidence is that they do have some effect upon relationships, and that they may influence patient care, especially where stereotyping occurs.

New roles and the organisation of nursing work

Sociological research on the nursing division of labour shows that how nurses negotiate their new roles and police the boundaries of their work within the wider division of labour and organisational constraints depends more upon pragmatic decisions about how to get their work done than upon philosophical principles.

Competing agendas

In her ethnographic study of nurses' assessment and care of older people admitted as emergencies to an acute medical unit, Latimer (2000) identified three competing agendas that shaped their work. First, to preserve the status of the hospital as one that delivered 'first class' acute medicine rather than other kinds of care. Secondly (as a result of working in a health system under strain), to respond to the demands for shorter lengths of patient stay and greater efficiency. Thirdly, to resolve the discrepancy between the demands of nursing theory to take all of the person's needs into consideration and the practical demands of nursing a large and ever changing flow of patients.

Her research shows that in practice the nurses worked within a bio-medical framework that focused upon clinical need, and effectively 'effaced' the social aspects of the patient during the admission process. This 'also reduces the patient to traits and parts . . . [and] ensures patients are non-participants' (Latimer 2000: 86). An important influence upon the way nurses worked was the organisational arrangements of the hospital that required them to move patients through the wards in a timely manner: success was measured by the managerial criterion of patient 'throughput' rather than by clinical criteria.

During their stay, the nursing care of patients focused upon their medical treatment, epitomised by drips, supportive machines, observations and charts, under the control of the medical consultants. Patients were categorised (and re-categorised during their stay) on the basis of their clinical needs. Very sick, 'high dependency', patients requiring the greatest amount of skilled nursing work were assigned to qualified nurses and placed in the bays nearest to the nursing station, where they could be most easily observed. Other patients requiring lower levels of clinical nursing expertise, such as long-term, terminally ill and convalescent patients were allocated to junior nurses (under supervision) and placed in bays and side wards further away from the nursing station. Such patients were not seen as 'medical' patients but were categorised as 'dependent', 'geriatric', 'social', 'demented' and 'disabled' (Latimer 2000: 36).

Although priority was given to medical need, the ultimate aim of the unit was to discharge its patients, which involved consideration of social factors. As Latimer puts it 'the medical domain relies on patients being returned to persons' (Latimer 2000: 191). Thus, social factors, such as relationships, attitude and morale, were important for future rehabilitation and discharge, and these were constantly assessed by the nurses. These were considered in nursing handovers, medical rounds and the 'social round' conducted by the geriatricians. For example, if an older person had been self-sufficient at home before her admission this suggested that she would be able to cope on discharge home. Similarly, the existence of family carers was a positive factor for discharge home. Sometimes 'medical' problems were reclassified as essentially 'social' problems. For example, a woman admitted with an injured leg following a road accident became reclassified from a medical patient in need of acute care to an old woman with orthopaedic problems at risk of prolonged immobility who should therefore be discharged. Latimer showed that while it appeared that medical decisions to discharge a patient were taken purely on a clinical basis, these depended upon nurses observing, exploring and interpreting the patient's social situation.

Latimer suggested that the doctors and nurses worked together to deliver the 'first class' acute medicine that the hospital is known for. However, the way the nurses conducted their work was not the direct effect of doctor's orders, nor were nurses dominated by doctors. She described the nurses as 'conductors of care', both in the sense of orchestrating the care of patients and in the sense of being the conduits of instructions and demands from management and doctors. Their main role appeared to be that of 'contextualising' patient care, especially patient's troubles, thereby influencing their diagnoses. However, the work of the nurses remained largely invisible, and this had three important consequences. First, it helped to maintain the appearance that diagnosis and discharge decisions were based solely on a clinical basis. Secondly, it maintained the supplementary rather than complementary status of their work. Thirdly, it presented nursing work as 'social' rather than clinical work. The effect of this pattern is to maintain the relative status of medicine and nursing, and to obscure the vital contribution that nurses make to achieving the managerial requirements of the organisation to 'pull patients through beds' in a timely and effective manner.

Blurred boundaries

In her qualitative research in a district general hospital, Allen (2001) examined the division of nursing labour, highlighting the 'jurisdictional ambiguity' that has been created by the introduction of new roles and blurred boundaries within nursing and between medicine and nursing. Within nursing, the shared belief that 'hands-on' care is central to nursing work and 'knowing the patient' generated strains between the senior staff, whose work mainly focused on ward management and bureaucratic tasks ('paperwork'), and the staff nurses who were responsible for the care of the patients on the ward. However, the other demands upon staff nurses themselves meant that they were not always able to engage in such work and that support staff (HCAs and auxiliaries) were involved more frequently in routine hands-on care. Allen concluded that the practical concerns of managing their work meant that there was considerable blurring of the nurse–support staff interface.

Allen found that although there were tensions between the devolution of doctors' work to nurses and the professional discourse of nursing stressing the re-integration of caring into the nursing role, the realignment of roles across the traditional medical–nursing boundary was taking place with very little explicit conflict. Nurses undertook what she calls purposive 'boundary blurring work' in order to improve the management of patient care. Examples of such boundary blurring were giving intravenous fluids which were not written up on a patient's chart, requesting standard blood tests so that they were ready for phlebotomists and to ensure that tests were carried out on time. Nurses (especially the more experienced ones) would make their own judgements about a patient's condition and act upon it; for example, requesting a blood test if a patient looked anaemic. They would also work within the spirit of one rule, even if this meant breaking another. For example, giving a saline flush (not prescribed by a doctor) after prescribed IV antibiotics had been given.

Nurses took such decisions to work across the traditional medical–nursing divide to benefit patient care and to increase their autonomy of practice. In general, they found it easier to 'do doctors' work', rather than to negotiate it with them, leading Allen to suggest that in some contexts it is more appropriate to refer to the *non*-negotiated, rather than the negotiated order of practice. Such flexible working contributed to clinical effectiveness, and she reported that the doctors recognised the skills of the nurses and were grateful when their initiatives eased the burden of work. Although doctors, nurses and support staff were concerned about risk management and the threat of litigation this did not stop them from blurring boundaries in order to complete the work of patient care. However, it is unsurprising that nurses were more likely to take such actions when working with a doctor they trusted.

The extent to which *negotiation* about roles is felt to be necessary, and the manner in which it takes place, seem to be strongly related to the organisational context of work and the demands of patient care. In the 'fast time frame' of the post-anaesthesia care unit (PACU) studied by Prowse and Allen (2002) medical and nursing tasks were overlapping and fluid, although there were legal boundaries preventing nurses from performing specialised activities such as tracheal intubation. PACU nurses had a wealth of experience that meant they were often more experienced and knowledgeable than junior doctors and, unlike the doctors, were always with the patient and used a range of strategies to influence interventions and to improve patient outcomes. For example, suggesting that a junior doctor ask for clarification about drug use from an anaesthetist.

Nurses were more likely to take on a directive role in emergency situations where unexpected, rapid, accelerating physiological change could result in death, if not immediately corrected. In such situations nurses were likely to become assertive and might independently start procedures such as administering oxygen and IV fluids to ensure that a patient's condition was not compromised when doctors were busy in the operating theatre or anaesthetic room. They might also challenge doctors' judgements.

Casualty and emergency departments are another type of fast-paced and changing environments where the roles of nurses may be blurred. Working as a team in order to cover each other's work with patients means that the nurses' work may often become fragmented and task-oriented, particularly when the mix of nursing grades and skills is poor. Research by Annandale *et al.* (1999) suggested that uncertainty and unpredictability in the number and case mix of patients in these environments has a significant impact on the kinds of roles that nurses are prepared to undertake. The extent to which nurses were willing and able to undertake 'new roles', such as venepuncture, taking blood gases, inserting venflons and cannulae, varied according to the 'busyness' of the unit. Contrasting strategies were employed. Nurses might decide to *do a task* such as taking blood or suturing in order to speed things up. Conversely, they might decide *not to do a task* when it was busy, falling back on more traditional nursing duties such as admitting patients and doing their basic observations. This made it difficult to know what nurses would, or would not, do at any one point in time, which sometimes caused confusion and problems with continuity of care.

Overview of nursing work

As we have seen above, nurses must manage and reconcile the contrary demands and expectations arising from competing clinical, management and patient care agendas. They have to manage and combine different types of information about their patients. They also have to manage the movement ('throughput') of patients through the various settings of care, and reconcile the needs of their patients with the needs of the organisation they work in. A considerable amount of nursing activity centres on creating and maintaining clinical documentation – often in the interests of doctors and other health staff and managers. Managing the work of others is also important, mainly by 'orchestrating' the work of doctors and also family carers. Paradoxically, qualified nurses seem to have little time to supervise the work of care assistants. Finally, as we have seen, it is often necessary for them to work flexibly in order to sustain the continuity and quality of care (Box 12.1).

Allen (2004) made the point that nurses occupy a central position within the division of clinical labour, supporting the clinical work of the medical profession and acting as intermediaries between doctors, therapists, other health workers and, to a lesser extent, patients and their relatives:

> . . . *the core nursing function is to mediate different agenda, articulate the work of different care providers around individual patients and fabricate patient identities from diverse information sources. It is nurses who reconcile the requirements of healthcare organisations with those of patients, and constitute and prioritise needs in response to available resources. It is nurses who broker, interpret, translate and communicate clinical social*

Box 12.1 What nurses do

- Manage and mediate the multiple agendas which shape contemporary health care systems.
- Manage patient throughput through their organisation.
- Bring the individual patient into the organisation through the use of routines and standard operating procedures.
- Manage the work of others, mainly by 'orchestrating' the work of doctors and family carers.
- Mediate occupational boundaries by working flexibly to sustain the continuity of care.
- Broker information by 'obtaining, fabricating, interpreting and communicating information'.
- Manage information flows; articulating different kinds of knowledge and thereby categorising, creating and recreating patient identities.
- Maintain records and clinical documentation, often in the interests of others.
- Prioritise patients' needs and the management and rationing of resources.

Source: derived from Allen, D. (2004) Re-reading nursing and re-writing practice: towards an empirically based reformulation of the nursing mandate. *Nursing Inquiry*, 11, 271–83.

and organisational information in ways that are consequential for patient diagnoses and outcomes. It is nurses who work flexibly to blur their juris-dictional boundaries with those of others in order to ensure continuity of care. In fulfilling these roles, it is nurses who weave together the many facets of the service and create order in a fast flowing and turbulent work environment (Allen 2004: 278–9).

She concluded that there is 'a mismatch between real life nursing work and the profession's occupational mandate with its emphasis on emotionally intimate therapeutic relationships with patients. Not only does this produce exaggerated expectations *of practice*, it fails to provide nurses with a know-ledge base to articulate what nurses do *in practice*' (Allen 2004: 279). She identified a number of ways in which the ideal of individualised care is com-promised, such as the standardisation and routinisation of their work, the introduction of new technologies and shorter face-to-face contacts. These mean that 'nurses are increasingly working in extended roles but the "black boxing" of the skills involved by medical and management driven protocols will only serve to limit their potential contribution' (Allen 2004: 281). At the same time, unqualified nursing staff are working closely with patients and providing most of their bedside care, but with minimal supervision from qualified nursing staff. Allen concluded that nursing should look at its con-tributions to how health care systems work rather than focusing upon the (unachieved) ideal of 'emotionally intimate' patient care.

The research evidence presented in this section suggests that rather than struggling to define nursing in terms of its knowledge base or in terms of philosophically based ideals of the 'holistic care' that it is claimed it should provide, it may be more fruitful to consider what nurses are actually doing. In particular, how are government policies and the blurring and re-drawing of boundaries and responsibilities between health professionals affecting the work that nurses do and their relationships with their patients?

Risk and regulation

New nursing roles are expected both to benefit patient care and to increase the autonomy of nurses and their job satisfaction. However, realising these objectives will vary according to the particular characteristics of the environ-ments in which nurses work. The new roles will also be influenced by wider pressures that cut across all settings, nurses' perceptions of risk and their attitudes to the increasing regulation of their work by government. Chapter 2 discussed the rise of *surveillance* as an increasingly important aspect of con-temporary health care and highlighted the possibly negative consequence of this for trust and consent between community nurses and their patients. However, one of the consequences of greater 'patient empowerment' in con-temporary Britain is that the work of nurses is also being monitored and assessed by others, including patients and their families. As Chapter 10 noted, the rise of consumerism has meant that patients are more willing to complain about health services.

Risk

Nurses feel increasingly that they are working in a climate of risk and uncertainty (Annandale 2002). The individual accountability that enhances the professional standing of nurses as a *profession* can also make them feel *personally* very vulnerable. *The Scope of Professional Practice* (UKCC 1997) indicated that in taking on new roles, nurses must be aware of any limits in their competence and decline duties unless they are able to perform them in a safe and skilled manner. Although this is very clear in principle and can be seen as a positive development that acknowledges the professional standing of nursing, in practice it can be difficult to realise. These requirements appear to heighten the concerns of individual nurses about their personal accountability and about the level of support that they might receive from colleagues and employers if something goes wrong.

There is evidence of confusion about the management of accountability for the scope of new roles and the standards that apply to them. In civil law, legal action is directed against the NHS Trust or employer rather than the individual nurse or doctor, and the Trust bears financial responsibility for damages. A nurse, like a doctor, has a 'duty of care' to use reasonable skill and care in their treatment of patients. If they are in breach of that duty and the patient suffers harm as a result, this is negligence. This is defined by deciding whether the nurse (or anyone else) had fallen below the standard of care that a patient can reasonably expect from a person of his or her professional standing in the circumstances. Thus a specific error from a junior nurse might not be 'negligent', whereas the same error by a senior nurse might be. However, because nurses' roles are so ill-defined there may be no obvious 'standard' for them to be judged from, thus creating uncertainty.

As we have seen above, there is also considerable blurring between 'nurses' work' and 'doctors' work'. This can be another source of difficulty because when crossing the boundary from traditional nursing work into the medical domain it may not be readily apparent what standard the nurse will be held to. Dowling *et al.* (2000) suggested that this is not the general standards of care expected of a nurse, but rather the standards that would be expected of the person, undertaking the task concerned – a doctor. It is therefore important that the legal context of new roles is clearly thought through and that clear guidelines on accountability if anything goes wrong are developed.

Although nurses are individually accountable, they work in a complex division of labour involving other nurses, doctors, managers and patients. The actions of others can enhance or compromise their ability to fulfil their duty of care. The decision to undertake or not undertake an aspect of patient care is often influenced by the perceptions of others, not only in terms of their skills and abilities, but also of the extent to which they can be trusted to support the nurse. As we have seen, Allen's research (2001) showed that this can influence the extent to which nurses are prepared to blur boundaries when working with doctors.

While many nurses feel that the new roles benefit practice, they also report downward pressure from management to take on roles to solve staffing problems. In this context individual accountability can be perceived more as a management tool to shift responsibility on to the individual nurse and away from management, than as part of autonomous practice. The pressures from management and feelings of vulnerability that can arise from the dependency on others in the division of labour may lead nurses to feel that they have responsibility for their work, but have little control over it (Annandale 2002).

Consumerism

Nurses' willingness to take on new roles is also influenced by patient consumerism (Chapters 2 and 10). There was a rapid rise in complaints about health care in the 1990s, with written complaints increasing by 10.9% between 1999/00 and 2000/01, although the number of written complaints has declined slightly since 2001. Significantly more written complaints were made against doctors (40,762 in 2004/05) than nurses (13,308 in 2004/05) (Department of Health 2006b) and there is no evidence that nurses in new roles are more likely to make mistakes than doctors in the same role. However, this has done little to allay nurses' fears. Comparable data are unavailable for subsequent years, primarily due to the introduction of new complaints procedures in 2005, but it is known that the number of written complaints has declined slightly.

Many nurses have mixed feelings about patient consumerism. They appreciate that patients want to know more and question more, but they may also experience the informed patient as a threat. Patients' increasing vigilance and lack of trust can feel like an attempt to 'catch nurses out' and hold them accountable when things go wrong, even when the nurse is not at fault. This sense of threat takes on particular significance when nurses do not feel supported by management.

These feelings can have an impact on nurses' willingness to undertake new roles. Annandale (2002) found that some nurses pulled back from undertaking some tasks because their confidence had been undermined by their perception that a patient or their relatives were likely to complain and they feared making a mistake. Nurses also reported the need to 'cover themselves' and to 'watch their back' all the time by, for example, constantly checking and re-checking their work and making sure that everything was documented. Documentation is very important since it is proof in a court of law. However, nurses feel that it has become excessive, especially when 'every little thing' is written down, irrespective of its relevance for patient care. Moreover, time spent on 'paperwork' is time away from patient care, and this can compromise care.

Personal vulnerability can also influence nurses' interactions with patients. While it may prompt good practice, such as making sure that patients and their relatives are fully informed, nurses may also shy away from giving information through fear of giving the wrong information, or because patients or relatives may misinterpret what they have said, with adverse consequences for the nurse. Annandale (2002) reported that 83% of the nurses and midwives in her study felt that their concern about legal accountability was influencing their communications in these ways.

Summary

Changes in nursing have been influenced by governmental initiatives to introduce greater flexibility of clinical practice and greater regulation and audit of that practice. Nursing practice has also been influenced by shortages in nursing and medicine, the demands for an increasingly skilled NHS workforce, the shifting balance in nursing's relationship to medicine and the professionalising strategies of nursing. Although these competing pressures have caused difficulties for nursing and for individual nurses, they have also provided opportunities for nurses to increase their autonomy and control of their work, albeit within tightly defined limits. In contemporary Britain nurses work in a wide range of settings, in a variety of different roles. For this reason it seems likely that new nursing roles will continue to emerge that embody *both* the development of new nursing roles *and* taking on what was previously defined as 'medical' work. While changes in the division of labour in the contemporary health care workforce offer nurses the opportunity to extend the scope of their practice, to increase their influence in clinical and management areas, and to practice more autonomously, government attempts to monitor the quality of health care and to regulate the work of health professionals sometimes work in the opposite direction. The result may be that although, historically, nursing work has become more self-directed, nurses may feel that they have less freedom and independence than previously.

References

Allen, D. (2001) *The Changing Shape of Nursing Practice*. Routledge, London.

Allen, D. (2004) Re-reading nursing and re-writing practice: towards an empirically based reformulation of the nursing mandate. *Nursing Inquiry*, 11, 271–83.

Annandale, E. (2002) Working on the front-line: risk culture and nursing in the new NHS, in S. Nettleton and U. Gustafsson (eds) *The Sociology of Health and Illness Reader*. Polity Press, Cambridge.

Annandale, E., Clark, J. and Allen, E. (1999) Interprofessional working: an ethnographic case study of emergency health care. *Journal of Interprofessional Care*, 13, 139–50.

Bradley, E., Campbell, P. and Nolan, P. (2005) Nurse prescribers: who are they and how do they perceive their role? *Journal of Advanced Nursing*, 51, 439–48.

Charles-Jones, H., Latimer, J. and May, C. (2003) Transforming general practice: the redistribution of medical work in primary care. *Sociology of Health and Illness*, 25, 71–92.

Colyer, H. (2004) The construction and development of health professions: where will it end? *Journal of Advanced Nursing*, 48, 406–12.

Davies, C. (2000) Care and the transformation of professionalism, in C. Davies, L. Finlay and A. Bullman (eds) *Changing Practice in Health and Social Care*. Open University/Sage, London.

Department of Health (2000) *A Health Service of All the Talents: Developing the NHS Workforce*. Stationary Office, London.

Department of Health (2005) NHS hospital and community health services non-medical staff in England: 1994–2004. *Statistical Bulletin*, March, available at www.dh.gov.uk

Department of Health (2006a) *Our Health, Our Care, Our Say; A New Direction for Community Services.* Available at www.dh.gov.uk/ourhealthourcareoursay (accessed June 2006).

Department of Health (2006b) *Data on Written Complaints in the NHS 2004–05.* Available at www.ic.nhs.uk/pubs/wcomplaints (accessed August 2006).

Dowling, S., Martin, R., Skidmore, P., Doyal, L., Cameron, A. and Lloyd, S. (2000) Nurses taking on junior doctors' work: a confusion of accountability, in C. Davies, L. Finlay and A. Bullman (eds) *Changing Practice in Health and Social Care.* Open University/Sage, London.

Hart, C. (2004) *Nurses and Politics.* Palgrave Macmillan, Basingstoke.

Latimer, J. (2000) *The Conduct of Care.* Blackwell Science, Oxford.

Latimer, J. and Rafferty, A.M. (1998) *Extension and Expansion. Emergent Roles in Nursing and Health Visiting.* Department of Health Nursing Executive, London.

Millard, L., Hallet, C. and Luker, K. (2006) Nurse–patient interaction and decision-making in care: patient involvement in community nursing. *Journal of Advanced Nursing,* 55, 142–50.

Nursing and Midwifery Council (2005) *Statistical Analysis of the Register 1st April 2004 to 31 March 2005.* Available at www.nmc-uk.org (accessed April 2006).

Peckham, S. and Exworthy, M. (2003) *Primary Care in the UK.* Palgrave, London.

Porter, S. (1995) *Nursing's Relationship with Medicine.* Avebury, Aldershot.

Prowse, M. and Allen, D. (2002) 'Routine' and 'emergency' in the PACU: shifting contexts of nurse–doctor interaction, in D. Allen and D. Hughes (eds) *Nursing and the Division of Labour in Healthcare.* Palgrave, London.

Royal College of Nursing (2002) *Defining Nursing.* RCN, London.

Royal College of Nursing (2005) *Past trends, future imperfect? A review of the UK Nursing Labour Market in 2004/2005.* Royal College of Nursing, London.

Salvage, J. (2002) The new nursing: empowering patients or empowering nurses? in J. Robinson, A. Gray and R. Elkan (eds) *Policy Issues in Nursing.* Open University Press, Buckingham.

Thornley, C. (2001) Divisions in health-care labour, in C. Komaromy (ed.) *Dilemmas in UK Health Care,* 3rd edition. Open University Press, Buckingham.

UKCC (1997 [1992]) *The Scope of Professional Practice.* UKCC, London.

Whittock, M., Edwards, C. and McLaren, S. (2002) 'The tender trap': gender, part-time nursing and the effects of 'family friendly' policies on career advancement. *Sociology of Health and Illness,* 24, 305–26.

Further reading

Allen, D. (2004) Re-reading nursing and re-writing practice: towards an empirically based reformulation of the nursing mandate. *Nursing Inquiry,* 11, 271–83.
A well-argued and provocative analysis of what nurses do and the future directions nursing should take.

Hart, C. (2004) *Nurses and Politics.* Palgrave Macmillan, Basingstoke.
An influential critical analysis of nursing in the UK.

Index